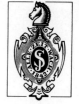

Short-Term Test Systems for Detecting Carcinogens

Edited by
K. H. Norpoth and R. C. Garner

With 211 Figures

Springer-Verlag
Berlin Heidelberg New York 1980

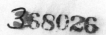

Professor Dr. K. H. NORPOTH
Institut für Staublungenforschung
und Arbeitsmedizin
der Westfälischen Wilhelms-Universität
Westring 10, 4400 Münster/FRG

Dr. R. C. GARNER
University of York
Cancer Research Unit
Heslington, York, YO1 5DD/Great Britain

ISBN 3-540-09203-X Springer-Verlag Berlin Heidelberg New York
ISBN 0-387-09203-X Springer-Verlag New York Heidelberg Berlin

Library of Congress Cataloging in Publication Data: Main entry under title: Short-term test systems for detecting carcinogens. Bibliography: p. Includes index. 1. Carcinogenicity testing–Congresses. 2. Chemical mutagenesis–Congresses. I. Norpoth, K.H., 1930–. II. Garner, R. Colin, 1944–. [DNLM: 1. Carcinogens–Analysis–Congresses. 2. Mutagens–Analysis–Congresses. 3. Toxicology–Methods–Congresses. QZ202 S559 1978]. RC 268. 65.S56   616.99'4071   80-10716.

Offsetprinting and bookbinding: Brühlsche Universitätsdruckerei, Giessen.
2121/3130-543210

Preface

The varying cancer incidence from country to country and region to region suggests that environmental factors play a considerable role in the aetiology of cancer. Whether these factors in the environment moderate the effect of carcinogenic chemicals or whether they might themselves be carcinogenic is not known at the present time. What is known is that there are various chemicals, both naturally occurring and man-made, which can induce cancer in man. In the Western world estimates vary as to how much cancer is occupational in origin; the figures range from 1% to 40%. It is our feeling that probably about 10% of cancer has a direct occupational origin. Nevertheless this number is considerable and it behoves us therefore to identify those chemicals which are carcinogenic and to reduce human exposure.

Recent work on the mode of action of carcinogenic chemicals suggests that the majority exert their effect through an activation step to give electrophilic metabolites. Such metabolites have as a common feature the ability to react with cellular nucleophiles to give covalently bound products. Such reaction will occur after carcinogen treatment of animals with nucleic acids particularly in target organs. It is reaction with nucleic acids that provides the basis of a number of short-term tests for carcinogens, since the basic composition of DNA is similar in micro-organisms and in human cells.

This symposium, of which the following pages are the proceedings, brought together a number of people who have been instrumental in developing and refining various short-term tests. There was considerable discussion on the role of mixed-function oxidase enzymes in activation as well as a novel enzyme-catalysed reaction in vitro of glutathione with dichloroethane. This reaction, like many of the others discussed, may not take place in vivo and it is this possibility which is currently of great interest in attempts to predict carcinogenic potency from in vitro assays. The conclusions of the symposium were that much remains to be understood in the area of short-term tests if we are going to be able to predict the carcinogenic hazard of a chemical to man. It is noteworthy that although various in vivo techniques were presented, all appear to be impractical for the routine screening of carcinogenic activity either because of their insensitivity or their expense. This symposium, like many others, perhaps raised more questions than answers, nonetheless it was a stimulating experience for all that. All the people who attended must have returned to their respective laboratories with the impression that this research area is not as simple as many would have one believe. For this reason alone it was a noteworthy occasion.

March, 1980   R.C. GARNER

Contents

VIII

Contributors

You will find the addresses at the beginning of the respective contribution

Opening

U. WÖLCKE[1]

Ladies and gentlemen, on behalf of the president of the Federal Institute of Occupational Safety and Accident Research, Prof. Hagenkötter, I welcome you in Dortmund to day on the occasion of the International Symposium on Short-Term Mutagenicity Test Systems for Detecting Carcinogens.

This is the first international symposium to be held within the walls of our new building into which we have moved only in January this year and which is the first part of a complex of buildings to be raised within the next few years. Behind me, that is behind the auditorium, a number of laboratories are currently being constructed.

Turning to the symposium ahead of us:

The problem of carcinogenic chemicals is of primary concern to everyone engaged in the field of occupational safety. After all, it is the worker who is generally exposed to a new chemical first and quite often most intensively in comparison with other people.

Presently, we are having a discussion in our country as to the percentage of cancer cases which must be ascribed to occupational causes. Similar discussions are in progress in other countries, in particular within the USA.

Undoubtedly it is difficult, and perhaps impossible, at present to establish the exact percentage. We more or less have to rely on what is generally called the "educated guess" of experts, a guess which is formed on the basis of all the epidemiologic information which we have today. I think it would be misleading, however, to discuss the problem of carcinogenic risk at the work place solely on the basis of a casuistic approach. We all know about the limitations of such an approach and the reasons for them. If one agrees to that, I think it is almost of secondary importance what the precise percentage on an epidemiologic basis would be. This becomes apparent when you transform any such percentages which are presently being discussed into absolute figures. They all turn out to be far too high to be acceptable, especially in view of the fact that most occupational cancer risks can be eliminated quite effectively.

---

[1]Bundesanstalt für Arbeitsschutz und Unfallforschung, Vogelpothsweg 50-52, 4600 Dortmund-Dorstfeld/FRG

Clearly, the identification of chemical carcinogens before there is human exposure is the most important prerequisite in protecting workers and the public at large.

The conventional mean to achieve this is long-term bioassays in animals. We all know about the merits of such bioassays, but we also know about the limitations in terms of time and money when too many chemicals must be tested.

The methodology of short-term mutagenicity testing is now hoped to lead the way out of the dilemma. This expectation may have at times resulted in undue optimism as far as the efficiency of the methods in question is concerned. On the other hand, it appears to me that the early optimism later turned into a partly irrational and unjustified pessimism.

I personally would therefore consider this symposium to be a success if it contributes to a balanced documentation of the present state of the art in this field, in particular with respect to the problem of interpretation of test results. In view of the outstanding participants, I am convinced that this objective can be achieved.

Section I

Significance and Validity of Short-Term Tests for Detecting Carcinogens – General Considerations

In Vitro Assays to Predict Carcinogenicity?

R. C. GARNER[1]

Abstract

With the acceptance of the idea that most, if not all, organic
chemical carcinogens are electrophiles, or must be converted to
such by metabolism, has come in the wake of this hypothesis, a
large number of screening tests which rely on the reaction of
the electrophilic species with DNA as a means of distinguishing
between carcinogens and non-carcinogens. Although this hypothesis is probably correct, it should be remembered that such
reactions must take place in whole cells, within an organ of a
whole animal for tumours to appear. Most in vitro assays do not
take these considerations into account, being unable to give an
idea of either pharmacokinetic or pharmacodynamic parameters.
Since these are often the sole reason for susceptibility or
resistance to a carcinogen, their importance cannot be overem-
phasized. In vitro assays at the present time can only give an
estimate of carcinogenic potential and not of potency. They also
cannot indicate whether man is susceptible or resistant to the
test substance. Examples of the various factors involved in
tumour initiation are presented using aflatoxins, aromatic amines
and some direct-acting carcinogens as models.

Introduction

The idea that most chemical organic carcinogens are electrophiles
(electron-deficient) or are converted in the body to such has
been proposed as a unifying mechanism for tumour initiation.
Since electrophiles readily react with nucleic acid bases along
with other macromolecules to give covalently bound adducts, the
biological effects of these reactions can be used as a monitor of
whether reaction has occurred or not. In Table 1 are listed a number of assays, which have been proposed, or are currently in use,
for studying carcinogen activation. In this paper attention to
two of these assays is stressed: (1) bacterial mutagenicity,
and (2) measurement of "unscheduled" DNA synthesis (UDS) in
HeLa cells. My research group has published a number of papers
(1-6) in these two areas which I wish to precis in order to
describe what short-term tests can and cannot do. In particular,
it is emphasized that UDS assays may be as good as, if not better
than, bacterial mutagenicity assays because activity can only
result as a consequence of the covalent binding of a carcinogen
to DNA.

---

[1]Cancer Research Unit, University of York, Heslington, York, YO1 5DD, United
Kingdom

Table 1. Possible rapid screening systems for carcinogens dependent on nucleic acid reaction

1. Mutagenicity

    a) Micro-organisms —bacteria, yeasts

    b) Tissue culture cells —mouse lymphoma, Chinese hamster, human fibroblasts etc.

    c) *Drosophila*

2. Cell transformation —morphological

    —growth in soft agar

    —tumours in animals

3. Repair studies

    a) Bacterial —repair deficient strains

    b) Mammalian cells —unscheduled DNA synthesis

    —sister chromatid exchange

    —alkaline sucrose gradient centrifugation

4. Macromolecular binding of labelled material

In Vitro Studies on the Activation of Aflatoxins and Benzidines

Aflatoxins

Much is known about the four naturally occurring aflatoxins, B_1, G_1, B_2 and G_2 (Fig. 1), in terms of their biological and carcinogenic activity. What is not well understood at the present is why aflatoxin B_1 (AFB_1) is such a potent carcinogen for the rat and yet is non-carcinogenic for the hamster and only a weak carcinogen for the mouse. In other words there is a great difference in susceptibility between these species. What is also not known is where man fits into this spectrum of activity, although there is now strong epidemiological evidence that primary liver cancer incidence in certain areas of the world can be related to aflatoxin contamination of foods (7, 8).

Aflatoxin B_2 (AFB_2), the dihydro analogue of AFB_1, is a much weaker carcinogen than AFB_1, suggesting that the vinyl ether group in AFB_1 is important for the biological activity of these compounds. Indeed, Swenson et al. have shown in an elegant experiment that AFB_2 may be carcinogenic by nature of it being dehydrogenated in the liver to AFB_1 which is subsequently activated to give the same DNA adducts as those found after AFB_1 administration (9). Aflatoxin G_1 (AFG_1) also seems to be activated in a similar manner to AFB_1, i.e. through epoxide production. AFG_1 is about one-third as potent a carcinogen as AFB_1 in the rat, suggesting that a slight difference in chemical structure renders less of the carcinogen available for epoxide formation. Aflatoxin G_2 (AFG_2) is the dihydro derivative of AFG_1 and, as far as I am aware, is a non-carcinogen.

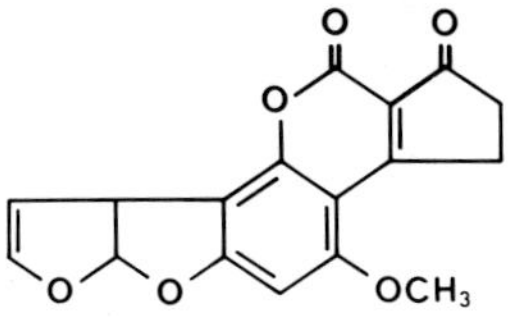

Aflatoxin B_1

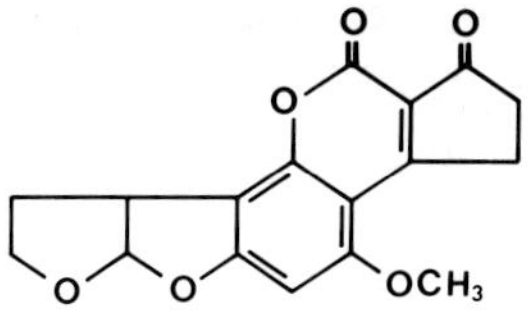

Aflatoxin B_2

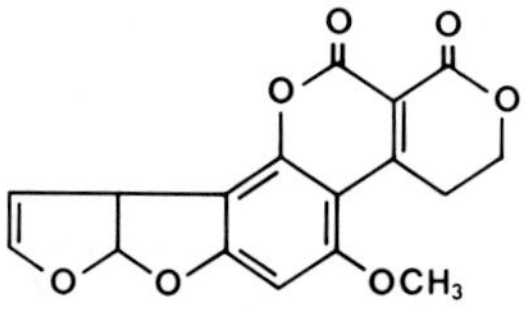

Aflatoxin G_1

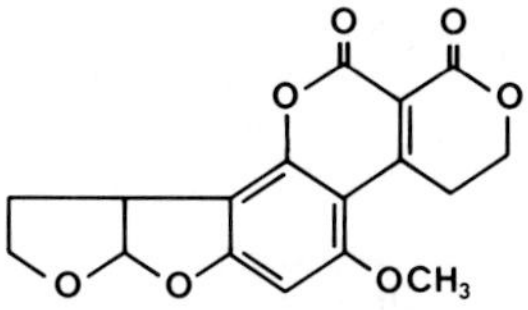

Aflatoxin G_2

Fig. 1. Chemical structure of the aflatoxins

Summarising what is known about the metabolism of AFB_1 (Fig. 2) in the rat, it would appear that activation through epoxide formation is a minor pathway in the total metabolism of AFB_1 and that other metabolites are produced to a much greater extent but these appear to be genuine detoxification products. However, it is the epoxide that is probably responsible for mutagenesis and tumour initiation by this compound. Epoxide formation occurs after mixed-function oxidase attack through cytochrome P-450 rather than P-448.

We have tested a number of aflatoxins and aflatoxin-related compounds for their ability to be activated to a metabolite which can inactivate *S. typhimurium* TA 1530 in a liquid suspension assay and the results of these studies are summarized in Table 2. Activity decreases from AFB_1 downwards, which to some extent parallels what is known about the carcinogenic potency of these compounds. A number have not been tested for carcinogenicity, including active compounds such as aflatoxicol. This compound has been reported by others to be nearly as active as AFB_1 in the *Salmonella* /microsome assay. Using the liquid suspension method we find AFG_1 to be the next most potent compound after AFB_1.

We have chemically synthesized a model of AFB_1 in which the vinyl ether function is retained (Table 3). Testing of this for mutagenicity showed it to have approximately 1/5000th the activity of AFB_1 after liver activation using *S. typhimurium* TA 100 as the tester strain, while it did not mutate strain TA 98 (3). Reduction of the vinyl ether linkage abolished biological activity, indicating that the model compound is also activated via epoxide

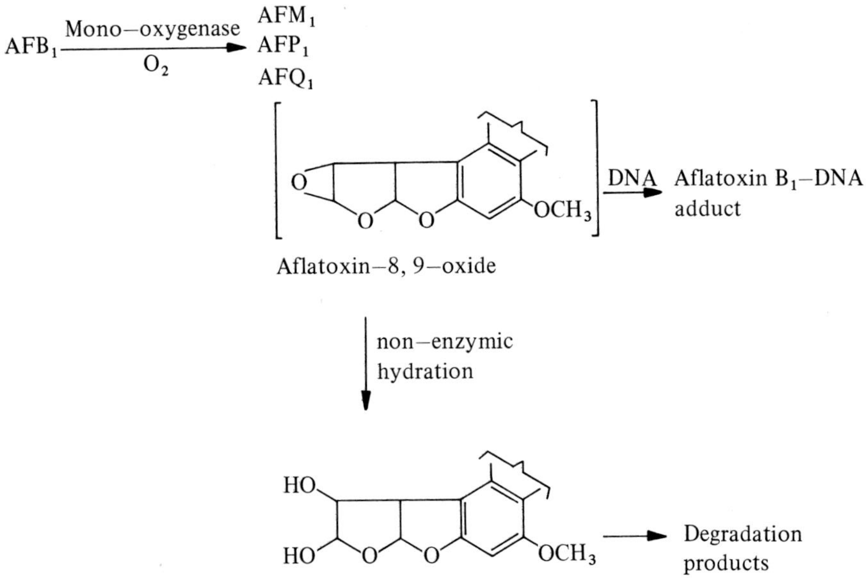

AFB$_1$ $\xrightarrow[\text{O}_2]{\text{Mono-oxygenase}}$ AFM$_1$
AFP$_1$
AFQ$_1$

$$\left[\begin{array}{c} \text{Aflatoxin-8,9-oxide structure with OCH}_3 \end{array} \right]$$ $\xrightarrow{\text{DNA}}$ Aflatoxin B$_1$–DNA adduct

Aflatoxin–8, 9–oxide

non–enzymic hydration

Degradation products

Fig. 2. Pathways for metabolism of aflatoxin B$_1$

Table 2. Activity of various aflatoxins, aflatoxin metabolites and aflatoxin-related compounds in inactivating *S. typhimurium* TA 1530

Compound	Lethality
Aflatoxin B$_1$	++++
Aflatoxin G$_1$	+++
Aflatoxin B$_2$	+
Aflatoxin G$_2$	−
Aflatoxin M$_1$	−
Aflatoxicol	+
Acetylaflatoxicol	+
Aflatoxin P$_1$	−
Aflatoxin B$_{2a}$	−
Parasiticol	++
O-Methylsterigmatocystin	+
5-Methoxysterigmatocystin	+
Versicolorin A	+
Versicolorin B	−

Lethality was measured in a liquid suspension assay with rat liver post-mitochondrial supernatant obtained from phenobarbitone-pretreated rats. For details see ref. 1.

Table 3. Mutagenicity of furobenzofurans towards *S. typhimurium* TA 98 and TA 100

Compound	Concentration (µg/plate)	Liver[a]	His$^+$ revertants/plate TA 98	TA 100
Aflatoxin B$_1$	0.05	+	*269*	*593*
		−	12	103
	0.10	+	*1174*	*980*
		−	17	108
	0.50	+	*1408*	*1564*
		−	17	129
	1.00	+	*1328*	*1372*
		−	14	126
Dihydrofurobenzofuran	20	+	23	118
		−	21	132
	50	+	14	*165*
		−	15	111
	100	+	28	*273*
		−	17	130
	200	+	17	*367*
		−	16	143
Dimethylsulphoxide (Control)		+	23	129
		−	15	123

Results are the mean of duplicate assays.

Numbers in italics indicate mutation considered significantly above background.

[a] Liver post-mitochondrial fraction   present +
                                                absent −

formation. It would appear, therefore, that compounds with a vinyl ether function are mutagenic after liver metabolism and that other vinyl ethers such as 2,3-dihydropyran or 2,3-dihydrofuran might also be active. We are currently working along these lines in our laboratory.

Benzidines

Benzidine, a human bladder carcinogen, is converted by mixed-function oxidase enzymes to a mutagen for *S. typhimurium* TA 98 (Table 4) (2). Substituted benzidines such as 3,3',5,5'-tetrafluorobenzidine and 3,3'-dichlorobenzidine are also active. 3,3',5,5'-Tetramethylbenzidine, on the other hand, in which all the *ortho* positions are substituted with methyl groups, is non-mutagenic and, as far as is known, non-carcinogenic. Other active benzidine analogues include dianisidine, *o*-tolidine and 2,2'-dichlorobenzidine. The mutagenicity of these compounds

Table 4. Mutagenicity of benzidine and its analogues to *S. typhimurium*

Compound	Concentration (µg/plate)	Liver	His[+]revertants/plate
Benzidine[a]	50	+	*430*
		−	5
	100	+	*640*
		−	15
3,3',5,5'-Tetrafluorobenzidine[a]	50	+	*560*
		−	20
	100	+	*1040*
		−	29
3,3',5,5'-Tetramethylbenzidine[a]	50	+	15
		−	5
	100	+	15
		−	9
3,3'-Dichlorobenzidine[a]	50	+	*3360*
		−	*114*
	100	+	*9520*
		−	*131*
2,2'-Dichlorobenzidine[b]	200	+	*44*
		−	24
	500	+	*54*
		−	15
Dianisidine[b]	20	+	*430*
		−	30
	100	+	*554*
		−	32
o-Tolidine[b]	20	+	*151*
		−	16
	100	+	*207*
		−	7

+ Liver present   [a]*S. typhimurium* TA 1538
− Liver absent   [b]*S. typhimurium* TA 98

Numbers in italics indicate a mutagenic effect. For experimental details see ref.2.

does differ and this does to some extent parallel what is known about their carcinogenicity. In other words, in a structural series, we can obtain some indication not only of carcinogenic potential but also of carcinogenic potency.

Turning away from bacterial mutagenicity as a short-term test, I wish to now discuss some results which have been obtained by my colleague, Dr. Carl Martin, using UDS in HeLa cells as a screen to distinguish between carcinogenic and non-carcinogenic

chemicals. In this assay, DNA S-phase synthesis in HeLa cells
in culture is much reduced by placing the cells in an arginine-
deficient medium for a number of days, followed by the addition
of hydroxyurea. Any incorporation of [^{3}H] thymidine under these
conditions can only be as a result of DNA repair synthesis. The
assay is performed by comparing the radioactivity of DNA extracted from cells which have been treated with the test chemical,
with or without a liver activation, in the presence of radiolabelled thymidine and control cells which have been solvent
treated only. A significant difference in radioactivity between
the two indicates that carcinogen activation has occurred with
subsequent covalent reaction with DNA and as a result the DNA
damage is repaired.

Using this technique we have tested a number of carcinogens and
non-carcinogens for DNA repair-stimulating activity. In Table 5
are listed the results obtained for benzidine and substituted
benzidines in the repair assay. All the carcinogenic compounds
were active whereas tetramethylbenzidine was not. As far as
trying to estimate carcinogenic potency using this test is concerned, this seems at the present time to be impossible unless
the compounds one is interested in are assayed at the same time
using cells from the same population and the same liver enzyme
fraction. One must also assume that the reaction products of
the different activated carcinogens with DNA are as effective
as each other in stimulating DNA repair, an unlikely possibility.

The DNA repair assay appears useful for distinguishing between
false-positive and false-negative results in the *Salmonella*/micro-
some assay (Table 6). For example, 9-aminoacridine is a potent
frameshift mutagen in *S. typhimurium* TA 98 and yet is inactive in
the DNA repair assay. The compound is also ineffective as a
mutagen in mammalian cells. Conversely, formaldehyde, a known
bacterial mutagen which can also induce mutations in *Drosophila
melanogaster*, was able to elicit UDS in the repair assay, suggesting that formaldehyde does react with DNA of cells in culture.
Urethane, a carcinogen, which is inactive in the *Salmonella*/micro-
some assay, also stimulates DNA repair synthesis after activation
by rat liver mixed-function oxidase enzymes. Similarly diethylstilboestrol, another compound inactive in the *Salmonella*/micro-
some assay, also stimulates UDS. Whether this occurs through
epoxide formation or through some other mechanism is not known,
nor is it known whether this synthetic hormone is a carcinogen
through electrophilic metabolite formation. Other results we have
found of interest are that sodium azide, a bacterial mutagen,
is inactive in the repair assay, and dimethylaminoazobenzene, a
carcinogen, inactive in the standard *Salmonella*/microsome assay
does stimulate UDS in HeLa cells. Many of the compounds requiring
liver activation in the repair assay have some effect in the absence of liver, showing that HeLa cells have some mixed-function
oxidase activity.

The results described above, together with others I have not
mentioned, lead me to suggest that this repair assay is one which
should be used in conjunction with bacterial mutagenicity in
any routine screening of chemicals for carcinogenic potential.

Table 5. UDS in HeLa cells induced by benzidine and its analogues

Compound	Liver	Active dose range (M)	Background dpm/µg DNA	Maximum dpm/µg DNA above background	Dose at highest activity (M)	P
Benzidine	P	$10^{-3} - 10^{-7}$	194 ± 25	54	10^{-6}	<0.05
2,2'-Dichlorobenzidine	P	$10^{-4} - 10^{-7}$	380 ± 34	158	10^{-4}	<0.01
3,3',5,5'-Tetrafluorobenzidine	P	$10^{-4} - 10^{-7}$	455 ± 50	181	10^{-4}	<0.01
3,3',5,5'-Tetrachlorobenzidine	P	$10^{-4} - 10^{-5}$	53 ± 6	59	10^{-4}	<0.01
3,3',5,5'-Tetramethylbenzidine	P	-	236 ± 34	8		
Dianisidine	P	10^{-7}	413 ± 30	101	10^{-7}	<0.05
o-Tolidine	P	$10^{-4} - 10^{-6}$	208 ± 4	43	10^{-6}	<0.05
3,3'-Dichlorobenzidine	P	$10^{-4} - 10^{-7}$	223 ± 2	109	10^{-5}	<0.05

P= phenobarbitone-induced rat liver PMS present. P= probability values calculated using Student's t-test with at least 5 df. For experimental details see ref. 6.

Table 6. Activity of some false-positive and false-negative compounds in bacterial mutagenicity assays in inducing UDS in HeLa cells

Compound	Liver	Active dose range (M)	Background dpm/µg DNA	Maximum dpm/µg DNA above background	Dose at highest activity (M)	P
9-Aminoacridine	-		93 ± 12	0		
Formaldehyde	-	$10^{-3} - 10^{-8}$	302 ± 16	56	10^{-3}	<0.05
Urethane	P	$10^{-3} - 10^{-5}$	228 ± 17	111	10^{-3}	<0.05
Diethylstilboestrol	P	10^{-6}	275 ± 25	140	10^{-6}	<0.05
Sodium azide			52 ± 5	4		
Dimethylaminoazobenzene		$10^{-5} - 10^{-8}$	127 ± 8	44	10^{-7}	<0.01

P= phenobarbitone-induced rat liver post-mitochondrial supernatant present. P= probability values calculated using Student's t-test with at least 5 df.

We have recently completed work using this assay, as well as testing for bacterial mutagenicity, in the MRC/ICI/NIEHS blind trial and we await the breaking of the code with interest.

In Vivo and Whole Cell Studies on the Activation of Aflatoxins

In 1971, while I was working with the Millers at the University of Wisconsin, I found that activation of AFB_1 in vitro by liver mixed-function oxidases was increased by prior phenobarbitone treatment (10). This was in contrast to the findings of McLean and Marshall that phenobarbitone decreased the carcinogenicity of AFB_1 (11). Similarly, hamsters, which are resistant to the carcinogenic action of AFB_1, had high levels of liver mixed-function oxidase enzymes for activating AFB_1 (12). More recent data, using mutagenicity rather than bacterial inactivation as an end point, are shown in Table 7. In order to investigate these discrepancies, we have examined the in vivo binding of $[^{14}C]$ AFB_1 to liver macromolecules in the rat, a susceptible species, and the hamster, a resistant species. These data have been presented elsewhere (13). Summarizing the results, we found that although similar amounts of AFB_1 were taken up in the liver by the two species, less $[^{14}C]$ AFB_1 was bound to hamster nucleic acids than to rat nucleic acids. There is a correlation between in vivo binding and carcinogenicity. Similar studies comparing the binding of AFB_1 in control or phenobarbitone-pretreated rats showed that phenobarbitone pretreatment decreased the binding of AFB_1 to nucleic acids, a result which paralleled the carcinogenicity data (14).

Table 7. Activity of control rat, phenobarbitone-pretreated rat and hamster liver in converting AFB_1 to a mutagen to *S. typhimurium* TA 100

Concentration (μg/plate)	Liver	His^+ revertants/plate		
		Control rat	PB rat	Hamster
0.5	+	137	193	190
	−	77	98	71
1.0	+	*340*	*397*	*415*
	−	100	105	102
2.0	+	*505*	*673*	*974*
	−	85	79	94

Numbers in italics indicate a mutagenic effect.
+ Liver present.
− Liver absent.

We have recently completed a project in which we have compared the liver macromolecular binding of AFB_1 and AFG_1 (AFG_1 is said to be only one-thirtieth as potent as AFB_1 in the *Salmonella/* microsome assay) (15). In our hands, we find that AFG_1 has about the same activity as AFB_1. This discrepancy we attribute to the fact that we use liver from phenobarbitone-pretreated rats whereas the other report used liver from Aroclor-1254-induced animals. AFG_1 is said to have about one-third the carcinogenic potency of AFB_1. After a single administration of either radiolabelled mycotoxin, the percentage uptake by the liver was similar. Macromolecular binding to nucleic acids, on the other hand, was lower for AFG_1 than for AFB_1 (Fig. 3a and b). Protein binding of both mycotoxins was similar. It is perhaps surprising that nucleic acid binding for the two mycotoxins is in the ratio of 3:1 for AFB_1 to AFG_1 mirroring the carcinogenic potency.

Examining the possible reasons for the difference in potency between AFB_1 and AFG_1 it seemed reasonable to look at whether the difference resided in how much of the mycotoxin partitioned into the endoplasmic reticulum membrane prior to metabolism by cytochrome P-450. Using various solvent/water mixtures which are said to simulate a lipid membrane, we found that in all cases more AFB_1 partitioned into the model membrane than AFG_1 (Table 8). n-Octanol/water is said to be the best model membrane system in terms of the distribution of phosphatidylcholine, a normal constituent of membranes. In this system about 1.5 times as much AFB_1 partitions into the octanol phase compared with AFG_1. It could be that distribution coefficients do play a role in determining carcinogenic potency for particular chemicals.

If one is not able to determine species susceptibility or resistance to carcinogens using in vitro subcellular fractionation methods, are there any other means of trying to determine human susceptibility? We have been exploring the use of liver slices to activate the aflatoxins to see whether a measure of susceptibility can be obtained. The end point we have used is DNA binding, since this correlated in vivo with carcinogenic susceptibility or resistance. In Table 9 is presented the amount of [^{14}C] AFB_1 bound to DNA in slices taken from male or female rats, rats pretreated with phenobarbitone, hamsters and mice. In all cases except for the male and female rat, a correlation was seen between DNA binding and carcinogen risk (the male rat is more susceptible than the female to AFB_1 carcinogenicity). It would appear that a whole cell system may reflect the in vivo situation better than subcellular systems. It should be possible to now examine human liver slices using this technique to attempt to estimate carcinogenic risk.

Conclusions

A number of points which arise from what has been presented which should be emphasized. First, that false-positive results in a bacterial mutagenicity assay may arise for the following reasons:
1. The chemical under study reacts with bacterial DNA but not mammalian cell DNA because in the latter there are a great number of detoxification processes.
2. Intercalating agents may mutate bacteria but may have no effect on mammalian cell DNA because they are not fixed into position by a covalent linkage.

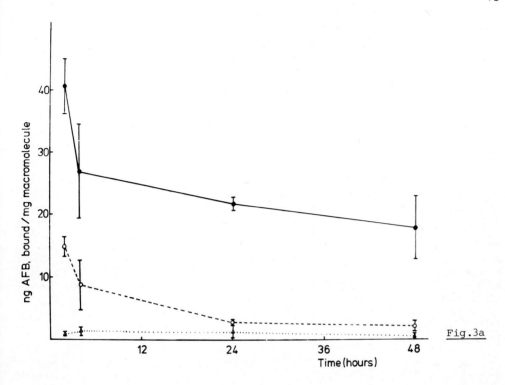

Fig.3a

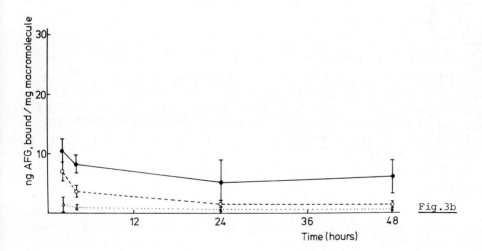

Fig.3b

Fig. 3. Binding of (a) [^{14}C] AFB$_1$, (b) [^{14}C] AFG$_1$ to macromolecules in rat liver after a single administration. ●——● rRNA; O – – – O DNA; Δ ·····Δ protein

Table 8. Distribution coefficients of
AFB_1 and AFG_1 in various model membrane
systems

Solvent	AFB_1	AFG_1
Isobutanol	11.06	2.87
Isoamylalcohol	14.02	9.75
n-Octanol	8.99	5.58
Ether	1.97	0.82

Distribution coefficient =

$$\frac{\text{concentration of mycotoxin in organic phase}}{\text{concentration of mycotoxin in water}} \; .$$

Assays were carried out in a 50:50 mixture
of water and the organic solvent.

Table 9. Binding of $[^{14}C]$ AFB_1 to DNA in
rat liver slices

Species	Sex	ng AFB_1/mg DNA
Rat	Male	31.7 ± 9.1
Rat	Female	35.7 ± 11.1
Rat (PB)	Male	14.3 ± 8.2
Hamster	Male	11.3 ± 3.4
Mouse	Male	1.3 ± 0.4

PB = phenobarbitone-pretreated. Binding to
DNA was measured after 120-min incubation
with 2.5 µg $[^{14}C]$ AFB_1 in 5 ml Hepes-Ringer
buffer.

3. Compounds are generated in vitro but not in vivo. It is possible that one metabolite may react with another or with the
   parent compound to give a new chemical which is mutagenic.
   This new chemical might not be formed in animals because
   dynamic processes are operating, preventing reaction.
4. The tester organism might produce mutagenic metabolites but
   not mammalian cells.
5. The concentration of compound tested could not be attained
   in vivo.
6. The assay is optimized for activation and not detoxification.

Some of the reasons for false-negative results in mutagenicity
assays are listed below:

1. Conditions for activation are not optimum.
2. A two or more step activation pathway and only the first
   step is operating (oxidation?).
3. The active metabolite might be too labile to react with
   bacterial DNA.
4. The chemical may be carcinogenic through a hormonal mechanism.

5. The chemical is active through a mechanism other than DNA reaction.

In summary, therefore, I think one should remember that the surface of an agar plate cannot be used as a model for a whole animal; in particularly, no account can be taken of pharmacokinetic and pharmacodynamic parameters. These two factors are responsible in many instances in determining carcinogenic susceptibility or resistance.

Mutagenicity assays are extremely valuable in determining carcinogenic potential but not in estimating carcinogenic potency. Among other tests which can be used in conjunction with bacterial mutagenicity assays, I feel that the DNA repair assay I have described is useful in that a positive result only occurs after reaction of the chemical with DNA.

Acknowledgments. I would like to thank Mark Tolson, Catherine Wright, Christine Pickering, Brian Coles, John Lindsay Smith and Carl Martin for providing most of the data I have described. Our own work is supported by grants from the Medical Research Council and the Yorkshire Cancer Research Campaign.

References

1. Garner RC, Wright CM (1973) Induction of mutations in DNA-repair deficient bacteria by a liver microsomal metabolite of aflatoxin B_1. Br J Cancer 28:544-551
2. Garner RC, Walpole AL, Rose FL (1975) Testing of some benzidine analogues for microsomal activation to bacterial mutagens. Cancer Lett 1:39-42
3. Coles BF, Lindsay Smith JR, Garner RC (1977) Mutagenicity of 3a,8a-dihydrofuro [2,3-b] benzofuran, a model of aflatoxin B_1, for *Salmonella typhimurium* TA 100. Biochem Biophys Res Commun 76:888-892
4. Garner RC, Nutman CA (1977) Testing of some azo dyes and their reduction products for mutagenicity using *Salmonella typhimurium* TA 1538. Mutat Res 44:9-19
5. Martin CN, McDermid AC, Garner RC (1977) Measurement of "unscheduled" DNA synthesis in HeLa cells by liquid scintillation counting after carcinogen treatment. Cancer Lett 2:355-360
6. Martin CN, McDermid AC, Garner RC (1978) Testing of known carcinogens and noncarcinogens for their ability to induce unscheduled DNA synthesis in HeLa cells. Cancer Res 38:2621-2627
7. Peers FG, Linsell CA (1973) Dietary aflatoxins and liver cancer —a population based study in Kenya. Br J Cancer 27:473-484
8. Peers FG, Gilman GA, Linsell CA (1976) Dietary aflatoxins and human liver cancer. A study in Swaziland. Int J Cancer 17:167-176
9. Swenson DH, Lin J-K, Miller EC, Miller JA (1977) Aflatoxin B_1-2,3-oxide as a probable intermediate in the covalent binding of aflatoxins B_1 and B_2 to rat liver DNA and ribosomal RNA *in vivo*, Cancer Res 37:172-181
10. Garner RC, Miller EC, Miller JA, Garner JV, Hanson RS (1971) Formation of a factor lethal for *S. typhimurium* TA 1530 and TA 1531 on incubation of aflatoxin B_1 with rat liver microsomes. Biochem Biophys Res Commun 45:774-780
11. McLean AEM, Marshall A (1971) Reduced carcinogenic effects of aflatoxin in rats given phenobarbitone. Br J Exp Pathol 52:322-329

18

12. Garner RC, Miller EC, Miller JA (1972) Liver microsomal metabolism of aflatoxin B_1 to a reactive derivative toxic to *Salmonella typhimurium* TA 1530. Cancer Res 32:2058-2066
13. Garner RC, Wright CM (1975) Binding of [^{14}C] aflatoxin B_1 to cellular macromolecules in the rat and hamster. Chem Biol Interact 11:123-131
14. Garner RC (1975) Reduction in binding of [^{14}C] aflatoxin B_1 to rat liver macromolecules by phenobarbitone pretreatment. Biochem Pharmacol 24:1553 -1556
15. Wong JJ, Hsieh DPH (1976) Mutagenicity of aflatoxins related to their metabolism and carcinogenic potential. Proc Natl Acad Sci USA 73:2241 -2244

Microbial Assays: Evaluation and Application to the Elucidation of the Etiology of Colon Cancer

H. S. Rosenkranz, G. Karpinsky, and E. C. Mc Coy[1]

Introduction

The value of short-term microbial assay procedures to screen for environmental agents possessing carcinogenic and/or genetic activity has been established, as evidenced by the plethora of recently published studies and critical reviews on this subject (1-14). Among the available tests, the *Salmonella* mutagenicity assay developed by Ames and his associates has achieved prominence, especially as its reliability as a predictor of carcinogenicity has been demonstrated in a number of studies (1, 7-9). Indeed, a number of investigators have suggested a quantitative relationship between mutagenic potency and carcinogenic potential (15,16; however see also 18-20).

Because of the wide acceptance of the *Salmonella* mutagenicity procedure, the need for careful standardization of the assay became evident so as to allow interlaboratory comparisons. As a matter of fact, questions have been raised (6,18,19) concerning the variability of the assay, which may reflect the nature and origin of the activation mixture as well as the condition of incubation.

In view of these uncertainties, we have undertaken a study of the effects of variables on the *Salmonella* mutagenicity assay and we have participated in a National Cancer Institute-sponsored collaborative study (21) to evaluate the reliability of this assay.

The present report is concerned with:

1. A systematic evaluation of the various factors which may influence the standard *Salmonella* mutagenicity assay or variations thereof.
2. A description of some of the results which were obtained when the assay was run under rigorously standardized conditions.
3. A summary of experiments which illustrate the usefulness of modified assay protocols in the elucidation of basic biologic phenomena such as the etiology of colon cancer.
4. An evaluation of the usefulness of the standard *E. coli* DNA repair assay using pol A$^+$ and pol A$^-$ strains and variations thereof for the detection of carcinogens.

---

[1]Department of Microbiology, New York Medical College, Valhalla, New York 10595, USA

Table 1. Effect of preparative procedure on the activity of the S-9 fraction

Mice	Procedure	Protein (mg/ml)	P-450 (nmol/mg protein)	Revertants		
				per plate	per mg protein	per nmol P-450
Araclor-induced	Potter-Elvehjem homogenizer	39.0	0.5	566	145	290
	Waring blendor	20.0	0.99	620	310	313
Uninduced	Potter-Elvehjem homogenizer	27.5	0.15	193	70	467
	Waring blendor	23.5	0.17	222	95	556
	Polytron homogenizer	21.5	0.20	157	73	365

Strain TA 1538;
1 µg 2-aminoanthrazene per plate;
used 0.1 ml of S-9 per plate

The *Salmonella* Mutagenicity Assay: Effect of Variables. Preparation and Protein Content of the S-9 Fraction

Currently, laboratories using the *Salmonella* mutagenicity assay follow the procedure described by Ames and his associates in 1975 (22). It should be mentioned, however, that the afore-mentioned procedure differs from the one described by the same laboratory in 1973 (23) with respect to the amount of S-9 in-corporated into the agar overlay. This is an important variable, as will be shown below. Moreover, although the procedure de-scribed by Ames et al. (22) indicates that the final S-9 protein yield is 40 mg/ml, there is some variability in the exact protein yield. Although Ames et al. (22) preferred a Potter-Elvehjem homogenizer, they indicated that for tissues other than liver, a Polytron homogenizer was preferable. Still, other laboratories including our own have, on occasion, used the Waring blendor (24).

An analysis of the method most suitable for cell disruption showed (Table 1) that the Potter-Elvehjem homogenizer was most efficient for the recovery of soluble proteins while the Waring blendor appeared to favor the "selective" extraction of cyto-chrome P-450. An analysis of the ability of these S-9 prepar-ations to activate 2-aminoanthracene to a mutagen revealed that the extract prepared with the Waring blendor was the most ef-ficient. This was verified further when mutagenicity was ex-pressed per unit cytochrome P-450 or protein.

A survey of the literature, as well as intra- and interlabor-atory comparisons, have revealed variations in the protein content of the S-9 fraction prepared, presumably, by the same procedures. This variation in protein content, which may aver-age 30%, is not usually apparent in the published literature, as reports often do not indicate the protein content of S-9 preparations. In view of the fact that protein level may well be an important variable in the assay, we have undertaken a study of the effect of a 33% increase in the S-9 protein con-tent on the expression of the mutagenic activity of a number of standard chemicals in the *Salmonella* mutagenicity assay.

With 2-aminoanthracene and S-9 derived from Araclor-induced as well as uninduced rat livers, it was found (Table 2, upper half) that:

1. The dose response obtained with S-9 from induced animals reached a higher plateau than for the corresponding prep-aration from uninduced rats.
2. Increasing the protein content by 33% had no significant effect on the mutagenic response when levels of 2-amino-anthracene in excess of 3.3 µg/plate were used.
3. At lower protein levels, "significant" mutagenicity was de-monstrated at a mutagen concentration of 1 µg/plate but the increased protein content resulted in an increased sensi-tivity, as evidenced by the finding that a significant re-sponse was obtained with 0.3 µg of the chemical per plate.

Table 2. Effect of rat liver S-9 concentration on mutagenicity of 2-aminanthracene in the "standard" and preincubation assays

Chemical	µg/Plate	No S-9	Uninduced +S-9	Uninduced 1.33 × S-9	Induced +S-9	Induced 1.33 × S-9
		Standard assay				
2-Aminoanthracene	0	6	15	13	15	11
	0.3	6	25	48	27	47
	1.0	5	51	123	103	179
	3.3	10	131	214	896	1090
	10	13	160	312	1946	1768
	33	19	230	282	1865	1760
	100	18	239	221	1931	1446
	333	27	186	468	1721	1573
		Preincubation assay				
2-Aminoanthracene	0		11	10	8	9
	0.3		26	43	32	153
	1.0		39	77	149	393
	3.3		63	128	718	701
	10		58	183	1439	1152
	33		124	166	927	1137
	100		165	224	1522	1037
	333		145	193	1067	1147

[a]*Salmonella typhimurium* TA 1538
NADP content was 2 µmol/tube. Preincubation was carried out in total volume of 0.65 ml for 30 min at 37°C.

Essentially similar results were obtained when the same test mutagen (2-aminoanthracene) was activated by preparations derived from induced and uninduced mouse liver (Table 3). In addition, the same results were obtained when rat liver S-9 was tested with a coded specimen (no. 23040, Table 4). The data indicate that the sensitivity of the mutagenic response was increased with the elevated protein content, i.e., mutagenic activity is evident with 0.3 µg/plate as in contrast to the 1.0 µg/plate required with the S-9 of lower protein content. The dose-response curve was generally more elevated with the protein-rich S-9. The same findings were made with a number of other coded as well as uncoded chemicals.

Some investigators (18,19,25) have used lower NADP levels in the S-9 mix than recommended by Ames et al. (22). These researchers in turn have obtained results which were critized by others because of these differences in the NADP concentration (16). These experimental discrepancies have led us to investigate the effect of NADP level on mutagenic expression. Our studies with 2-aminoanthracene and 2-aminofluorene have shown that S-9 derived from uninduced rat liver was more sensitive to NADP level than a preparation from induced rats (Fig. 1).

Table 3. Effect of mouse liver S9 concentration on the mutagenicity[a] of 2-aminoanthracene

| | | Revertants per plate | | | | |
| | | | Uninduced | | Induced | |
Chemical	μg/Plate	No S-9	S-9	1.33 × S-9	S-9	1.33 × S-9
2-Aminoanthracene	0	5	7	12	8	7
	0.3	8	8	18	16	40
	1.0	6	12	40	52	93
	3.3	8	30	46	265	328
	10	14	37	84	454	342
	33	16	38	76	506	401
	100	11	69	82	715	481
	333	24	80	104	500	457
2-Nitrofluorene	100	291				

[a]*Salmonella typhimurium* TA 1538
In each instance the mix contained 2 μmol NADP and 1 μmol glucose-6-phosphate per plate; however, the mix designated 1.33 × S-9 and the one designated S-9 contained 1.6 and 1.2 mg protein per plate, respectively.

Table 4. Effect of rat liver S9 concentration on the mutagenicity of compound no. 23040

| | | | Revertants per plate | | | |
| | | | Uninduced | | Induced | |
Chemical	μg/Plate	Strain	1.33 × S-9	S-9	1.33 × S-9	S-9
23040	0	TA 98	37	18	46	18
	0.3	TA 98	56	19	70	34
	1.0	TA 98	617	147	133	77
	3.3	TA 98	1037	287	339	188
2-Aminoanthracene	1	TA 98	850	111	870	171
23040	0	TA 1538	19	12	33	12
	0.3	TA 1538	214	31	43	41
	1.0	TA 1538	583	102	349	39
	3.3	TA 1538	1076	258	783	172
2-Aminoanthracene	1	TA 1538	712	95	374	146
23040	0	TA 100	93	184	92	210
	0.3	TA 100	236	183	187	276
	1.0	TA 100	360	217	244	191
	3.3	TA 100	594	291	317	233
	10	TA 100	992	420	494	431
2-Aminoanthracene	10	TA 100	1018	445	2184	830

In order to ascertain the role of the composition of the S-9 mix on routine testing of coded specimens, such a chemical was tested using S-9 preparations prepared at different times; the mixes were reconstituted at different times. The results indicate that the 1.33 × S-9 preparation increases the sensitivity. NADP content: 2 μmol/plate.

24

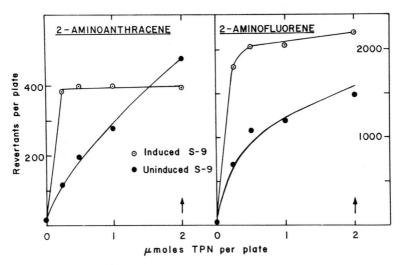

Fig. 1. Effect of NADP content on mutagenic expression. The S-9 preparations were derived from the livers of Araclor-induced and uninduced rats. The *arrow* indicates the level of NADP (2 μmol/plate) which is part of the standard plate incorporation assay described by Ames et al. (22). The levels of 2-aminoanthracene and 2-aminofluorene were 1 and 250 μg/plate, respectively. The tester strain was *S. typhimurium* TA 1538

Thus, for induced S-9 the response reached a maximal value with a NADP level between 0.25 and 0.5 μmol/plate. Contrariwise, with uninduced S-9 the response was not saturated, even with levels of 2 μmol of NADP, which is the NADP concentration used in the "standard" *Salmonella* assay (22). The basis of these findings remains to be determined. It is unlikely, however, that they reflect an increased NADP content of microsomal preparations from induced livers. They could, however, reflect a more efficient conversion of NADP to NADPH by induced S-9 preparations.

As it is conceivable that investigators who used decreased NADP levels in their S-9 mix also had the usual (30%) variations in protein content, an investigation was undertaken to determine the effect of varying both protein and NADP contents simultaneously.

Studies with mice (uninduced, Table 5) and induced as well as uninduced hamsters (Fig. 2) indicated that the increase in protein content of the hepatic S-9 more than compensated for any decreased response due to suboptimal NADP level. As a matter of fact, it was observed that after a minimum NADP level had been reached, the determining factor for maximal mutagenic response was the protein content of the S-9.

Glucose-6-phosphate was not limiting under these experimental conditions (Table 6). The complete omission of this cofactor had no effect on the mutagenic response. A similar observation was made by Ames et al. (22,23).

Table 5. Effect of composition of microsomal activation mixture on mutagenicity

Addition	µg/Plate	No S-9	"Standard" S-9	2 × S-9	1.33 × S-9
		Revertants per plate			
None	0	9	7	14	12
2-Nitrofluorene	100	430			
2-Aminofluorene	250	9	1599	2547	1734
2-Aminoanthracene	1	5	197	930	360
Composition of mix					
Protein mg/plate		0	1.2	2.4	1.6
NADP µmol/plate		0	2.0	2.0	0.32
Glucose-6-phosphate µmol/plate		0	2.6	2.6	1.0

Strain TA 1538. The S-9 was derived from the livers of uninduced mice.

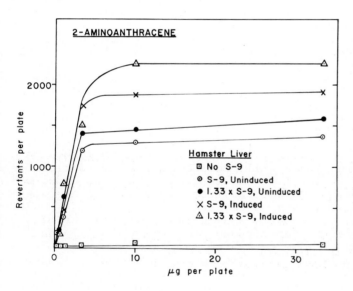

Fig. 2. Effect of protein content and NADP level on the mutagenic expression of 2-amino-anthracene. The S-9 preparations were derived from the livers of Araclor-induced and uninduced hamsters. The mix designated as S-9 contained per plate 1.2 mg protein and 2 µmol NADP while the preparation designated 1.33 × S-9 contained 1.6 mg protein and 0.32 µmol NADP per plate. The tester microorganism was *S. typhimurium* TA 1538

Although the present results indicate that the protein content and the cofactor level influence the extent of the mutagenic response, the findings also indicate that when complete dose-response determinations are carried out (rather than a spot test at a single test chemical concentration), that within limits, the variations in the assaying conditions will not influence whether a test chemical will be scored as a mutagen. Not considered in the above discussion, but of prime importance to the ultimate validation and acceptance of the *Salmonella*/microsome assay procedure, are a number of additional factors related to S-9 activation:

Table 6. Effect of glucose-6-phosphate content in microsomal activation mixture on mutagenicity

Glucose-6-phosphate (µmol/plate)	Mix	No addition	2-Aminoanthracene	2-Aminofluorene
0	-	18	14	96
0	A	14	1125	2223
1	A	22	1215	2142
3	A	21	1127	2022
5	A	17	1114	2135
0	B	19	559	2086
1	B	14	1009	1589
3	B	19	917	1432
5	B	18	650	1941

Mix A and mix B contained 2 µmol NADP per plate but the protein content of mix A was 2 mg protein per plate while for mix B it was 2.4 mg protein per plate. The levels of 2-aminoanthracene and 2-aminofluorene were 1 and 250 µg/plate, respectively. The S-9 was derived from uninduced mouse liver. TA 1538.

1. Known intraspecies variations in S-9 activity. This has been documented for man (1), our ultimate concern.
2. The ability of S-9 to quench (or detoxify) reactive mutagens (24,26,27). This may be directly affected by the protein content of the S-9 (24,26).
3. The species of origin of the S-9 will have a bearing on the ability of such preparations to activate premutagens. Such effects have been amply documented (6,18-20,28-30). Undoubtedly, the current collaborative study (21) sponsored by the National Cancer Institute will provide cogent information on this subject, as it involves the testing of several hundred coded specimens with S-9 derived from the livers of Araclor-induced and uninduced rats, mice, and hamsters.
4. Obviously the mode of hepatic enzyme induction will be of crucial importance. It has already been shown (18,31) that certain chemicals will be activated only with preparations derived from animals induced with specific inducers (18,31; and McCoy and Rosenkranz, unpublished results).
5. It is known that the ultimate in vitro mutagenic expression of premutagens (and precarcinogens) will be the result of several competing "activating" and "inactivating" enzymes, e.g., monooxygenase, epoxide hydratases (18,19,30). In addition to the known differences in the levels of these enzymes among species, the stability of these enzymes is not known; it is therefore conceivable that some of them are more readily inactivated upon incubation at 37°C or storage in the cold.

Salmonella Mutagenicity Assays: Procedural Variations

Although the procedure described by Ames et al. (22) is the most
widely used of the *Salmonella* mutagenicity assays, a number of
modifications of this procedure may be preferable under certain
experimental conditions.

The Preincubation Assay

Nitrosamines are an important class of carcinogens, yet they
present a problem when assayed by the standard plate incorporation procedure, presumably due to the labile nature of the
metabolic intermediates which may be capable of reacting with
the excess agar present in the standard assay. To overcome this
deficiency, Yahagi and colleagues (12-14,32) have modified the
standard assay wherein the chemical, S-9 and cofactors are preincubated at 37°C for 30 min; the reaction mixture is then added
to molten agar and spread onto the surface of the agar plate. The
plates are incubated and enumerated in the usual manner. Using
this assay, increased reliability in detecting the mutagenicity
of nitrosamines has been reported (12-14). In our hands (24,33
-35), the procedure was satisfactory for demonstrating the
mutagenicity of a series of volatile chemicals (Table 7) as well
as the mutagenicity of labile chemicals such as glycidaldehyde
(see Fig. 12).

Table 7. Effect of procedure on the mutagenicity of labile chemicals

Compound	Amount per plate	Revertants per plate[a]	
		Standard	Preincubation
Dimethylcarbamyl chloride	0	22	29
	0.3 µg	18	24
	1.0 µg	22	27
	3.3 µg	19	25
	10 µg	23	56
	33 µg	33	138
	100 µg	57	517
	333 µg	98	644
Allyl chloride	0	14	20
	1 µl	13	42
	2 µl	19	56
	5 µl	15	82
	10 µl	15	60

[a]Strain TA 1535 was used in all experiments

In view of the fact that a number of mutagens undetectable by the standard assay give positive responses in the preincubation procedure, it has been suggested (12-14) that the preincubation assay be used routinely in preference to the standard plate incorporation method. However, it has been reported that the stability of the microsomal enzymes may be affected by the preincubation conditions (36). Indeed, we found that incubation of S-9 at 37 C for 30 min could result in reduced enzyme activity (Table 8). It would seem, therefore, that the preincubation assay does not necessarily combine the advantage of detectability of labile and volatile chemicals with the ability of the standard assay to activate chemicals over prolonged periods. It appears that in the standard procedure the agar may exercise a stabilizing effect on enzyme activity.

Finally, until such time as the preincubation procedure has been validated under the same rigorous conditions as the standard plate incorporation assay (i.e., the use of coded samples analyzed in multiple laboratories), it would seem that it should be used only when the test chemical is known to be volatile or when it is uniformly negative in the standard assay procedure. Still, because of the potential usefulness of the preincubation assay, and in order to establish criterial for standardizing and subsequently validating it, we have undertaken a study of some of the factors influencing this assay. We have also compared its sensitivity in a number of instances with that of the standard plate incorporation procedure.

Table 8. Effect of preincubation on microsomal activity

Preincubation	S-9	Revertants per plate		
		No addition	2-Aminofluorene[a]	2-Aminoanthracene[a]
−	−	7	26	14
+	−		29	9
−	Rat, uninduced	6	520	818
+	Rat, uninduced		81	39
−	−	4	36	
−	Mouse, induced	12	1218	
+	Mouse, induced		1444	

[a]The final contents of 2-aminofluorene and 2-aminoanthracene were 250/plate and 1 μg/plate, respectively

The preincubation S-9 + cofactors were incubated for 30 min at 37°C whereupon the test chemical and 2 ml of soft agar were added and upon mixing the contents were spread onto the surface of agar plates. Bacterial strain TA 1538. Note that only the preparation from uninduced rat liver was inactivated by preincubation.

When comparing the mutagenic response of microorganisms with certain levels of test agents by the standard plate incorporation procedure and by the preincubation modification thereof, it must be realized that even though results are expressed as mutants per microgram of test agent added per plate, during the actual preincubation period the test chemical is in 0.65 ml, to which subsequently 2 ml of soft agar are added. On the other hand, in the standard procedure of 0.05-0.1 ml of the test agent is added directly to 2 or 2.4 ml of soft agar which are poured onto 25-30 ml of 1.5% agar. Hence in the preincubation modification, if it be assumed that the entire reaction takes place during the 30 min of preincubation, the actual concentration of the test agent is at least 3.8-fold greater than in the standard plate incorporation assay.

With these facts in mind, data derived from preincubation and standard plate incorporation assays can be examined. For direct-acting agents (Table 9) which demonstrate little bactericidal activity, the results are variable. Thus, 9-aminoacridine and sodium azide at nonsaturating levels yield, reproducibly, more mutants per dose of chemical added in the preincubation assay. However, when saturating levels of the test chemical are reached, the two assays may give very similar results (see 9-aminoacridine, Table 9). On the other hand, with 2-nitrofluorene no great difference between the two procedures was seen at any of the levels tested (Table 9). For strongly bactericidal agents, i.e., nitrofuran (AF-2, Fig. 3), the tester strain responds over a much narrower dose range in the preincubation assay, presumably reflecting: (a) the greater actual concentration of the test agent during the initial period of incubation (see above), (b) the lower survival rate of the bacteria under these conditions, and (c) the increased lethal effect of these batericidal agents under the conditions of enhanced growth that are prevalent in the liquid medium.

Because 2-aminoanthracene causes frameshift as well as base-substitution mutations, it is frequently used as the model for chemicals requiring metabolic activation. With enzymes from induced as well as uninduced *mouse* liver, it was found that the sensitivity of the assay was increased in the preincubation procedure (i.e., lower levels of the test agents were detectable) (Table 10). However, no such effect was observed with enzymes from induced as well as uninduced *rat* livers. As with the standard plate incorporation procedure, an increase in the protein content of the S-9 resulted in an increased sensitivity of the assay (Table 2).

The relevance of the above results to the data obtained during routine screening conditions remains to be elucidated. However, the findings thus far indicate that the two modifications cannot be used interchangeably to obtain quantitatively similar results which could then be used for potency comparisons. Rather, the results indicate that the preincubation assay, at this time, should be used only to determine the mutagenicity of chemicals that do not react in the standard assay procedure.

Table 9. Sensitivity of "standard" and "preincubation" assay procedures for direct-acting mutagens

Chemical	µg/Plate	Strain	Revertants per plate Standard	Revertants per plate Preincubation
None	0	TA 1537	4	5
9-Aminoacridine	50	TA 1537	461	800
9-Aminoacridine	100	TA 1537	2221	2349
2-Nitrofluorene	0	TA 1538	8	9
	0.3		10	18
	1.0		34	24
	3.3		68	77
	10		149	236
	33		275	293
	100		354	
	333		460	418
Sodium azide	0		14	18
	0.3	TA 1535	16	85
	1.0		57	176
	3.3		168	678
	10		460	1035
	33		843	1474
	100		913	1873

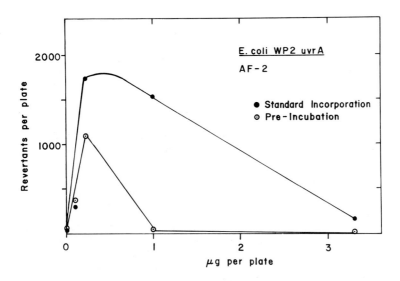

Fig. 3. Demonstration of the mutagenicity of the nitrofuran AF-2 by the standard plate incorporation and the preincubation assays. The data shown in the figure were obtained with *E. coli* WP2 uvrA (87-89), but similar results are obtained with *S. typhimurium* TA 100. The purpose of the above example is to illustrate the fact that *E. coli* WP2 uvrA can be evaluated in a manner similar as the *S. typhimurium* strains

Table 10. Comparison of "standard" and "preincubation" assays using 2-aminoanthracene

Chemical	µg/Plate	Strain Enzyme	Revertants per plate	
			Standard	Preincubation
2-Aminoanthracene	0	TA 1538 MI	11	8
	0.3		37	118
	1.0		143	460
	3.3		613	802
	10		1188	1001
	33		1146	815
	100		1277	1032
	333		746	760
2-Aminoanthracene	0	TA 1537 MU	4	5
	2.5		18	90
2-Aminoanthracene	0	TA 1538 RU	15	1
	0.3		25	26
	1.0		51	39
	3.3		131	63
	10		160	58
	33		230	124
	100		239	165
	333		186	145
2-Aminoanthracene	0	TA 1538 RI	15	8
	0.3		27	32
	1.0		103	149
	3.3		896	718
	10		1946	1439
	33		1865	
	100		1931	1522
	333		1721	1067

Pre-incubation was for 30 min at 37°C. MI and MU: S-9 from induced and uninduced mouse liver, respectively; similarly for RI and RU: S-9 from induced and uninduced rat liver.

The Liquid Suspension Assay

Classically, the genetic effects of chemical and physical agents have been expressed as mutation frequency (mutants per survivors). Obviously, this procedure is more tedious and time-consuming than the plate incorporation assay, as it requires serial dilutions followed by the enumeration, on selective media, of mutants and of survivors. A preliminary determination of the optimal level of test agents and optimal period of incubation for appropriate survival is also required. The survival rate should be at least 25%-40% to permit the enumeration of a sufficient number of mutants. Obviously, the main advantage of the standard plate incorporation assay is circumvention of these tedious and time-consuming maneuvers. It must be realized, however, that in the standard assay, results are expressed as

revertants per plate and that no adjustment is made for bactericidal agents which may cause decreases in the survival rate
(26,37). Thus, it was found that mutagens that were also strongly
bactericidal could not be scored by the standard plate incorporation assay because of low survival rates and a coincidence of
minimal bactericidal concentrations with optimal mutagenic
levels. The genetic activity of such chemicals was, however,
readily demonstrated (26,37-41) in liquid suspension assays
wherein results are expressed as mutants per survivors. This was
accomplished upon adjusting conditions of exposure to allow for
adequate survival, thereby permitting the survival and subsequent enumeration of sufficient mutants. This can be done by
limiting exposure in contrast to the 48 h of incubation in the
presence of test chemicals which is part of the standard protocol.

The liquid suspension assay has the added advantage that it can
be used to study the properties of chemicals requiring metabolic
activation when for technical reasons this metabolic conversion
cannot be achieved in the plate incorporation assay. This may
be either because the active intermediate is labile and may not
reach the bacteria and, hence, may react preferentially with the
agar, or it may be volatile. As a matter of fact, the liquid
suspension assay for *Salmonella* in conjunction with metabolic
activation has been pioneered by Malling and his associates, who
investigated the mutagenicity of nitrosamines (42,43).

We have acquired considerable expertise with the liquid suspension
assay coupled to microsomal activation mixtures and we have found
that the assay can give reproducible results only when it is
rigorously standardized with respect to the age of the culture,
the bacterial density, the composition of the reaction mixture,
the S-9 mix, the age of the S-9, and the ionic strength of the
media and buffers.

Although, we have identified a number of bactericidal agents
whose mutagenicity was expressed only in the liquid suspension
assay, we have as yet not found a nonbactericidal agent requiring
metabolic activation whose genetic activity was demonstrable
only in the liquid suspension assay coupled to S-9. All such
chemicals were also positive either in the standard plate incorporation assay or in the preincubation modification thereof.
Still it was evident from all of our studies that the liquid
assay procedure was the most sensitive of the *Salmonella* assays
studied in our laboratory. Much lower levels of test agents
were required to demonstrate genetic activity. Moreover, because
the volume of the incubation mixture can be adjusted, the absolute amount of chemical required per test may be quite low.
The sensitivity of the liquid assay procedure compared with that
of the standard assay is illustrated in Table 11 with respect
to the activity of nitrosomorpholine.

Table 11. Relative sensitivity of "standard" and "liquid suspension" procedures

Nitrosomorpholine

µg/Assay	µg/ml	Liquid suspension Revertants/10^8 survivors	Standard assay Revertants per plate
0	0	0.34	11
0.25	0.083	0.68	6
2.5	0.83	2.5	17
25	8.3	10	24
250	83	9.4	118
2500	833	13.4	244

TA 1535. S-9 from uninduced mouse liver, diluted 1/10. In the liquid assay the exposure time was 90 min, whereupon dilutions of the treated cultures were plated for the determination of the number of revertants to histidine independence and of survivors.

Bactericidal Activity of Microsomal Preparations

Although it has been recognized that S-9 preparations are toxic to mammalian cells growing in tissue culture, the possible inhibitory effect of such preparations on bacterial cells has neither been considered nor reported. Indeed, in view of the already wide use of the microbial assays coupled to microsomal activation mixtures, such an effect would have been detected. However, in the course of our studies on the *Salmonella* liquid suspension assay, we became aware of the fact that during the standard period of incubation (90 min, 37°C) there was a considerable loss of bacterial viability (Table 12) that frequently interfered with the interpretation of the experimental results. Further investigations revealed that this bactericidal effect of the S-9 mix was independent of the presence of cofactors (NADP, glucose-6-phospphate) but that it was abolished by heating at 56°C for 30 min (Table 12), which suggested that perhaps this bactericidal activity was mediated by complement (which, classically, is inactivated by heating at 56°C for 30 min).

The bactericidal effect of the S-9 could be decreased by a reduction in the protein content (Table 13), but this in turn resulted in a suboptimal S-9 concentration which was no longer able to allow expression of the mutagenic potential of the test agent. Additional studies indicated that inactivation of the bactericidal activity by heating at 56°C for 30 min also destroyed the enzymatic activity of the S-9 (Table 14), as evidenced by the inability of such a heated preparation to activate nitrosomorpholine to a mutagen.

The exact nature of this bactericidal principle remains to be investigated. It does on occasion, however, interfere with the liquid assay procedure, and its effect on the standard plate incorporation procedure as well as on the preincubation assay remains to be established. Such an investigation is currently under way in our laboratory.

Table 12. Evidence for heat-labile* bactericidal activity
in mouse microsomal preparations

| Conditions | Fractional survival | |
	TA 1535	TA 98
I Control	1.41	1.23
+ S-9 mix	0.33	0.15
+* Heated S-9 mix	1.82	1.40
II Control	1.33	
+ S-9 (no cofactors)	0.32	
+ S-9 mix (+ cofactors)	0.47	
+* Heated S-9 (no cofactors)	1.88	
+* Heated S-9 mix (+ cofactors)	1.45	

Heating of S-9 was for 30 min at 56°C. Conditions of incubation: 90 min at 37°C, as for standard liquid assay
procedure. The S-9 was prepared from uninduced mouse liver.

Table 13. Effect of S-9 concentration on bacterial survival and
on mutagenicity

| Strain | | Fractional survival | | |
		S-9	0.6 × S-9	
TA 1535		0.24	1.30	
TA 1537		0.16	0.51	
TA 98		0.08	1.03	
		0.09	1.04	
Chemical	µg/Plate	Frequency of mutations[a]		
		S-9	0.6 × S-9	No S-9
2-Aminoanthracene	0	7.1	2.1	
	167	8.1	1.7	
	250	11.8	1.7	
2-Nitrofluorene	33			53.1

[a]Strain TA 98. Revertants per 10^7 survivors
In each instance incubation was for 90 min at 37°C. S-9 from
uninduced mouse liver.

Table 14. Effect of heating at 56°C on microsomal activation

| Chemical | µg/ml | Revertants per 10^8 survivors | |
		+S-9	+heated S-9
Nitrosomorpholine	0	1.7	1.5
	208	19.0	3.0
	417	35.2	2.9
	833	53.4	2.3

Heating: 56°C, 30 min. S-9 was derived from the livers of
uninduced mice. Strain TA 1535.

Results Obtained When the Standard Plate Incorporation Assay Is Carried Out Under Rigorously Standarized Conditions

Most laboratories using the *Salmonella* mutagenicity assay follow the directions provided by Ames et al. (22). Still, in a collaborative study (21) it was found that using the same chemical (same lot) and the same strains (freshly received from Dr. Ames at the beginning of the investigation), interlaboratory variations were found (Fig. 4), even with direct-acting chemicals. Further inquiry revealed that intralaboratory variations, although less dramatic, were also common (Fig. 5).

These findings led the collaborating laboratories to institute carefully controlled conditions pertaining to the growth and physiologic state of the indicator bacteria at the time of their addition to the agar (only exponentially growing bacteria were used), the composition and source of the media, the storage of the agar plates, the age, protein content, and mode of preparation of the S-9 and cofactor mix, etc.

Using such standardized conditions, the reproducibility of the assay was greatly improved, although variations still occurred. Some intralaboratory results obtained over a 1-year period for sodium azide and 2-nitrofluorene are shown in Figs. 6 and 7. It is to be noted that the plasmid-containing strains (TA 98 and TA 100) appear to be less variable than the corresponding non-plasmid-containing strains (TA 1538 and TA 1535, respectively). Good interlaboratory reproducibility was also observed (21).

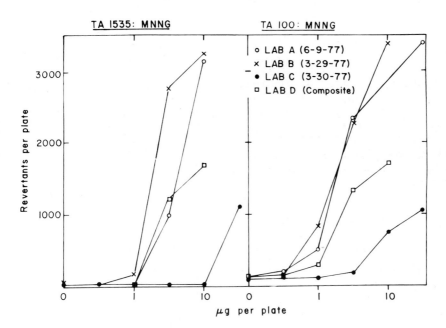

Fig. 4. Mutagenicity of MNNG (N-methyl-N'-nitro-N-nitrosoguanidine) for *S. typhimurium*: interlaboratory comparisons. The standard plate incorporation assay was used. *Left*, TA 1535; *right*, TA 100

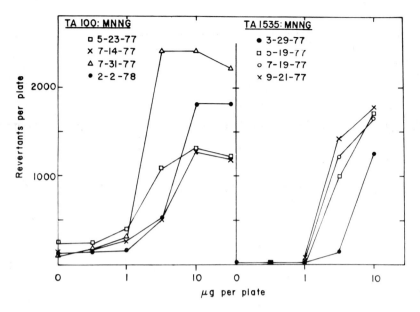

Fig. 5. Mutagenicity of MNNG for *S. typhimurium* TA 100 and TA 1535. Intra-laboratory variation. The standard plate incorporation assay was used. The *numbers* next to the symbols indicate the dates on which the assays were carried out

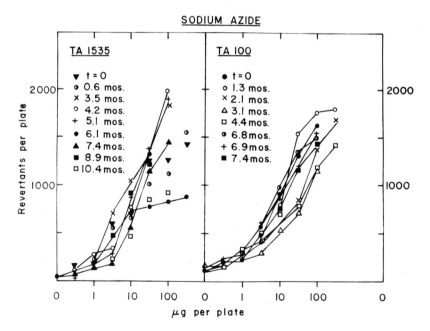

Fig. 6. Mutagenicity of sodium azide for *S. typhimurium* TA 100 and TA 1535: intralaboratory variation. The procedure (standard plate incorporation) was rigorously standardized; however, at intervals different persons carried out the assays

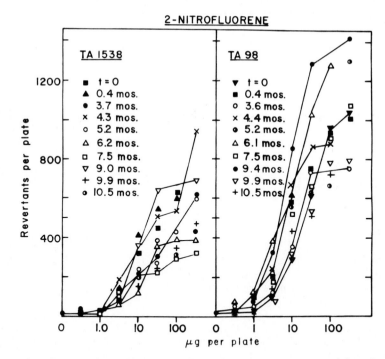

Fig. 7. Mutagenicity of 2-nitrofluorene for *S. typhimurium* TA 98 and TA 1538; intralaboratory variation. The procedure (standard plate incorporation) was rigorously standardized; however, at intervals the assay was carried out by different persons

In an attempt to determine the causes of these variations, which were observed even when conditions were carefully standardized, the background (spontaneous frequency) and the number of mutants induced by a standard amount of a mutagen were analyzed. It was found that each tester strain appeared to have intrinsic variability. Thus strain TA 1535 (Fig. 8) exhibited a narrow range of spontaneous revertants, but the presence of a standard dose of a mutagen (10 μg sodium azide per plate) resulted in a rather heterogeneous mutagenic response. A further analysis of these data (Fig. 9) indicated that these variations did not appear to reflect the age of the culture, nor did a subculture with a high spontaneous frequency result in an enhanced mutagenic response to the mutagen, i.e., the ratio of mutagenic response-background value was not constant.

Even though strain TA 1535 had a narrow range of spontaneous mutants (Fig. 8), its plasmid-containing derivative TA 100 exhibited a broader range of spontaneous mutants (Fig. 10). On the other hand, the mutagenic response of TA 100 to sodium azide was over a much narrower range (Fig. 10). In this respect, therefore, strains TA 100 and TA 1535 appeared to have opposite reactions.

The addition of S-9 to TA 100 increased the heterogeneity of the spontaneous response, and the presence of S-9 and of 2-aminoanthracene (2 μg/plate) resulted in a broad mutagenic response (Fig. 10).

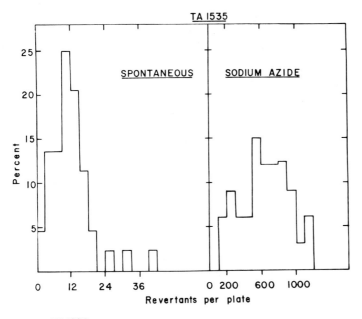

Fig. 8. Characteristics of the tester strain TA 1535: distribution of spontaneous revertants and of sodium azide (10 μg/plate) induced revertants. (Note the change in scale of the *abscissa* for the two histograms.)

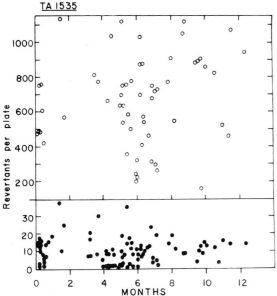

Fig. 9. Historical response of *S. typhimurium* TA 1535 under standard conditions as a function of time. *Upper portion*, response to 10 μg sodium azide per plate; *lower portion*, spontaneous frequency. Each *point* is the mean of three individual plates. (Note the change in scale of the *ordinate*.)

The variability in the response of TA 100 did not derive from the age of the culture and, as with TA 1535, a high spontaneous background did not result in an enhanced mutagenic response (Fig. 11).

The present findings indicate that standardization of testing procedure increases reproducibility. However, in view of the variations which occur even under the most stringent of conditions

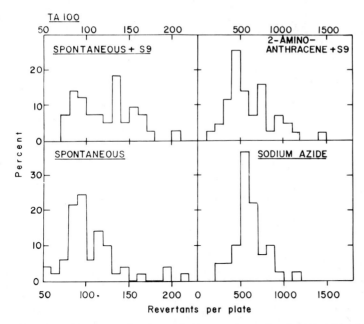

Fig. 10. Characteristics of the tester strain TA 100: distribution of spontaneous revertants in the presence (*upper left*) and absence (*lower left*) of S-9, of sodium azide (10 µg/plate) induced revertant (*lower right*), and of revertants induced by 2-aminoanthracene (2.5 µg/plate) in the presence of S-9 (*upper right*). (Note the change in scale of the *abscissa* between the histograms on the left and those on the right.)

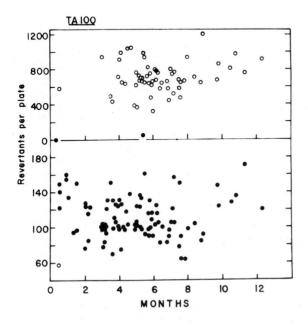

Fig. 11. Historical response of tester strain TA 100 under standard conditions as a function of time. *Upper portion*, response to 10 µg sodium azide per plate; *lower portion*, spontaneous frequency. (Note the change in scale of the *ordinate*.)

it would appear that the *Salmonella* mutagenicity assay, as currently used for routine screening, cannot yield *exact* specific mutagenicity activity values (i.e., mutants per nanomole). The basis of these variations remains unexplained and surely deserves further investigation.

As part of this study of the reproducibility of the assay procedure, the variations intrinsic to the preincubation assay were also investigated. Under carefully controlled conditions (Fig. 12), it was found that the reproducibility of this procedure was in the same range as that observed for the standard plate incorporation assay.

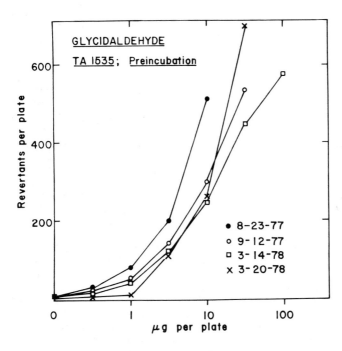

Fig. 12. Mutagenicity of glycidaldehyde. Intra-laboratory variation of the preincubation procedure. The *numbers* next to the symbols refer to the date on which the assay was run. The procedure was carried out under rigorously standardized conditions; however, at the intervals indicated different individuals carried out the assay

Finally, it may well be that intra- as well as interlaboratory variabilities reflect seemingly minor changes in protocol or differences in the impurities present in the major constituents of the assay. Thus the lack of genetic activity of saccharin in several microbial systems was reported (44). However, making some apparently minor alterations in the protocol, Batzinger and colleagues (45) were able to demonstrate the mutagenicity of this sweetener for *Salmonella typhimurium*.

Microbial Assays and the Etiology of Colon Cancer

Even while the use of microbial assays for the systematic identification of environmental mutagens and carcinogens must be standardized rigorously to achieve reproducible results, there are certain experimental conditions in which the flexibility of the microbial assays is a great asset to the investigator in the study of basic phenomenon.

Thus, using nitroreductase-deficient *Salmonella* tester strains in the standard assay, we were able to demonstrate (46,47) the mutagenic activation of therapeutically important nitro-containing chemicals by hepatic microsomes, thereby establishing that these chemicals were not dependent upon microbial enzymes for activation to mutagenic and/or carcinogenic substances. Additional studies demonstrated that nonmicrosomal activation systems could be readily coupled to the microbial assays. We were able to demonstrate that photoactivation of premutagens could be linked to the assay procedures (34,35,48,49). Also, it was possible to show that urines from anesthesiologists (50) and from patients undergoing certain therapeutic maneuvers (51) contained mutagenic chemicals. These activities could be fractionated using the microbial assays to monitor the purification of the mutagenic chemicals.

These findings led us to apply these procedures to a systematic evaluation of the factors responsible for colon cancer. First of all, it must be realized that the colon provides an anaerobic environment. Moreover, epidemiologic studies have implicated diets rich in meats and fat in the induction of colon cancer in human populations. Such diets have been shown to result in an enhanced production of bile acids and in an increase in the anaerobic colonic flora. Furthermore, the anaerobic bacterial flora have been shown to be capable of metabolizing bile acids to structures which bear structural relationships to known carcinogens (52-65). Finally, bile metabolites have been implicated as promoters of colon cancer and as comutagens (66-68,70,71).

These hypotheses and findings led us to undertake a number of preliminary studies designed to develop assay systems which would mimic the colonic environment. While most in vitro systems seeking to elucidate the role of certain organ-specific carcinogens are performed under aerobic conditions (see 72,73), the situation with colon cancer requires that anaerobic conditions be established wherein metabolites that are formed and that may be oxygen-sensitive can be evaluated. Accordingly, experimental conditions were devised for determining the mutagenic potential under conditions which included a period of anaerobic incubation (74). It was demonstrated (Table 15) that chemicals which do not include an oxygen-labile intermediate in their metabolism are not affected by these conditions, while agents which were biotransformed to metabolites, which are potentially unstable in the presence of oxygen, exhibited a greatly increased mutagenic potential under these conditions (26,37,74).

It is not often realized that the colonic flora is predominantly anaerobic and that it is presumably very active in the bioconversion of metabolites to active intermediates. Accordingly, we investigated procedures for preparing cell-free extracts derived from anaerobic bacteria which could be incorporated into the microbial assay in place of (or in addition to) the S-9 microsomal preparation. A method for preparing such cell-free prep-

Table 15. Effect of anaerobiosis on mutagenicity for *Salmonella typhimurium*

				Revertants per plate	
Group	Additions	Strain	μg/Plate	Aerobic	Anaerobic
I	Ethyl methanesulfonate	TA 100	7	5000	5000
	2-Bromoethanol	TA 100	5.5	690	710
	1,2-Epoxybutane	TA 100	14	390	410
	Propyleneimine	TA 100	1.4	7000	7000
II	Azathioprine	TA 100	0	109	107
			25		114
			100		239
			250	165	375
			400		553
			500	149	659
III	6-Nitrosopurine	TA 1535	0	28	21
			10	24	33
			25	28	34
			100	28	61
			250	44	79
	2-Nitrofluorene	TA 1538	5 μg	700	1220
	2-Nitronaphthalene	TA 1535	100 μg	480	816

Anaerobiosis was achieved by placing the Petri plates into Gas Pak jars (BBL, Cockeysville, Maryland) which were incubated (37°C) in the dark for 14 h, whereupon the plates were removed from the jar and incubated aerobically for an additional 34 h. It should be noted that chemicals in group I were not affected significantly by anaerobic incubation. They do not yield oxygen-sensitive intermediates. The mutagenicity of azathioprine could only be demonstrated under anaerobic conditions. The mutagenicity of chemicals in group II was enhanced significantly when incubated anaerobically. The metabolic intermediates of the chemicals in groups II and III are presumably the corresponding oxygen-labile hydroxamates.

arations and for including them in their *Salmonella* assay was devised (75) (Table 16). Such preparations which required an anaerobic environment were capable of activating 2-aminofluorene to a mutagenic metabolite, presumably the corresponding 2-hydroxylaminofluorene. This ability to perform an oxidative conversion of a premutagen to an active intermediate is an important requirement of the system, for, although in the anaerobic milieu there is no oxygen, still the bacteria must be capable of such an oxidative conversion if they are to be active in the transformation of procarcinogens. Presumably, this can be accomplished through mixed fermentation reactions such as the Stickland reaction.

Finally, another factor that must be considered is the metabolic activity of the colonic mucosa. Thus, although the hepatic enzymes are presumably very active in the conversion of procarcinogens and promutagens, other studies have already indicated that tissue specificity in the activation of specific carcinogens

Table 16. Activation of 2-aminofluorene by cell-free extracts from anaerobic bacteria

Source of extract	Amount of extract (mg protein per plate)	Condition of incubation	Mutants per plate	
			No 2-amino fluorene	+2-amino fluorene[a]
Clostridium perfringens	1.0	Anaerobic		288
Clostridium perfringens	2.0	Anaerobic	5	505
Heated *C. perfringens*	1.0	Anaerobic		21
Heated *C. perfringens*	2.0	Anaerobic	12	16
Bacteroides fragilis	1.0	Anaerobic		345
Bacteroides fragilis	2.0	Anaerobic	5	549
Heated *B. fragilis*	1.0	Anaerobic		14
Heated *B. fragilis*	2.0	Anaerobic	9	17
None	0	Anaerobic	10	18
None	0	Aerobic	4	34
B. fragilis	0.5	Anaerobic	4	533
B. fragilis	0.5	Aerobic	9	68
C. perfringens	0.8	Anaerobic	5	424
C. perfringens	0.8	Aerobic	8	56

[a] 25 µg 2-aminofluorene
Note that maximal activity was achieved only when incubation was in the absence of oxygen. Heating of the extracts (80°C) destroyed the activity.

may be very important (72,73). Previously it was found (26,37) in our laboratory that microsomes derived from the epidermal tissues of the newborn rat metabolized the flame retardant Tris [= tris(2,3-dibromopropyl)phosphate] to a different mutagenic intermediate than did the hepatic S-9 derived from the same animals. It is, therefore, probable that the colonic mucosa is endowed with its own metabolic potential which may intervene in the carcinogenic event that triggers colon cancer. Accordingly, we investigated the optimal conditions for preparing and demonstrating the activation of promutagens by S-9 derived from colonic mucosa (Table 17). Current studies in our laboratory are concerned with the ability of cell-free bacterial extracts and of the microsomes from the colonic mucosa to convert separately or in concert candidate colon-specific carcinogens to mutagens.

However, in parallel with these we have investigated the mutagenic potential of human bile in view of the proposed role of bile in the induction of colonic (see above) and extracolonic cancer (75). Preliminary studies have been most promising. Thus, although human bile is without mutagenic activity both in the presence and absence of S-9 preparations (derived from Araclor-induced rat livers) (Table 18), exposure of such preparations

Table 17. Activation of 2-aminoanthracene to a mutagen by S-9 from colonic mucosa

Additions	Revertants	
	per Plate	per mg Protein
None	3	6
2-Aminoanthracene (10 µg)	34	83

Strain *Salmonella typhimurium* TA 1538.

Table 18. Presence of a mutagenic component in a human bile

Addition	Amount per plate	Revertants per plate	
		-S-9	+S-9
None	0	7	
Bile	0.001 µl	3	9
	0.01 µl	7	4
	0.1 µl	7	8
	1 µl	10	4
	10 µl	6	6
Picrolonic acid	250 µg	786	
2-Aminofluorene	100 µg	117	557
		After cycling in anaerobes	
None	0	2	4
Bile	5 µl	218	1006
	10 µl	382	1543
	15 µl	313	1604

Tester strain *Salmonella typhimurium* TA 1538

to actively growing selected bile-tolerant microorganisms resulted in the formation of mutagenic compounds. The genetic activity of this preparation was increased even further by incubation with hepatic S-9 preparations (Table 18). The results indicate that bile may well contain a precarcinogen which can be metabolized to a carcinogen by the sequential metabolic action of bacterial and mucosal enzymes. This appears to be the first evidence for the role of bile as a "classic" carcinogen rather than as a tumor promoter.

It must be stressed that these findings which are being investigated further in our laboratory were made possible by the availability of a simple and readily adaptable microbial assay system, in the absence of which such a study could not have been undertaken by our group. The same microbial system is now being used to monitor the isolation of the active principle(s).

The Detection of DNA-Modifying Activity with the *E. coli* Pol A/Pol A Assay System

As is evident both from the published literature as well as from the above discussion, the *Salmonella* mutagenicity assay developed by Ames et al. (22) is very useful for the detection of important environmental chemicals. Moreover, given the variability of the test, it is quite possible that the reliability of the assay may be extended even further when used under strictly standardized conditions and employing S-9 preparations from more than one species. As has been mentioned previously, however, a number of agents of known as well as unknown carcinogenicity are negative in the standard *Salmonella* assay system but give reproducibly positive results in another microbial assay, the *E. coli* pol A^+/pol A^- system (24,26,34,35,37-40,76).

The DNA-repair assay is predicated upon a different principle: the preferential inhibition of the DNA polymerase-deficient *E. coli* pol A_1^- by mutagens and carcinogens (11,76). The chemicals in this group include bactericidal agents (povidone-iodine (37,40), hydroxylamino-O-sulfonic acid (77), sodium hypochlorite (39), halogenated hydrocarbons [1,1,2,2-tetrabromoethane (38,78)], some intercalating agents [auramine O, *p*-rosaniline, Miracil D, chloroquine (24,34,35,79,80)], and others [N-hydroxyurethan (34, 81)].

The demonstration of the preferential inhibition of the pol A_1^- strain can be accomplished by three experimental procedures:

I) The determination of the viability of the bacterial cultures as a function of time and of dose (concentration) (Figs. 13 and 14) (79,82-86).

II) A disk diffusion spot test in which DNA-modifying agents can be shown to inhibit preferentially the pol A^- strain as evidenced by larger zones of growth inhibition (Fig. 15 and Table 19) (26,37,76,81).

III) A modification of procedure I in which specimens of pol A^+ and pol A^- are exposed to a single or a multiple dose of the test agents for a predetermined period of time (90 min) whereupon survivors are enumerated (37,76). Results are expressed as fractional survivors. Values below 1.0 are taken to indicate a preferential inhibition of the pol A^- strain.

In practice, for the routine screening of environmental agents, chemicals are first tested by procedure II and, in the event that neither strain is inhibited (i.e., a "no test" result), the chemicals are tested by procedure III.

In order to evaluate the pol A assay and to compare its reliability for predicting carcinogens with the *Salmonella* mutagenicity assay, a series of representative carcinogens and noncarcinogens was tested in both assays. The results summarized (Tables 21-23) are presented in greater detail elsewhere (24,76). They indicate that in the present group of chemicals no substance was positive in the *Salmonella* assay but negative in the pol A procedure. Conversely, however, some chemicals were positive only in the pol A assay.

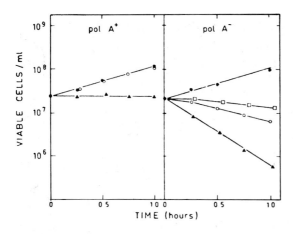

Fig. 13. Effect of acridine orange (AO) on viability of *E. coli* pol A and pol A$_1^-$. Bacteria were brought to the exponential growth phase, at which time portions of the cultures were distributed into flasks containing premeasured amounts of AO. At intervals portions of each culture were removed for enumeration of viable cells. Symbols: o, □, o, and Δ bacteria exposed to 0, 20, 60, and 100 µg AO/ml, respectively

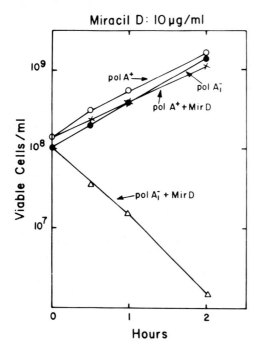

Fig. 14. Preferential killing of *E. coli* pol A$_1^-$ by Miracil D. Bacteria were brought to the exponential growth phase, at which time portions of the cultures were supplemented with Miracil D (final concentration: 10 µg/ml). The cultures were incubated with aeration at 37°C and at intervals portions of the cultures were withdrawn and processed for the determination of the number of viable cells

In this series, 56% of carcinogens were detected as mutagens in the *Salmonella* assay and 79% with the pol A assay. It must be stated, however, that in the study referred to above, the newer *Salmonella* tester strains TA 98 and TA 100 were not included. Had these newer strains been used, approximately 80% of carcinogens would have been detected as mutagens (24). However, some of those detected by the pol A assay would still have remained undetected by the *Salmonella* system and hence if the two systems had been used in tandem in excess of 95% of the test chemicals would have been detected correctly.

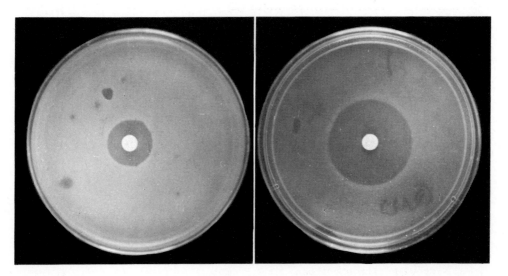

Fig. 15. Effect of 4-nitroquinoline-N-oxide on the growth of *E. coli* pol A$^+$ (*left*) and pol A$\bar{1}$ (*right*). Each disk contained 10 µg of the test agent

The present data indicate that the pol A assay (procedure II and occasionally procedure III, see above) is by itself a reliable indicator of carcinogenic potential; when used in tandem with the *Salmonella* system which includes the newer tester strains, the two assays have great reliability in correctly predicting carcinogenicity. In view of the increasing reliance on short-term assay procedures, and because of the simplicity and low cost of the pol A assay, it would appear wise to include this procedure in a battery of short-term microbial assays for the detection of environmental mutagens and carcinogens.

Acknowledgments. These studies were supported by the National Cancer Institute, the National Institute of Environmental Health Sciences, and the U.S. Environmental Protection Agency. This study would not have been possible without the enthusiastic collaboration of Monika Anders, Linda Biuso, Carol Cheli, Donna DeFrancesco, George DeMarco, Ilse Hochroth, and Lynn Petrullo.

Table 19. Effects of various agents on the growth of a DNA polymerase-deficient strain (standard assay)

Group	Agent	Amount	Size of zone of inhibition (mm) Pol A$^+$	Pol A$_1^-$
I	Penicillin	3 units	9	8
	Erythromycin	15 µg	9	9
	Cycloserine	50 µg	62	62
	Chloramphenicol	30 µg	30	30
	Kanamycin	30 µg	18	18
II	Methyl methanesulfonate	10 µl	44	60
	Ethyl methanesulfonate	10 µl	0	20
	N-Methyl-N-nitrosourea	0.5 µmol	45	85
	N-Ethyl-N-nitrosourea	0.5 µmol	0	13
	N-Methyl-N-nitrosourethan	0.1 µmol	2	46
	N-Ethyl-N-nitrosourethan	0.5 µmol	0	16
	Formaldehyde	10 µl	59	62
	N-Hydroxyurethan	20 µmol	12	21
	Nitrosofluorene	0.5 µmol	0	15
	N-Hydroxylaminofluorene	0.5 µmol	0	12
	1,2-Dimethylhydrazine	250 µg	0	12
	NFTF	60 µg	25	38
	1-Phenyl-3,3-dimethyl-triazine	250 µg	24	47
	Natulan	250 µg	16	22
	Chloroquine	0.2 µmol	9	15
	Acridine orange	250 µg	7	9
	Miracil D	1 µmol	7	19
	Auramine O	250 µg	9	14
	p-Rosaniline	250 µg	6	10

NFTF, N-[4-(5-nitro-2-furyl)thiazolyl] formamide.

Table 20. The preferential inhibition of the pol A strain: modified procedure

	Amount	S-9	Survival index
Chloramphenicol	20 µg/ml	−	1.02
Nalidixic acid	20 µg/ml	−	0.14
Miracil D	10 µg/ml	−	0.06
Vapona (DDVP)	6.4 × 10^{-3} M	−	0.11
Captan	20 µg/ml	−	0.66
	40 µg/ml	−	0.37
Acridine orange	20 µg/ml	−	0.60
	60 µg/ml	−	0.44
	100 µg/ml	−	0.04
Formamidoxime	0.08 M	−	0.05
Hydroxyurea	0.2 M	−	0.40
Ethyl methanesulfonate	0.02 M	−	0.09

Table 20 (continued)

Formaldehyde	0.3%	–	0.21
Mitomycin C	0.05 µg/ml	–	0.01
N-Methyl-N'-nitro-N-nitrosoguanidine	2.5 µg/ml	–	0.07
Natulan	2 µg/ml	–	0.64
Epichlorohydrin	0.01 µl/ml	–	0.05
Myleran	2 µg/ml	–	0.50
Cyclophosphamide	10 µg/ml	+	0.67
Diethylnitrosamine	0.1 µg/ml	+	0.58
Dimethylnitrosamine	0.1 µg/ml	+	0.49
Vinyl chloride	0.1% (v/v, gas)	+	0.73

The strains (pol A_1^- or pol A^+) were exposed to the test agents for 90 min and then processed for the determination of the number of viable bacteria. Results are expressed as survivors pol A_1^-/% survivors pol A^+.

Table 21. Comparison of mutagenic, carcinogenic, and DNA-modifying activity of test chemicals

Aromatic amines	Carcinogenicity	Mutagenicity (*Salmonella*)	Pol A assay
N-Acetoxy-N-2-fluorenyl-acetamide	UC	+	+
4-Aminoazobenzene	PC	–	–
2-Aminobiphenyl	NC	–	–
4-Aminobiphenyl	PC	+	+
Aniline	NC	–	–
1-Anthramine	NC	+	±
2-Anthramine	PC	+	+
Auramine O	UC	–	+
Bis-(*p*-dimethylamino) diphenylmethane	PC	–	+
o-Chloraniline	NT	–	+
p-Chloraniline	NC	–	+
N,N-Dimethyl-4-amino-azobenzene	NC	–	–
2,3-Dimethyl-4-aminobiphenyl	PC	+	+
2-Fluorenamine	PC	+	+
N-2-Fluorenylacetamide	PC	+	+
N-4-Fluorenylacetamide	NC	–	–
N-Hydroxy-N-2-fluorenyl-acetamide	PC	+	+
1-Hydroxy-2-fluorenyl-acetamide	NC	–	–
3-Hydroxy-2-fluorenyl-acetamide	NT	–	–
5-Hydroxy-2-fluorenyl-acetamide	NT	+	+
7-Hydroxy-2-fluorenyl-acetamide	NC	+	+
3-Methoxy-4-aminoazobenzene	PC	+	+

Table 21 (continued)

2-Methyl-4-dimethylamino-azobenzene	PC	−	−
3'-Methyl-4-dimethylamino-azobenzene	PC	−	−
1-Naphthylamine	NC	+	+
2-Naphthylamine	PC	+	+
1-Naphthylhydroxylamine	UC	+	+
2-Naphthylhydroxylamine	UC	+	+
α-Naphthylisothiocyanate	NC	−	−
4-Nitrobiphenyl	PC	−	+
2-Nitrofluorene	PC	+	+
2-Nitronaphthalene	PC	+	+
p-Rosaniline	PC	−	+
o-Toluidine	PC	−	+
p-Toluidine	PC	−	−
4-*o*-Tolylazo-*o*-toluidine	PC	+	+
Aromatic polycyclic hydrocarbons			
Anthracene	NC	−	−
Benz(a)anthracene	PC	−	−
Benzo(a)pyrene	PC	+	+
Benzo(e)pyrene	PC	−	−
7-Bromoethyl-12-methyl-benz(a)anthracene	UC	+	+
Chrysene	PC	−	−
4,5-Dihydrobenzo(a)pyrene-4,5-epoxide	UC	+	+
7,12-Dimethylbenz(a)anthracene	PC	+	±
3-Hydroxybenzo(a)pyrene	PC	−	+
7-Hydroxymethyl-12-methyl-benz(a)anthracene	PC	−	+
Phenanthrene	NC	−	−
Heterocyclic compounds			
1'-Acetoxysafrole	UC	−	+
Acridine orange	PC	−	+
Aflatoxin B$_2$	PC	−	−
3-Amino-1,2,4-triazole	PC	−	−
7,9-Dimethylbenz(c)-acridine	PC	−	+
4-Hydroxylaminoquinoline-N-oxide	UC	+	+
1'Hydroxysafrole	PC	−	−
N-[4-(5-Nitro-2-furyl)thiazolyl]formamide	PC	−	+
4-Nitroquinoline-N-oxide	PC	+	+
Safrole	PC	−	+
Alkylating agents			
Benzyl chloride	UC	+	+
Bromobenzene	NT	−	±
Butane sultone	UC	+	+
ε-Caprolactone	NT	−	−
1,2,3,4-Diepoxybutane	UC	+	+

51

Table 21 (continued)

1,2-Epoxybutane	NC	+	+
Ethyl-*p*-toluenesulfonate	UC	+	+
Glycidaldehyde	UC	+	+
Glycidol	NC	+	+
Methylazoxymethanol acetate	PC	+	+
Methyl iodide	UC	+	+
Propane sultone	UC	+	+
β-Propiolactone	UC	+	+
Propyleneimine	UC	+	+
Uracil mustard	UC	+	+

Nitrosamines, hydrazines, and related substances

1,2-Dimethylhydrazine	PC	−	+
Diphenylnitrosamine	NC	−	−
Hydrazine sulfate	PC	+	+
N-Methyl-N'-nitro-N-nitrosoguanidine	UC	+	+
Natulan	PC	−	+
N-Nitrosodiethylamine	PC	−	+
N-Nitrosoethylurea	UC	+	+
1-Phenyl-3-dimethyltriazene	PC	+	+

Amides, ureas, and acylating agents

Acetamide	PC	−	−
Dimethylcarbamyl chloride	UC	−	+
Methyl carbamate	NC	−	−
Succinic anhydride	NT	−	−
Thioacetamide	PC	−	−
Thiourea	PC	−	−
Urethan	PC	−	−
N-Hydroxyurethan	PC	−	+

Antimetabolites

5-Bromodeoxyuridine	NC	−	No test
Ethionine	PC	−	No test
5-Fluorodeoxyuridine	NC	−	−
5-Iododeoxyuridine	NC	−	No test
Methotrexate	NC	−	No test

Inorganics

Beryllium sulfate	−	No test
Hydroxylamine hydrochloride	−	+
Lead acetate	−	No test
Titanocene dichloride	−	No test

Promoters

Phorbol	−	No test
12-O-Tetradecanoyl-phorbol-13-acetate	−	No test
1,8,9-Trihydroxyanthracene	+	+

NC, noncarcinogen; PC, procarcinogen; UC, ultimate carcinogen; NT, not tested.
Although, in our hands, dimethylcarbamyl chloride was not mutagenic in the standard *Salmonella* assay, a mutagenic response was obtained when it was tested under conditions which prevented evaporation.

Table 21 (continued)

For the pol A assay, chemicals were first tested in the standard disk diffusion assay and results recorded as positive (preferential inhibition of
pol A_1 strain) or negative (equal inhibition of both tester strains). Chemicals inhibiting neither strain ("no test" result) were then tested in the
modified liquid suspension assay. Chemicals not showing preferential inhibition of the pol A_1 strain were retested in the presence of S-9 and cofactors. In the above table a "no test" result indicates that the test agent
was tested only by the plate diffusion assay and that in that assay, neither
strain was inhibited.

Table 22. Mutagenicity and DNA-modifying activity of representative chemical classes

Classes	Carcinogenicity	N	M^+P^+	M^+P^-	M^-P^+	M^-P^-
Aromatic amines (33)	UC	4	3	O	1	O
	PC	19	11	O	4	4
	NC	10	3	O	1	6
Aromatic polycyclic	UC	3	3	O	O	O
hydrocarbons (12)	PC	7	2	O	2	3
	NC	2	O	O	O	2
Heterocyclic compounds (10)	UC	2	1	O	1	O
	PC	8	2	O	3	3
	NC	O				
Alkylating agents (13)	UC	10	10	O	O	O
	PC	1	1	O	O	O
	NC	2	2	O	O	O
Nitrosamines hydrazines	UC	2	2	O	O	O
and related (8)	PC	5	2	O	3	O
	NC	1	O	O	O	1
Amides, ureas, and	UC	1	O	O	1	O
acylating agents (7)	PC	5	O	O	1	4
	NC	1	O	O	O	1
Antimetabolites (5)	UC	O				
	PC	1	O	O	O	1
	NC	4	O	O	O	4
Metals (3)	Carcinogens	3				3

Number in parenthesis indicates the number of chemicals tested in that class.
For abbreviations, see Tables 21 and 23.

Table 23. Correlation between mutagenicity (*Salmonella*) and DNA-modifying activity (pol A$^+$/pol A$_1^-$)

Classes	N	Percent			
		M$^+$P$^+$	M$^+$P$^-$	M$^-$P$^+$	M$^-$P$^-$
All carcinogens	71	56	O	23	21
Ultimate carcinogens	25	88	O	12	O
Procarcinogens	46	39	O	28	33
Noncarcinogens	20	25	O	5	70
Unknown carcinogenicity	6	17	O	33	50

M, mutagenicity in *Salmonella typhimurium*; P, ability to preferentially inhibit *E. coli* pol A$_1^-$.

References

1. Bartsch H (1976) Predictive value of mutagenicity tests in chemical carcinogesis. Mutat Res 38:177-190
2. Bridges BA (1976) Short-term screening tests for carcinogens. Nature 261:195-200
3. Serres FJ de (1976) The utility of short-term tests for mutagenicity. Mutat Res 38:1-2
4. Serres FJ de (1976) Prospects for a revolution in the methods of toxicological evaluation. Mutat Res 38:165-176
5. Serres FJ de (1976) Mutagenicity of chemical carcinogens. Mutat Res 41:43-50
6. Maugh TH (1978) II. Chemical carcinogens: the scientific basis for regulation. Science 201:1200-1205
7. McCann J, Choi E, Vamasaki E, Ames BN (1975) Detection of carcinogens as mutagens in the Salmonella/microsome test: assay of 300 chemicals. Proc Natl Acad Sci USA 72:5135-5139
8. McCann J, Ames BN (1976) Detection of carcinogens and mutagens in the Salmonella/microsome test: assay of 300 chemicals: discussion. Proc. Natl Acad Sci USA 73:950-954
9. McCann J, Ames BN (1977) The *Salmonella*/microsome mutagenicity test: predictive value for animal carcinogenicity. In: Hiatt HH, Watson JD, Winsten JA (eds). Origins of human cancer, Book C. Cold Springer Harbor Laboratory, pp 1431-1450
10. Purchase IFH, Longstaff E, Ashby J, Styles JA, Anderson D, Lefevre DA, Westwood FR (1976) Evaluation of six short-term tests for detecting organic chemical carcinogens and recommendations for their use. Nature 264:624-627
11. Rosenkranz HS (1973) Aspects of microbiology in cancer research. Annu Rev Microbiol 27:383-401
12. Sugimura T, Sato S, Nagao M, Yahagi T, Matsushima T, Seino Y, Takeushi M, Kawachi T (1976) Overlapping of carcinogens and mutagens. In: Magee PN et al. (eds) Symposium, Princess Takamatsu Cancer Research Fund. University of Tokyo Press, Tokyo, pp 191-213
13. Sugimura T, Kawachi T, Matsushima T, Nagao M, Sato S, Yahagi T (1977) A critical review of submammalian systems for mutagen detection. In: Scott D, Bridges BA, Sobels FH (eds) Progress in genetic toxicology. Elsevier/North-Holland Biomedical Press, Amsterdam, pp 125-140
14. Sugimura T, Nagao M, Kawachi T, Honda M, Yahagi T, Seino Y, Sato S, Matsukura N, Mutsushima T, Shirai A, Sawamura M, Matsumoto H (1977)

Mutagen-carcinogens in food, with specific reference to highly mutagenic pyrolytic products in broiled foods. In: Hiatt HH, Watson JD, Winsten JA (eds) Origins of human cancers. Book C. Cold Spring Harbor Laboratory. pp 1561-1577

15. Meselson M, Russell K (1977) Comparisons of carcinogenic and mutagenic potency. In: Hiatt HH, Watson JD, Winsten JA (eds) Origins of human cancer, Book C. Cold Springer Harbor Laboratory, pp 1473-1481

16. Ames BN, Hooper K (1978) Does carcinogenic potency correlate with mutagenic specificity in the Ames assay? —A reply. Nature 274:19-20

17. Coombs MM, Kissonerghis AM, Allan JA (1976) Evaluation of the mutagenicity of compounds of known carcinogenicity belonging to the benz(a)-anthracene, chrysene, and cyclopenta(a)phenanthracene series using Ames's test. Cancer Res 36:452-4529

18. Ashby J, Styles JA (1978) Does carcinogenic potency correlate with mutagenic potency in the Ames assay? Nature 271:452-455

19. Ashby J, Styles JA (1978) Factors influencing mutagenic potency in vitro. Nature 274:20-22

20. McGregor DB (1978) Cotton rat anomaly. Nature 274:21

21. Dunkel V (1979) Collaborative studies on microbial mutagenicity assays. J Assoc Off Anal Chem 62:874-882

22. Ames BN, McCann J, Yamasaki E (1975) Methods for detecting carcinogens and mutagens with the *Salmonella*/mammalian microsome mutagenicity test. Mutat Res 31:347-364

23. Ames BN, Durston E, Yamasaki E, Lee FD (1973) Carcinogens as mutagens: a sample test system combining liver homogenates for activation and bacteria for detection. Proc Natl Acad Sci USA 70:2281-2285

24. Rosenkranz HS, Poirier LA (1979) An evaluation of the mutagenicity and DNA-modifying activity in microbial systems of carcinogens and non-carcinogens. J Natl Cancer Inst 62:873-892

25. Ashby J, Styles JA, Anderson D (1977) Selection of an in vitro carcinogenicity test for derivatives of the carcinogen hexamethylphosphoramide. Br J Cancer 36:564-571

26. Rosenkranz HS, Gutter B, Speck WT (1976) Microbial assay procedures: experience with two systems. In: Serres FJ de, Fouts JR, Bends JR, Philpot RM (eds) In vitro metabolic activation in mutagenesis testing. North-Holland, Amsterdam, pp 337-363

27. Flora S de (1978) Metabolic deactivation of mutagens in the *Salmonella*-microsome test. Nature 271:455-456

28. Bartsch H, Malaveille C, Montesano R, Tomatis L: Tissue-mediated mutagenicity of vinyledene chloride and 2-chlorobutadiene in *Salmonella typhimurium*. Nature 255:641-643

29. Selkirk JK (1977) Divergence of metabolic activation systems for short-term mutagenesis assay. Nature 270:604-607

30. Oesch F, Raphael D, Schwind H, Glatt HR (1977) Species differences in activating and inactivating enzymes related to the control of mutagenic metabolites. Arch Toxicol (Berl) 39:97-108

31. Gold MD, Blum A, Ames BN (1978) Another flame retardant, Tris-(1,3-dichloro-2-propyl) phosphate and its expected metabolites are mutagens. Science 200: 785-787

32. Nagao M, Suzuki E, Yasuo K, Yahagi T, Seino Y, Sugimura T, Okada M (1977) Mutagenicity of N-butyl-N-(4-hydroxybutyl)nitrosamine, a bladder carcinogen, and related compounds. Cancer Res 37:399-407

33. McCoy EC, Burrows L, Rosenkranz HS (1978) Genetic activity of allyl chloride. Mutat Res 57:11-15

34. Rosenkranz HS, McCoy EC, Anders M, Speck WT, Bickers D (to be published) The use of microbial assay systems in the detection of environmental mutagens in complex mixtures. In: Waters MD et al. (eds) Applications

of short-term bioassays in the fractionation and analysis of complex environmental mixtures. US Environmental Protection Agency, Research Triangle Park, NC EPA-600/9-78-027

35. Rosenkranz HS, McCoy EC, Biuso L, Speck WT (to be published) Short-term assays in the assessment of carcinogenic risk
36. Malaveille C, Planche G, Bartsch H (1977) Factors for efficiency of the *Salmonella*/microsome mutagenicity assay. Chem Biol Interact 17:129-136
37. Rosenkranz HS, Gutter B, Speck WT (1976) Mutagenicity and DNA-modifying activity: a comparison of two microbial assays. Mutat Res 41:61-70
38. Brem H, Stein AB, Rosenkranz HS (1974) The mutagenicity and DNA-modifying effect of haloalkanes. Cancer Res 34:2576-2579
39. Wlodkowski TJ, Rosenkranz HS (1975) Mutagenicity of sodium hypochlorite for *Salmonella typhimurium*. Mutat Res 31:39-42
40. Wlodkowski TJ, Speck WT, Rosenkranz HS (1975) Genetic effects of povidone-iodine. J Pharm Sci 64:1235-1237
41. Green MHL, Rogers AM, Muriel WJ, Ward AC, McCalla DR (1977) Use of a simplified fluctuation test to detect and characterize mutagenesis by nitrofurans. Mutat Res 44: 139-143
42. Malling HV (1971) Dimethylnitrosamine: formation of mutagenic compounds by interaction with mouse liver microsome. Mutat Res 13:425-429
43. Frantz CN, Malling HV (1975) The quantitative microsomal mutagenesis assay method. Mutat Res 31:365-380
44. U.S. Congress, Office of Technology Assessment (1977) Cancer Testing Technology and Saccharin. Superintendent of Documents, U.S. Government Printing Office, Washington, D.C. (Stock No. 052-003, 00471-2)
45. Batzinger RP, Ou S-YL, Bueding E (1977) Saccharin and other sweeteners: mutagenic properties. Science 198:944-946
46. Rosenkranz HS, Speck WT (1975) Mutagenicity of metronidazole: activation by mammalian liver microsomes. Biochem Biophys Res Comm 66:520-525
47. Rosenkranz HS, Speck WT (1976) Activation of nitrofurantoin to a mutagen by rat liver nitroreductase. Biochem Pharm 25:1555-1556
48. Gutter B, Speck WT, Rosenkranz HS (1977) A study of the photoinduced mutagenicity of methylene blue. Mutat Res 44:177-182
49. Gutter B, Speck WT, Rosenkranz HS (1977) Light-induced mutagenicity of neutral red (3-amino-7-dimethylamino-2-methylphenanzine hydrochloride). Cancer Res 37:1112-1114
50. McCoy EC, Hankel R, Rosenkranz HS, Guiffrida JG, Bizzari DV (1977) Detection of mutagenic activity in the urines of anesthesiologists: a preliminary report. Environ Health Perspect 21:221-223
51. Speck WT, Stein AB, Rosenkranz HS (1976) Mutagenicity of metronidazole: presence of several active metabolites in human urines. J Natl Cancer Inst 56:283-284
52. Hill MJ (1974) Bacteria and the etiology of colon cancer. Cancer 34:815-818
53. Hill MJ (1975) Metabolic epidemiology of dietary factors in large bowel cancer. Cancer Res 35:3398-3402
54. Hill MJ (1975) Role of colon anaerobes in the metabolism of bile acids and steroids, and its relation to colon cancer. Cancer 36:2387
55. Hill MH (1977) The role of unsaturated bile acids in the etiology of large bowel cancer. In: Hiatt HH, Watson JD, Winsten JA (eds) Origins Of human cancer, Book C. Cold Spring Habor Laboratory, pp 1627-1640
56. Moore, WEC, Holdeman LV (1975) Discussion of current bacteriological investigations of the relationship between intestinal flora, diet and colon cancer. Cancer Res 35:3418-3420
57. Finegold SM, Sutter VL, Sugihara PT, Elder HA, Lehmann SM, Phillips RL (1977) Fecal microbial flora in Seventh-day Adventist population and control subjects. Am J Clin Nutr 30:1781-1792

58. Slemrova J, Edenharden R (1977) Die Bedeutung des bakteriellen Steroid-abbau für die Ätiologie des Dickdarmkrebses. VII. Zur Methodik der Identifizierung von Gallensäureabbauprodukten. Zentralbl Bakteriol (Orig B) 164:236-249

59. Goldin B, Gorbach SL (1977) Alteration in fecal microflora enzymes related to diet, age, Lactobacillus supplements and dimethylhydrazine. Cancer 40:2421-2426

60. Wynder EL (1976) Nutrition and cancer. Fed Proc 35:1309-1315

61. Reddy BS, Narisawa T, Maronpot R, Weisburger JH, Wynder EL (1975) Animal models for the study of dietary factors and cancer of the large bowel. Cancer Res 35:3421-3426

62. Reddy BS, Mastromarino A, Wynder EL (1975) Further leads on metabolic epidemiology of large bowel cancer. Cancer Res 35:3403-3406

63. Reddy BS, Weisburger JH, Wynder EL (1975) Effect of high and low risk diets for colon carcinogenesis on fecal microflora and steroids in man. J Nutr 105:878-884

64. Reddy BS, Mangat S, Sheinfil A, Weisburger JH, Wynder EL (1977) Effect of type and amount of dietary fat and 1,2-dimethylhydrazine on biliary bile acids, fecal bile acids, and neutral sterols in rats. Cancer Res 37:2132-2137

65. Lowenfels AB, Anderson ME (1977) Diet and cancer. Cancer 39:1809-1814

66. Narisawa T, Magadia NE, Weisburger JH, Wynder EL (1974) Promoting effect of bile acids on colon carcinogenesis after intrarectal instillation of N-methyl-N'-nitro-N-nitrosoguanidine in rats. J Natl Cancer Inst 55:1093-1097

67. Reddy BS (1975) Role of bile metabolites in colon carcinogenesis. Cancer 36:2401-2406

68. Reddy BS, Narasawa T, Weisburger JH, Wynder EL (1976) Promoting effect of sodium deoxycholate on colon adenocarcinoma in germfree rats J Natl Cancer Inst 56:441-442

69. Lowenfels AB (1978) Does bile promote extra-colonic cancer? Lancet 7/29:239-241

70. Reddy BS, Watanabe K, Weisburger JH, Wynder EL (1977) Promoting effect of bile acids in colon carcinogenesis in germ-free and conventional F33 rats. Cancer Res 37:3238-3242

71. Silverman SJ, Andrews AW (1977) Bile acids, co-mutagenic activity in the *Salmonella*-mammalian microsome mutagenicity test. J Natl Cancer Inst 59:1557-1559

72. Brusick D, Bakshi K. Jagannath DR (1976) The application of in vitro mutagenesis techniques to investigations of comparative metabolism in mice. In: Serres FJ de, Fouts JR, Bend JR, Philpot RM (eds) In vitro metabolic activation in mutagenesis testing. Elsevier/North-Holland Biomedical Press, Amsterdam, pp 125-141

73. Weekes U, Brusick D (1975) In vitro metabolic activation of chemical mutagens. II. The relationship amoung mutagen formation, metabolism and carcinogenicity for dimethylnitrosamine, diethylnitrosamine in the liver, kidney and lungs of BALB/C J, C57 BL/6J and RF/J mice. Mutat Res 31:175-183

74. Speck WT, Rosenkranz HS (1976) Mutagenicity of azathioprine. Cancer Res 36:108-109

75. McCoy EC, Speck WT, Rosenkranz HS (1977) Activation of a procarcinogen to a mutagen by cell-free extracts of anaerobic bacteria. Mutat Res 46:261-264

76. Rosenkranz HS (1980) Determining the DNA-modifying activity of chemicals using DNA polymerase-deficient *Escherichia coli*. In: Serres FJ de (ed) Chemical mutagens, Vol. 6. Plenum Press, New York, pp 109-147

77. Rosenkranz HS (1973) Hydroxylamine-O-sulfonic acid: in vitro and possible in vivo reaction with DNA. Chem Biol Interact 7:195-204

78. Rosenkranz HS (1977) Mutagenicity of halogenated alkanes and their derivatives. Environ Health Perspect 21:79-84

79. Rosenkranz HS (1973) Miracil D: inhibition of deoxyribonucleic acid polymerase-deficient *Escherichia coli*. Antimicrob Agents Chemother 3:530-531

80. Rosenkranz HS, Southwick FS (1971) Preferential inhibition by chloroquine and quinacrine of *E. coli* deficient in DNA polymerase. Environ Mutat Soc Newslett 5:38

81. Slater EE, Anderson MD, Rosenkranz HS (1971) Rapid detection of mutagens and carcinogens. Cancer Res 31:970-973

82. Ishii Y, Kondo S (1975) Comparative analysis of deletion and base-change mutabilities of *Escherichia coli* B strains differing in DNA repair capacity (*wild type, uvr A$^-$, pol A$_1^-$, rec A$^-$*) by various mutagens. Mutat Res 27:27-44

83. Lucia P de, Cairns J (1969) Isolation of an *E. coli* strain with a mutation affecting DNA polymerase. Nature 224:1164-1166

84. Mullinix KP, Rosenkranz HS (1971) Recovery from N-hydroxyurethan-induced death. J Bacteriol 105:565-572

85. Rosenkranz HS (1973) Preferential effect of dichlorvos (Vapona) on bacteria deficient in DNA polymerase. Cancer Res 33:458-459

86. Southwick FS, Carr HS, Carden GA III, D'Alisa RM, Rosenkranz HS (1972) Effects of acridine orange on the growth of *Escherichia coli*. J Bacteriol 110:439-441

87. Bridges BA (1972) Simple bacterial systems for detecting mutagenic agents. Lab Pract 21:413-419

88. Bridges BA, Mottershead RP, Rothwell MA, Green MHL (1972) Repair-deficient bacterial strains suitable for mutagenicity screening: tests with the fungicide captan. Chem Biol Interact 5:77-84

89. Green MHL, Muriel WJ (1976) Mutagen testing using trp+ reversion in *Escherichia coli*. Mutat Res 38:3-32

Validity of Bacterial Short-Term Tests for the Detection of Chemical Carcinogens[1]

H. Bartsch, C. Malaveille, A.-M. Camus, G. Brun, and A. Hautefeuille[2]

Summary

Terms used to describe the validity of screening tests are discussed and include *specificity*, *sensitivity*, and *predictive value* (*PV*). Therefore the results from any short-term tests should only be considered fully acceptable for the prediction of the potential carcinogenicity of chemicals if certain criteria have been met: a high *specificity* and *sensitivity* is required and adequate animal data should have been used for its validation. Experimental data which do or do not support a correlation between potency of a chemical as an animal carcinogen and its activity as a mutagen in the *Salmonella*/microsome assay or in other short-term tests are briefly summarized. Using some examples, the utility of mutagenicity tests to identify both man-made or naturally occurring mutagens in the environment, or to study mechanisms in chemical carcinogenesis, is illustrated. To select therapeutically effective drugs without adverse biologic effects, confidence is increased when several tests are combined and results are uniformly obtained. At present, short-term assays cannot replace long-term tests in predicting the carcinogenicity of new chemicals; their stature in future will depend on further demonstration of consistency of carcinogenicity experiments in rodents and with human data.

Introduction

Most of the short-term tests which are at present widely used for the detection of potential carcinogens are assays for the mutagenic activity of chemicals, or of their ability to interact with genetic material (1). A good correlation between chemicals causing cancer and those causing mutation has been demonstrated (2-6), which suggests that a common molecular event may be shared by the two processes. But even without direct proof that neoplasms arise through somatic mutations, such tests can already be used as predictors for the carcinogenicity of chemicals (7). In this article, the current status of such short-term tests and their potential application in the field of primary cancer prevention is briefly reviewed.

---

[1]Presented in part at the XII International Cancer Congress, Buenos Aires, 1978

[2]Unit of Chemical Carcinogenesis, International Agency for Research on Cancer, F-69372 Lyon/France

Methods

Most of the studies mentioned in this text have been carried out with *Salmonella typhimurium;* two methods were used:

Plate Incorporation Assay (Method A). Each plate contained $1-2 \times 10^8$ cells of *S. typhimurium* TA 1530, $9000 \times g$ supernatant from rat or human liver, an NADPH-generating system and the test compound dissolved in 100 µl acetone or DMSO per plate (8). The number of revertant colonies was determined in triplicate after 48 h of incubation.

Assays for Volatile Compounds (Method B). Mutagenicity assays for vinyl chloride and other volatile halo-olefins were carried out in assays adapted to test volatile compounds (9). Plates containing $1-2 \times 10^8$ bacteria of TA 1530 strain and other ingredients mentioned in method A were exposed to a gaseous mixture of vinyl chloride or other halo-olefins in air at $37^{\circ}C$ in the dark. The concentration of the halo-olefins in the aqueous phase was determined by gas-liquid chromatography. After exposure, the halo-olefin was removed and replaced by air. Incubation of the plates was continued for up to 48 h and the number of revertants scored.

Terms Used to Describe the Validity of Screening Tests

Because mutagenicity tests do not have the production of tumors in animals as an end point, such tests have to be validated, using a number of known carcinogens (C^+) and noncarcinogens (C^-) as a standard for validation. As an increasing number of such tests are becoming available, it is necessary to judge the utility of a given test system, which of course depends on its ability to be used generally and how practical it is. But apart from these factors, there are terms which can describe the validity of screening tests (5,10,11), which are: *sensitivity, specificity,* and *predictive value* (PV) of a test, and the definitions are explained in Table 1. If a mutagenicity test used for the detection of carcinogens has correctly identified a certain number of carcinogens as mutagens, this figure is termed C^+M^+, those chemicals which were found both noncarcinogenic and nonmutagenic are C^-M^-, those chemicals which are "false negatives" are C^+M^-, and those which are "false positives" are C^-M^+. As expressed in Table 1, the *sensitivity* of a test depends on its capacity to identify carcinogens as mutagens, the *specificity* reflects its resolution power to discriminate between the noncarcinogens and carcinogens, and the *predictive value* (PV) is defined as the ratio of correctly identified carcinogens-mutagens (C^+M^+) over all the test compounds which have been found to be mutagenic ($C^+M^+ + C^-M^+$). This predictive value is also dependent on the *proportion of carcinogens* (Table 1) among the total number of reference compounds tested (n_{total}) as explained in Table 3.

These terms describing the validity of screening tests are illustrated with two examples, such as the validation of the widely used *Salmonella*/microsome mutagenicity test with 300 chemicals (4,12) in Table 2. The sensitivity of this test can

Table 1. Terms[a] used to describe screening tests

Sensitivity	$= C^+M^+/(C^+M^+ + C^+M^-)$
Specificity	$= C^-M^-/(C^-M^+ + C^-M^-)$
Predictive value (PV)	$= C^+M^+/(C^+M^+ + C^-M^+)$
Proportion of carcinogens	$= (C^+M^+ + C^+M^-)/n_{total}$

[a]Multiplied by 100 and expressed as %

Table 2. Validation of the *Salmonella*/microsome mutagenicity test with 300 chemicals (4)

Sensitivity	$= 157/175$ (90%)
Specificity	$= 94/108$ (87%)
Predictive value (PV)	$= 157/(157 + 14)$ (92%)
Proportion of carcinogens	$= 175/(175 + 108)$ (62%)

be calculated according to the terms given in Table 1 to be 90%, the specificity as 87%, and the predictive value as 92%. The proportions of carcinogens among the total number of compounds tested was 62%. It is important to emphasize that a good test should have both a high sensitivity and a high specificity. The predictive value, however, which for the *Salmonella* test has been established independently or by different groups to be about 90% (5,6,12), is often incorrectly equated with the percentage of carcinogens which can actually be identified as mutagens in any given number of test chemicals.

This is not the case, as shown in Table 3. Assuming that 1000 chemicals containing 10 carcinogens, i.e., 1%, are assayed with the *Salmonella*/ microsome test and using the results from the validation studies listed in Table 2, i.e., the sensitivity and specificity of this test are both 90%, then the predictive value has dropped to 8.3%, meaning that among 1000 chemicals this test would predict 108 chemicals as being carcinogens, whereas only 9 true carcinogens would be among these false-positive results. Therefore, it should be kept in mind that the predictive value is a function of the proportion of carcinogens among the series of test chemicals. This issue was also discussed by Purchase et al. (5).

Table 3. Screening of 1000 chemicals containing 1% carcinogens with the *Salmonella*/microsome test

Sensitivity	$=$ (90%)
Specificity	$=$ (90%)
Predictive value (PV)	$= 9/108$ (8.3%)
Proportion of carcinogens	$= 10/1000$ (1%)

Although there is no direct proof, there may be little hope that mutagenicity tests can be improved to give both 100% sensitivity and specificity, and there may always be a finite level of false-positive and false-negative results. Therefore, in order to assign a definite carcinogenicity to chemicals, it is implied that none of these tests can at present replace long-term animal experiments. Accordingly, among other useful applications, they can serve as prescreens to select chemicals which have to be submitted with priority at present to bioassays in experimental animals.

The predictive value, of course, is also influenced by the quality of the animal data for the selected chemicals used as a standard for validation. For a further examination of the obtainable level of correlation between mutagenicity tests and carcinogenicity results from animal bioassays, a list of about 200 chemicals from the IARC Monograph Programme on "The Evaluation of the Carcinogenic Risk of Chemicals to Humans" is available, for which sufficient evidence of carcinogenicity in animals exists (13,14).

Quantitative Correlations Between Carcinogenic Potency and Activity of Chemicals in Short-Term Tests

Apart from qualitative correlations between the two biologic phenomena, carcinogenesis and mutagenesis, interest has focused on whether a quantitative correlation exists between in vivo and in vitro data (for a review, see 15). It is quite evident that if such a correlation could be established, for example between mutagenic activity of a chemical in vitro and its potency as a carcinogen in animals (or man), it would be extremely beneficial (16,17); for example, it would allow a better risk estimation of pure chemicals and complex carcinogenic mixtures found in man's environment in case insufficient animal data are available. It would also aid the design of carcinogenicity tests in terms of the number of animals required, for example in order to detect weakly active carcinogenic chemicals. Several published studies (18-22) have already attempted to examine the possible quantitative correlation between in vivo carcinogenicity and in vitro experiments; Meselson and Russel (23) calculated the carcinogenic potency of several chemicals using IARC Monographs, volumes 1-8 (24-31). In this study, the carcinogenic potency was expressed as the daily animal dose which gives 50% cumulative single risk incidence of induced cancer after 2 years' exposure in experimental animals, usually referred to as D_{50} or TD_{50}. Mutagenic activity was defined as the reciprocal number of micrograms of a compound which gives 100 revertant colonies in the *Salmonella*/microsome test. In a log-log plot between the mutagenic activity and carcinogenic potency for 10 compounds, both variables span a range of approximately 10^4. Although most of the compounds agreed with a linear correlation, some N-nitroso compounds showed an exception. According to the author's statements, more compounds are needed to test the generality that there is a proportionality between mutagenic and carcinogenic potency.

Data from the IARC laboratory using mutagenicity results obtained with a series of N-nitrosamines and published data on
the carcinogenic potency (32,33) revealed no such correlation
if all compounds were considered (Fig. 1). Mutagenic activity
is given as the number of revertants/µmol of nitroso compound
on the abscissa and carcinogenicity on the ordinate as $[D_{50}]^{-1}$
values. Although many more attempts are being made to examine
the correlation between quantitative aspects of mutagenicity and
carcinogenicity, it is reasonable to state at present that the
existence of such a relationship, as it has been suggested (23),
is not sufficiently well established for all classes of carcinogens to allow its general use.

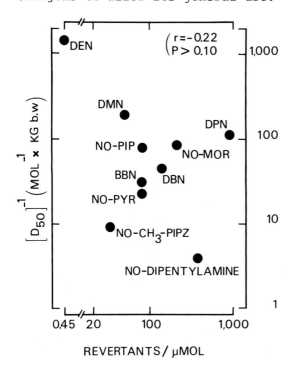

Fig. 1. Mutagenic activity (re-
vertants/µmol) in the *Salmonella*/
microsome assay of a series of
N-nitrosamines versus their
carcinogenic potency $[D_{50}]^{-1}$
(Bartsch et al., unpublished
data). Mutagenicity was determined in plate assays (procedure A, Methods) and calculated
from linear portions of the
dose-response curves using the
most sensitive *Salmonella* strain
and optimal conditions with regard to liver S-9 concentration
and type of pretreatment of
rats. D_{50} values in rats were
taken from Druckrey et al. (32)
and Wishnok et al. (33).
BBN, *N*-nitroso-*n*-butyl-(4-hydroxyl-
butyl)amine; DBN, *N*-nitroso-di-
n-butylamine; DEN, *N*-nitroso-
diethylamine; DMN, *N*-nitroso-
diethylamine; DPN, *N*-nitroso-
di-*n*-propylamine; NO-Dipentyl-
amine, *N*-nitroso-di-*n*-pentyl-
amine; NO-CH$_3$-PIPZ, *N*-nitroso-
-N'-methyl-piperazine; NO-MOR,
N-nitrosomorpholine; NO-PIP,
N-nitrosopiperidine; NO-PYR,
N-nitroso-pyrrolodine

Results on the mutagenicity of 149 chemicals, which had been
tested in the *Salmonella*/ microsome assay with its adapted procedures in the IARC laboratory, are summarized in Fig. 2 and included drugs, industrial chemicals, mycotoxins, pesticides, and
halo-olefins (9,21,34,35,40,41). Among 71 tested chemicals, for
which no data on carcinogenicity exist in the literature, 34
were found to be mutagenic. Using the terms described in Table 1,
the following analysis of the interim results is obtained: 52
compounds (C+M+) for which evidence of carcinogenicity exists
in the literature have been found mutagenic. Sixteen compounds
(C+M-) which are described as carcinogenic were not detected as
mutagens. Five false-positive results were obtained (C-M+) and

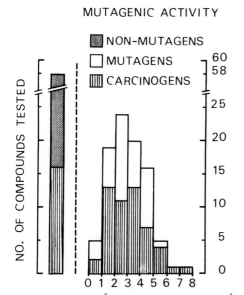

Fig. 2. Frequency distribution of 149
chemicals which had been tested in the
Salmonella/microsome assay (8) according to their mutagenic activity (re-
vertants/µmol) in a semilog plot
(Bartsch et al., unpublished date).
Mutagenicity was determined as described
in the legend to Fig. 1, using the plate
incorporation assay with its adapted
procedures (procedures A and B, Methods).
For more details, see text

five chemicals for which there was negative evidence for carcinogenicity were also not mutagenic (C⁻M⁻). Accordingly, the sensitivity of the test was 76%, the specificity 50%, and the predictive value 91%, when 78 compounds are considered for which
data from long-term animal tests exist and which contained a
proportion of 87% of carcinogens.

Most interesting, however, is the finding that the range of
mutagenic activities in these 78 compounds tested (Fig. 2)
varied over a millionfold range, which has also been previously
reported by McCann and Ames (16) and Nagao et al. (55). In the
peak of the (nearly Gaussian) distribution curve shown in
Fig. 2, a proportion of 26% of all the chemicals tested displayed
a mutagenic activity ranging from 100-1000 revertants/µmol of
test compound.

From our mutagenicity studies on 149 chemicals (Bartsch et al.,
unpublished data), we tried to classify mutagenic chemicals
also according to structural classes (in parenthesis, the number
of compounds) which are shown in Fig. 3, such as aromatic amino
compounds (6), polycyclic aromatic hydrocarbons (25), direct-
alkylating agents (11) *N*-nitrosamines (26), and halo-olefins
(11), to see whether, the (geometric) mean mutagenic activity
of all compounds from each class, which is given in a log plot
as revertants/µmol in the most sensitive *Salmonella* strain on the
abscissa, is distinctly different. A statistical analysis of
the data showed that differences between modal positive values
(*m*) for the selected classes of compounds are significantly different. Further analyses are required to prove whether this interesting relationship holds true also for a larger number of
mutagens belonging to chemically different structural classes.

64

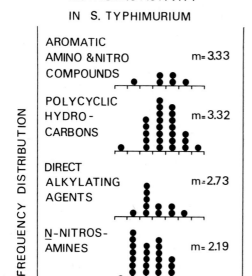

MUTAGENIC ACTIVITY
IN S. TYPHIMURIUM

AROMATIC AMINO & NITRO COMPOUNDS   m= 3.33

POLYCYCLIC HYDRO- CARBONS   m=3.32

DIRECT ALKYLATING AGENTS   m=2.73

N-NITROS- AMINES   m= 2.19

HALO- OLEFINS   m=1.09

FREQUENCY DISTRIBUTION

0 1 2 3 4 5 6 7

LOG [REVERTANTS/ μMOL]

Fig. 3. Frequency distribution of the mutagenic activity (logarithm of the numbers of revertants/μmol) of chemicals grouped into different structural classes (Bartsch et al., unpublished data). Mutagenicity was determined as described in the legend to Fig. 1. Each solid circle represents an individual chemical; m, modal positive values of the (geometric) mean mutagenic activity for the compounds in each different class; for details see text

Attempts to obtain good correlations between carcinogenesis and mutagenesis would appear to be more successful if the pattern and relative proportion of mutagenic metabolites produced in vitro is similar to that for metabolites which are relevant to carcinogenic processes in vivo. Some recent studies on aromatic hydrocarbons, e.g., benzo[α]pyrene and methylbenz[α]anthracene derivatives, have indicated that the mutagens produced by rat liver microsomal systems in vitro may be different from those which are generated by enzymes in intact cells (38-40). Such an explanation may be valid for understanding the lack of correlation between mutagenicity of certain hydrocarbons and their carcinogenicity index in vivo (19).

Table 4 lists some of our own studies (41) on three hydrocarbons: benz[α]anthracene, 7-methyl[α]anthracene, and 7,12-dimethylbenz[α] anthracene, concerning their mutagenicity in the *Salmonella*/ microsome test and their carcinogenicity as expressed in terms of the Iball index in mice or rats [for definition see footnote (d) in Table 4]. The results in Table 4 indicate that the mutagenic activities of the hydrocarbons were in the order: benz[α] anthracene > 7-methylbenz[α]anthracene > 7,12-dimethylbenz[α] anthracene. An attempt was made to compare the carcinogenicities of the three hydrocarbons in terms of Iball indices with the mutagenicities of both of the hydrocarbons and of their 3,4-dihydro-

Table 4. Comparisons between the carcinogenicities of benz[α]anthracene,
7-methylbenz[α]anthracene, and 7,12-dimethylbenz [α] anthracene, their
binding indices, and the mutagenicities in $S.$ $typhimurium$ TA 100 of the
hydrocarbons and of their 3,4-dihydrodiols (41)

Hydrocarbons	Mutagenicity (revertants/nmol)		Binding indices of hydrocarbons[c]	Carcinogenicity indices of hydrocarbons[d]
	of hydrocarbons[a]	of 3,4-dihydrodiols[b]		
Benz[α]anthracene	6.5	8.5	0.8	5
7-Methylbenz[α] anthracene	5.5	33	16	45
7,12-Dimethyl- benz[α]anthracene	2.5	80	170	95

[a]Mutagenicity data are calculated at a 25 μM concentration in $S.$ $typhimurium$
TA 100 in the presence of liver microsomes from 3-methylcholanthrene-
treated rats
[b]Mutagenicity data are expressed as the slope of the linear regions of the
dose-response curves
[c]Binding indices are defined as the extents of covalent reaction with DNA
of cultured mouse embryo cells (μmol/mol phosphorus) divided by the nmol
of hydrocarbon metabolized per ml of medium (from Duncan et al., 42)
[d]Carcinogenicity indices taken from Arcos and Argus (43) correspond to the
average of the Iball indices for sarcoma, epithelioma, and papilloma
formation in mice

diols. There was a positive correlation(r = 0.994; P < 0.01)
between the carcinogenicity indices of the hydrocarbons and the
mutagenicities of the 3,4-dihydrodiols, but an inverse correlation between the carcinogenicity indices and the mutagenicities
of the hydrocarbons. A positive correlation (r = 0.966; P < 0.05)
between the binding indices of the three hydrocarbons to cellular DNA of mouse embryo cells [for definition see footnote
(c) in Table 4] and the mutagenicities of the 3,4-dihydrodiols,
but not of those of the parent hydrocarbons, was also observed.

The data listed in Table 4 are consistent with the assumption
that liver microsomes in vitro produce predominantly simple
oxides which are mutagenic, while cells are apparently capable
of carrying out a three-step activation process involving the
sequential formation of epoxides, diols, and diol-epoxides;
the latter are now the assumed ultimate carcinogens for polycyclic hydrocarbons (44). But, on incubation of liver microsomes
with the appropriate diol precursor, microsomes catalyze the
formation of vicinal diol-epoxides. Such results indicate that
in vitro subcellular activation systems may be improved in order
that bacterial mutagenicity tests can not only be used qualitatively for the mass screening of chemicals.

General Applications of Mutagenicity Tests

Mutagenicity tests with bacterial or mammalian cells have been
most successfully applied in the following areas: (a) tracing
carcinogens/mutagens in complex environmental mixture, (b) prescreening compounds, (c) carrying out mechanistic studies in
chemical carcinogenesis, and (d) monitoring exposure of the
human population by measuring mutagens in body fluids (45).
Some examples of how these tests have been applied for these
purposes are discussed in the following.

Some chemical carcinogens initially detected as microbial mutagens include the antibacterial food additive furyl furamide,
AF-2 (46), the industrial chemicals ethylene dichloride and
ethylene dibromide (3), the latter being used as a gasoline additive, and a flame-retardant, *tris*(2,3-dibromopropyl)phosphate
(47). All three of these compounds have been detected as mutagens in several microbial systems, including the *Salmonella*
test system. In the IARC laboratory, we were able to demonstrate
mutagenic activity for vinylidene chloride (9) and vinyl bromide
(48), analogues of the well-known human and animal carcinogen
vinyl chloride (50). Subsequently performed tests in rodents
provided evidence that all these microbial mutagens are also
carcinogenic (49-51,56).

Another possible application of this test is to study species
differences in pathways or rates of carcinogen metabolism and
the magnitude of interindividual variations using tissue samples
from different human subjects. Such studies may provide additional
knowledge, which may aid the extrapolation of animal data to
man.

Figure 4 lists some of our studies on four cyclic *N*-nitrosamines,
for which the formulae are listed, such as *N*-nitrosomorpholine
and *N*-nitrosopiperidine, *N*-nitrosopyrrolidine and *N*-nitroso-*N*'-
methylpiperazine. All the liver samples obtained from different
human subjects, which are represented by solid bars, were able
to convert these *N*-nitrosamines into alkylating and mutagenic
intermediates. Relative mutagenicity as compared with liver
microsomal fractions from untreated rats is given on the ordinate.
Although large interindividual variations were observed, the
average activity ($\bar{m}$) of the human samples was in general close
to that of rat liver (36). However, *N*-nitroso-*N*'-methylpiperazine
showed an exception, as the average human liver activity was
more than 10 times, and in some individuals even 100 times, higher
than that of rat liver. These data reveal interindividual and
species differences and suggest that man may not be resistant
to such carcinogenic *N*-nitrosamines.

A similar picture was seen when the mutagenicity of several halo-
olefins was studied in the presence of human liver fractions
(Fig. 5) when the resulting activities were compared with mouse
or rat liver controls; the average mutagenic activity ($\bar{m}$) of
the human samples was lower or close to that seen in a rodent
control, indicating the potential biologic hazard of this class
of chemicals to man (35).

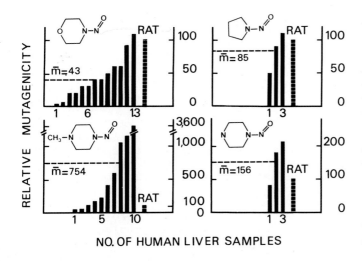

Fig. 4. Enzymic capacities of individual human liver specimens (*solid bars*) to convert N-nitrosopyrrolidine, N-nitrosomorpholine, N-nitroso-N'-methylpiperazine, and N-nitrosopiperidine into electrophiles, mutagenic to S. *typhimurium* TA 1530. Mutagenic activity (method A) is expressed relative to that obtained in assays using liver fraction from untreated rats (*dashed bars*) which is given as 100. Mean activity ($\bar{m}$) of all human samples measured is listed (36)

NO. OF HUMAN LIVER SAMPLES

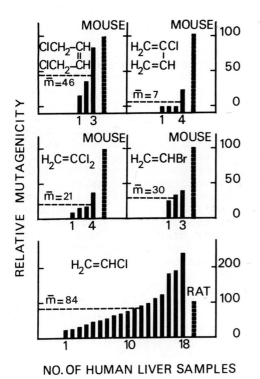

NO. OF HUMAN LIVER SAMPLES

Fig. 5. Enzymic capacities of individual human liver specimens (*solid bars*) to convert 1,4-dichlorobutene-2, 2-chlorobutadiene, vinylidene chloride, vinyl bromide, and vinyl chloride into electrophiles mutagenic to S. *typhimurium* TA 1530. Mutagenic activity was calculated from the linear region of dose- and/or time-dependent assays and is expressed relative to that obtained in assays using liver fractions from untreated rats or mice (*dashed bars*) which are given as 100. Mean activity ($\bar{m}$) of all human samples measured is listed. Mutagenicity of 1,4-dichlorobutene-2 was determined according to method A, whereas other volatile halo-olefins were assayed by method B (Methods) (From Bartsch et al., 36)

Bacterial mutagenicity tests have been particularly helpful in identifying mutagenic principles present in complex environmental mixtures and there are many reports now available. For example, Sugimura et al. (37) and Yamamoto et al. (52) succeeded in isolating mutagenic principles from pyrolysis products of tryptophane, called *Trp*-P-1 and *Trp*-P-2 and of *L*-glutamic acid, *GLu*-P-1 and *GLu*-P-2. These mutagens are also formed when fish or meat are cooked by direct exposure to flames (55). All the compounds are to a certain extent related to the hepatocarcinogenic 2-aminofluorene, and the latter two compounds are aza analogues, showing extremely high mutagenicity in *Salmonella*. The role of these mutagens in the etiology of human cancer is under investigation.

In a collaborative study, we investigated pyrrolyzed substances which are consumed in two areas where oesophageal cancer is frequent, that is, in north-east Iran and in areas of the Transkei (53). Mutagenic activity in *Salmonella* strains was found in samples of *sukhteh*; (this is the local name for opium pipe residues) or in the Transkei tobacco pipe residues; both products are chewed or eaten in the two areas. Whether these mutagenic opium and tobacco pyrolysis products are the etiologic factors involved in the cause of oesophageal cancer in these two areas needs to be demonstrated. These studies, however, leave no doubt that mutagens are consumed by the two populations, demonstrating another successful application of bacterial mutagenicity tests to trace hitherto unknown mutagens in man's environment. The elucidation of the structure of the active mutagenic principles is under way.

Finally, an example of where a battery of short-term tests was used to assay a new, effective antischistosomal drug, *Praziquantel* (for formula, see Fig. 6), which had not so far been tested for carcinogenicity in rodents, is summarized in Table 5. Because of certain limitations of the individual systems, for example the *Salmonella* test described in references (4,6) does not detect certain carcinogenic chemicals or certain chemical classes, confidence in positive or negative results is increased when the data are confirmed in different test systems using either different biologic end points or genetic indicator organisms or different activation systems. Praziquantel was tested in a collaborative study (34) in different indicator organisms, such as *Salmonella* yeast, mammalian cells, in the presence of different activation systems, such as microsomes, in vitro or host-mediated assays. The biologic end points were reverse and forward mutations, gene conversions, mitotic recombination, or unscheduled DNA repair. This compound was further tested in V79 Chinese hamster cells and in *Drosphila* using either microsomal or cell-mediated activation or in vivo feeding studies. The biologic end points included thioguanine, azaguanine-, and ouabain-resistant mutants, sister chromatid exchanges, and X-linked recessive lethals in *Drosophila melanogaster*. No detectable genetic activity in the various short-term tests was found for Praziquantel, while hycanthone, a well-known schistosomicide, which was included as a positive control, was active. The absence of genetic activity of Praziquantel uniformly obtained also confirms the assumption that the antischistosomal effect of this drug is not related to mutagenic activity. These negative results have encouraged the implementation of extensive clinical and field trials on this effective antischistosomal drug (54) for which carcinogenicity tests are under way (U. Mohr, personal communication).

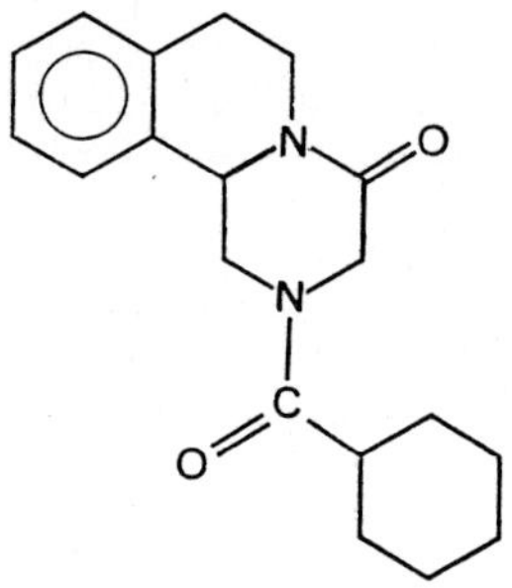

Fig. 6. Chemical formula of Praziquantel

Table 5. Evaluation of the biologic effects of Praziquantel in various short-term tests (from 34)

Genetic indicator	Metabolic activation system	Biologic end point
S. typhimurium TA 100 and 98	Liver (S-9) from 3-MC or aroclor, 3-MC + PB-treated rats or mice[a]	His[+] reversion
S. cerevisae	None	Gene conversion
S. pombe	Mouse liver (S-10)	Forward mutation
S. pombe	Host-mediated assay (mice)	Forward mutation
Human heteroploid cell line	Mouse liver (S-10)	Unscheduled DNA repair
V79 Chinese hamster cells	Mouse liver (S-10)	6-Thioguanine resistance
V79 Chinese hamster cells	Mouse liver (S-10)	Sister chromatid exchanges
V79 Chinese hamster cells	Rat liver (S-15) PB-induced	8-Azaguanine and ouabain resistance
V79 Chinese hamster cells	Cell-mediated system	8-Azaguanine and ouabain resistance
Drosophila melanogaster	In vivo	X-linked recessive lethals

[a]S-9, 9000 g supernatant fraction, 3-MC, 3-methylcholanthrene, PB, phenobarbital

In summary, attention was drawn to the fact that certain criteria should be met before results of any short-term tests can be considered fully acceptable for the prediction of potential carcinogenicity of chemicals. Among those, a high *specificity* and *sensitivity* is required and adequate animal data should have been used for its validation. The utility of mutagenicity tests to identify both man-made or naturally occurring mutagens in the environment, or to study mechanisms in chemical carcinogenesis, was illustrated. To select therapeutically effective drugs without adverse biologic effects, confidence may be increased when several tests are combined. Whether short-term assays will eventually reach the stature of long-term tests in predicting the carcinogenicity of new chemicals will depend on a further demonstration of consistency of carcinogenicity experiments in rodents and with the human data.

Acknowledgments. The author's research activities in this area were in part supported by contract No 1-CP-55630 from the National Cancer Institute of the USA; the help of Dr. N.E. Day, Unit of Biostatistics, IARC, in carrying out statistical analyses is gratefully acknowledged.

References

1. IARC Scientific Publications, No. 12, Screening tests in chemical carcinogenesis. Lyon, 1976
2. Miller JA, Miller EC (1971) Chemical carcinogenesis: mechanisms and approaches to its control. J Natl Cancer Inst 47:V
3. McCann J, Simmon V, Streitwieser D, Ames BN (1975) Mutagenicity of chloroacetaldehyde a possible metabolic product of 1,2-dichloroethane, chloroethanol, vinyl chloride and cyclophosphamide. Proc Natl Acad Sci USA 72:3190-3193
4. McCann J, Choi E, Yamasaki E, Ames BN (1975) Detection of carcinogens as mutagens in the *Salmonella*/microsome test: assay of 300 chemicals. Proc Natl Acad Sci USA 72:5135-5139
5. Purchase IFH, Longstaff E, Ashby J, Styles JA, Anderson D, Lefevre PA, Westwood FR (1978) An evaluation of 6 short-term tests for detecting organic chemical carcinogens. Br J Cancer 37:873-959
6. Sugimura T, Sata S, Nagao M, Yahagi T, Matsushima T, Seino Y, Takeuchi M, Kawachi T (1976) Overlapping of carcinogens and mutagens. In: Magee PN, Takayama S, Sugimura T, Matsushima T (eds) Fundamentals in cancer prevention. University of Tokyo Press, Tokyo University Park Press, Baltimore, pp 191-215
7. Bartsch H (1976) Predictive value of mutagenicity tests in chemical carcinogenesis. Mutat Res 38:177-190
8. Ames BN, McCann J, Yamasaki E (1975) Methods for detecting carcinogens and mutagens with the *Salmonella*/mammalian-microsome mutagenicity test. Mutat Res 31:347-364
9. Bartsch H, Malaveille C, Montesano R (1975) Human rat and mouse liver-mediated mutagenicity of vinyl chloride in *S. typhimurium* strains. Int J Cancer 15:429-437
10. Malaveille C (1977) Methodologie de mise en évidence des effets mutagènes de substances organiques. Nature des relations entre mutagenicité et cancérogénicité. Proceedings of the "Comité Additifs alimentaires du Centre National de Coordination des Etudes et Recherches sur la Nutrition et l'Alimentation (CNCERNA", Paris, pp 8-10
11. Cooper JA, Saracci R, Cole P (1979) Describing the validity of carcinogen screening tests. Br J Cancer 39:87-89
12. McCann J, Ames BN (1976) Detection of carcinogens as mutagens in the *Salmonella*/microsome test: assay of 300 chemicals: discussion. Proc Natl Acad Sci USA 73:950-954
13. IARC Internal Technical Report No. 78/003, International Agency for Research on Cancer, Lyon 1978
14. Tomatis L, Agthe C, Bartsch H, Huff J, Montesano R, Saracci R, Walter E, Wilbourn J (1978) Evaluation of the carcinogenicity of chemicals: A review of the Monograph Program of the International Agency, a Research on Cancer (1971-1977) Cancer Res 38:877-885

15. Bartsch H (1978) Carcinogenic activity and biological effects in short-term tests; quantitative aspects. Staub Reinhalt Luft 38:240-243
16. McCann J, Ames BN (1977) The *Salmonella*/microsome mutagenicity test: predictive value for animal carcinogenicity. In: Hiatt HH, Watson JD, Winsten JA (eds) Origins of human cancer. Cold Spring Harbor, pp 1431-1450
17. Ames BN, Hooper K (1978) Does coarcinogenic potency correlate with mutagenic potency in the Ames assay? A reply. Nature 274:19-20
18. Druckrey H, Kruse H, Preussmann R, Ivankovic S, Landschütz Ch (1970) Cancerogene alkylierende Substanzen. III. Alkyl-halogenide, -sulfate, -sulfonate und ringgespannte Heterocyclen. Z Krebsforsch 74:241-270
19. Coombs MM, Dixon C, Kissonerghis A-M (1976) Evaluation of the mutagenicity of compounds of known carcinogenicity, belonging to the benz[α] anthracene, chrysene and cyclopental[α]phenanthrene series, using Ames's test. Cancer Res 36:4525-4529
20. Teranishi K, Hamada K, Watanabe H (1975) Quantitative relationship between carcinogenicity and mutagenicity of polyaromatic hydrocarbons in *Salmonella typhimurium* mutants. Mutat Res 31:97-102
21. Bartsch H, Malaveille C, Stich HF, Miller EC, Miller JA (1977) Comparative electrophilicity, mutagenicity, DNA repair induction activity and carcinogenicity of some *N*- and *O*-acyl derivatives of *N*-hydroxy-2-aminofluorene. Cancer Res 37:1461-1467
22. Krahn DF, Heidelberger C (1977) Liver homogenate-mediate mutagenesis in Chinese hamster V79 cells by polycyclic aromatic hydrocarbons and aflatoxins. Mutat Res 46:27-44
23. Meselson M, Russel K (1977) Comparisons of carcinogenic and mutagenic potency. In: Hiatt HH, Watson JD, Winsten JA (eds) Origins of human cancer. Cold Spring Harbor, pp 1473-1481
24. IARC Monographs on the Evaluation of the Carcinogenic Risk of Chemicals to Man. Vol 1. Some inorganic substances, chlorinated hydrocarbons, aromatic amines, *N*-nitroso compounds and natural products. Lyon 1972
25. IARC Monographs on the Evaluation of the Carcinogenic Risk of Chemicals to Man. Vol 2. Some inorganic and organometallic compounds. Lyon 1973
26. IARC Monographs on the Evaluation of the Carcinogenic Risk of Chemicals to Man. Vol 3. Certain polycyclic aromatic hydrocarbons and heterocyclic compounds. Lyon 1973
27. IARC Monographs on the Evaluation of the Carcinogenic Risk of Chemicals to Man. Vol 4. Some aromatic amines, hydrazine and related substances, *N*-nitroso compounds and miscellaneous alkylating agents. Lyon 1974
28. IARC Monographs on the Evaluation of the Carcinogenic Risk of Chemicals to Man. Vol 5. Some organochlorine pesticides. Lyon 1974
29. IARC Monographs on the Evaluation of the Carcinogenic Risk of Chemicals to Man. Vol 6. Sex hormones. Lyon 1974
30. IARC Monographs on the Evaluation of the Carcinogenic Risk of Chemicals to Man. Vol 7. Some anti-thyroid and related substances, nitrofurans and industrial chemicals. Lyon 1974
31. IARC Monographs on the Evaluation of the Carcinogenic Risk of Chemicals to Man. Vol 8. Some aromatic azo compounds. Lyon 1975
32. Druckrey H, Preussmann R, Ivankovic S, Schmähl D (1967) Organotrope carcinogene Wirkung bei 65 verschiedenen *N*-Nitroso-Verbindungen an BD-Ratten. Z Krebsforsch 69:103-201
33. Wishnok JS, Archer MC, Edelman AS, Rand WM (1978) Nitrosamine carcinogenicity: a quantitative Hansch-Taft structure activity relationship. Chem Biol Interact 20:43-54
34. Bartsch H, Kuroki T, Malaveille C, Loprieno N, Barale R, Abbondandolo A, Bonatti S, Rainaldi G, Vogel E, Davis A (1978) Absence of mutagenicity

of Praziquantel, a new, effective anti-schistosomal drug, in bacteria, yeasts, insects and mammalian cells. Mutat Res 58:133-142

35. Bartsch H, Malaveille C, Barbin A, Planche G (1979) Mutagenic and alkylating metabolites of halo-ethylenes, chlorobutadienes and dichlorobutenes produced by rodent or human liver tissues; evidence for oxirane formation by P450-linked microsomal mono-oxygenases. Arch Toxicol 41:249-277

36. Bartsch H, Sabadie N, Malaveille C, Camus A-M, Richter-Reichhelm HB (1979) Carcinogen metabolism with human and experimental animal tissues: Interindividual and species differences. Proc. XII Int Cancer Congr, Buenos Aires. Pergamon Press, Oxford

37. Sugimura T, Kawachi T, Nagao M, Yahagi T, Seino Y, Okamoto T, Shudo K, Kosuge T, Tsuji K. Wakabayashi K. Iitaka Y, Itai A (1977) Mutagenic principle(s) in tryptophan and phenylalanine pyrolysis products. Proc Jpn Acad 53:58-61

38. Selkirk JK (1977) Divergence of metabolic activation systems for short-term mutagenesis assays. Nature 270:604-607

39. Bigger CAH, Tomaszewski JE, Dipple A (1978) Differences between products of binding of 7,12-dimethylbenz[a]anthracene to DNA in mouse skin and in a rat liver microsomal system. Biochem Biophys Res Commun 80:229-235

40. Malaveille C, Tierney B, Grover PL, Sims P, Bartsch H (1977) High microsome-mediated mutagenicity of the 3,4-dihydrodiol of 7-methylbenz-[a]anthracene in S. typhimurium TA 98. Biochem Biophys Res Commun 75:427-433

41. Malaveille C, Bartsch H, Tierney B, Grover PL, Sims P (1978) Microsome-mediated mutagenicity of the 3,4-dihydrodiol of benz[a]anthracene (BA), 7-methyl-BA and 7,12-dimethyl-BA correlates with the carcinogenic activity of the parent hydrocarbons. Abstracts of 7th Int. Congr. Pharmacol., Paris No 402, p 160, Pergamon Press, Oxford

42. Duncan M, Brookes P, Dipple A (1969) Metabolism and binding to cellular macromolecules of a series of hydrocarbons by mouse embryo cells in culture. Int J Cancer 4:813-819

43. Arcos JC, Argus MF (1968) Molecular geometry and carcinogenic activity of aromatic compounds. New perspectives. Adv Cancer Res 11:305-471

44. Jerina DM, Lehr R, Schaefer-Ridder M, Yagi H, Karle JM, Thakker DR (1977) Bay-region epoxides of dihydrodiols: a concept explaining the mutagenic and carcinogenic activity of benzo(a)pyrene and benzo(a)anthracene. In: Hiatt HH, Watson JD, Winsten JA (eds) Origins of human cancer. Cold Spring Harbor, pp 639-658

45. Yamasaki E, Ames BN (1977) The concentration of mutagens from urine by XAD-2-adsorption: cigarette smokers have mutagenic urine. Proc Natl Acad Sci USA 74:3555-3559

46. Kada T (1973) E. coli mutagenicity of furyl furamide. Jpn J Genet 48:301-305

47. Blum A, Ames BN (1977) Flame retardant additives as possible cancer hazards. Science 195:17-23

48. Bartsch H, Malaveille C, Barbin A, Planche G, Montesano R (1976) Alkylating and mutagenic metabolites of halogenated olefins produced by human and animal tissues. Proc Am Assoc Cancer Res 17:17

49. IARC Monographs on the Evaluation of the Carcinogenic Risk of Chemicals to Man. Vol 15. Some fumigants, the herbicides 2,4-D and 2,4,5-T, chlorinated dibenzodioxins and miscellaneous industrial chemicals. Lyon 1977

50. IARC Monographs on the Evaluation of the Carcinogenic Risk of Chemicals to Humans. Vol 19. Some monomers, plastics and synthetic elastomers, and Acrolein. Lyon 1979

51. IARC Monographs on the Evaluation of the Carcinogenic Risk of Chemicals to Humans. Vol 20. Halogenated hydrocarbons. Lyon (to be published)

52. Yamamoto T, Tsuji K, Kosuge T, Okamoto T, Shudo K, Takeda K, Iitaka Y, Yamaguchi K, Seino Y, Yahagi T, Nagao M, Sugimura T (1978) Isolation and structure determination of mutagenic substances in L-glutamic acid pyrolysate. Proc Jpn Acad 54:248-250
53. Hewer T, Rose E, Ghadirian P, Castegnaro M, Bartsch H, Malaveille C, Day N (1978) Ingested mutagens from opium and tobacco pyrolysis products and cancer of the oesophagus. Lancet II:494-496
54. Davis A (1977) Initial experiences with Praziquantel in the treatment of human infections due to *Schistosoma haematobium*. Kurzfassungen der Tagung deutschsprachiger tropenmed Gesellschaften 24:3-26.3.77, Lindau, p 45
55. Nagao N, Sugimura T, Matsushima T (1978) Environmental mutagens and carcinogens. Ann Rev Genet 12:117-159
56. Nomura T (1975) Carcinogenicity of the food additive furyl furamide in foetal and young mice. Nature 258:610-611

The Significance and Interpretation of in Vitro Carcinogenicity Assay Results

J. ASHBY[1]

Introduction

The major implication of discovering a new chemical carcinogen, whether synthetic of natural, is that it may present a carcinogenic risk to exposed populations. Only in cases where significant manufacturing or environmental human exposure to that chemical exists will a possible human carcinogenic hazard exist. It is therefore desirable that a system of hazard assessment should be devised. The above approach assumes that chemical carcinogens are easily and clearly definable —but such, of course, is not the case. One of the major causes of confusion in this area is the fear felt by many that insufficient or circumstantial evidence of carcinogenicity will be used to stimulate the response usually reserved for established human carcinogens. For example, few people would disagree with attempts to remove a recognizable source of potential hazard, such as the presence of a potent animal carcinogen in drinking water, but many would question whether abrupt action should be taken on finding that hamburgers contain chemicals mutagenic to *S. typhimurium*.

The results of lifetime studies in animals are usually taken as the surest indication of carcinogenicity, but even this technique often gives inconclusive results. Quite apart from the cases where it is unclear whether a genuine carcinogenic effect has been produced, there are two more fundamental concerns. The first is that the degree of carcinogenicity of a chemical often depends upon such variables as the species, strain, age, sex, diet and route of administration of the test animal. These uncertainties are generally accepted because it is not usually possible to predict which set of experimental conditions most closely resemble man. The second concern is that animal carcinogenicity data generated for a chemical using levels of exposure far in excess of those likely to be encountered by man, and demonstrated via an effective but perhaps unrepresentative route of administration, may be defining a carcinogenic potential unlikely to be realized under the actual conditions of human exposure.

Until recently the only method of anticipating a potential human carcinogen was to demonstrate a carcinogenic effect for that chemical in animals. On occasions, this approach was supplemented by structural analysis — the visual recognition of carcinogens by chemical structure. For example, dimethoxybenzidine (Fig. 1),

---

[1] Imperial Chemical Industries, Ltd., Central Toxicology Laboratory, Alderley Park, Macclesfield/United Kingdom

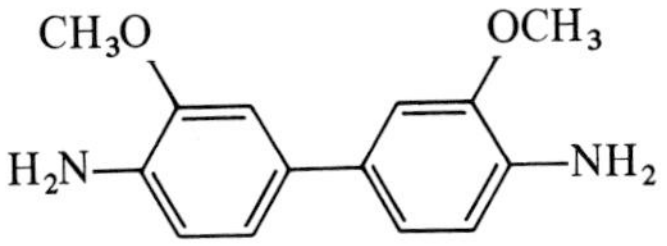

Fig. 1. Dimethoxybenzidine

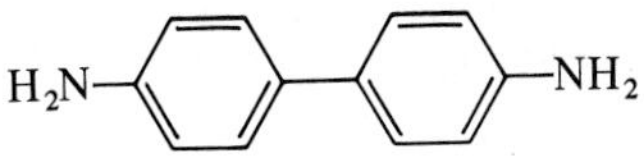

Fig. 2. Benzidine

could be considered as a possible carcinogen simply by virtue
of its structural similarity to the carcinogen benzidine (Fig. 2).

In Vitro Tests for Carcinogenicity

The advent of short-term in vitro "carcinogenicity" assays has
presented the prospect of a short-cut to carcinogen definition,
and thereby challenged the position previously held by long-
term animal tests. Many in vitro carcinogenicity assays are now
available, most of which are based upon either bacterial mutation or mammalian cell transformation effects, and several
provide an impressive correlation between carcinogenicity and
the end-point of the assay. If these tests were completely reliable (i.e., 100% predictive of carcinogenic activity), few
problems would remain; but they are not. Incorrect predictions
are made, both false positive and false negative, and although
these appear to be few they cannot be neglected.

The incorrect predictions made by in vitro assays, which are
often minimized by supporters and emphasized by opponents of
such tests, should be approached logically. First, however, it
is necessary to emphasize the immense usefulness of these tests
as they undoubtedly represent a major advance in cancer research.

Figure 3 lists the type of question that these assays can answer
rapidly. Compounds on the left are established carcinogens and
those on the right are compounds which are structurally related
to them but of unknown carcinogenicity. The final column lists
the predictions of activity made by in vitro assays, and several
similar predictions have now been confirmed in vivo. If such
predictions are assessed within the total context of biochemical,
pharmacokinetic, and chemical considerations, a confident assessment of the carcinogenicity of such test compounds can be made.
This is, indeed, progress considering that not long ago, several
years and large amounts of money would have had to be expended
to obtain similar answers from animal studies.

Faced with such impressive, and potentially valuable assays, the
relevant issue is perhaps "implications of short-term tests"
rather than "implications of carcinogenicity." All that separ-
ates these two phrases are the "false predictions," so a study
of how and why the latter arise should be profitable.

The advantages to be gained by directly studying false predictions are several. The first is that when we know why such mistakes are made we will be in a better position to anticipate

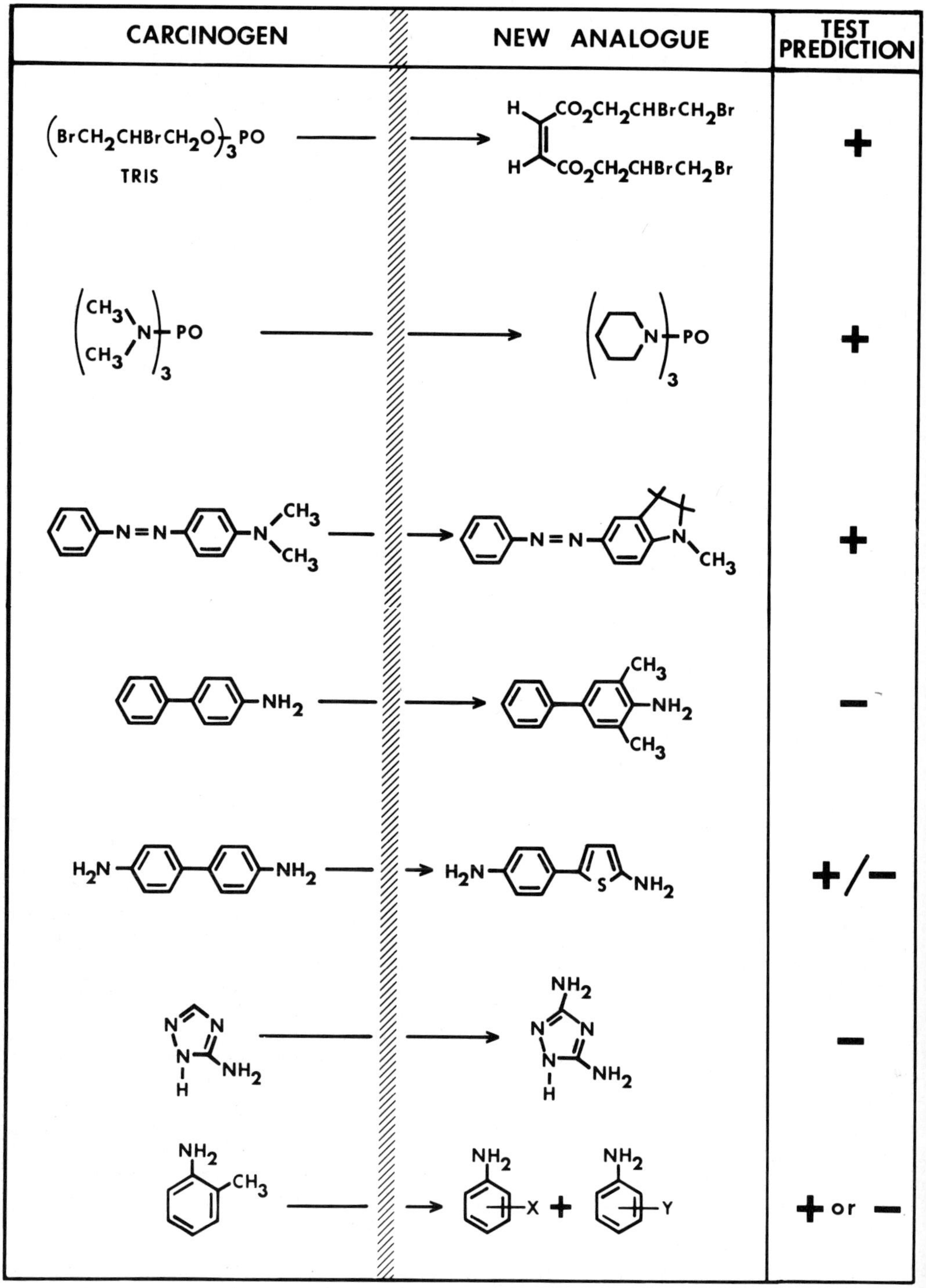

Fig. 3. In vitro test predictions of possible carcinogenicity produced for the novel analogues shown on the *right* of the established carcinogens listed

and avoid further similar mistakes. Secondly, a knowledge of
these mistakes will enable a clearer picture to be drawn of
what validation figures of ~90% predictivity really mean. Why,
for example, are these assays not 100% predictive of carcinogenicity, and could they appear to be of low predictivity if different chemicals were to be studied?

Based upon theoretical, conceptual and experimental considerations, at least four types of "false" predictions can be anticipated, the genesis of which are shown diagrammatically in
Fig. 4 and described below:

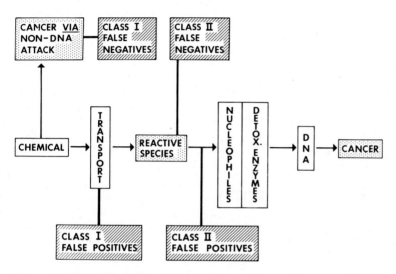

Fig. 4. Simplified diagram of the progress of a chemical from administration
in vivo to tumour production. The areas in which false results could arise
are shown as *cross-hatched boxes*

Class I False Negatives (Mechanism; Fig. 5). The possibility that some
carcinogens may elicit their effect via a non-mutagenic mechanism
has been discussed for many years and has still not been finally
resolved. Clearly, a carcinogen which causes cancer without
reacting with the DNA of cells will be negative in any assay
based on DNA modification. Some possible examples of this type
of compound are shown in Fig. 5. These compounds can elicit
tumours in some experimental animals, under some conditions of
testing, but they are negative in most of the mutation-based
assays. If these compounds truly operate by an *epigenetic* mechanism,
no amount of technical modification of a mutation-based test
will secure their detection. Assays with some form of cellular
disturbance, as opposed to genetic change, as their end-point
may be best equipped to detect such compounds.

Class II False Negatives (Activation; Fig. 6). Most carcinogens/mutagens
require to be transformed into active (electrophilic) species
before they can react with DNA. In a living animal this activation is achieved at various metabolic centres, such as the

78

Class I **False negatives** (mechanism).

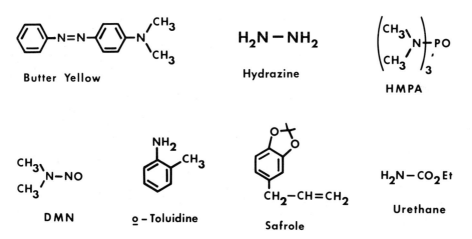

CHCl₃

Chloroform

DDT

DES

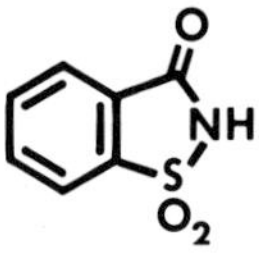

saccharin

Fig. 5. Animal carcinogens which may give false-negative results in in vitro assays due to the fact that they may produce cancer via a mechanism which does not require an initial chemical attack on DNA (see Fig. 4 for key)

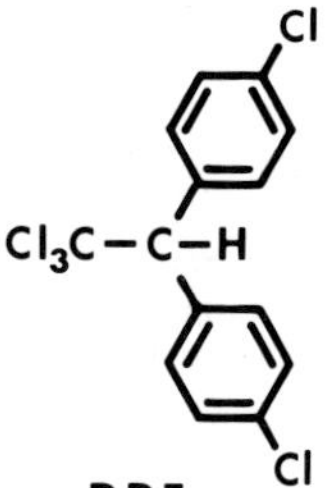

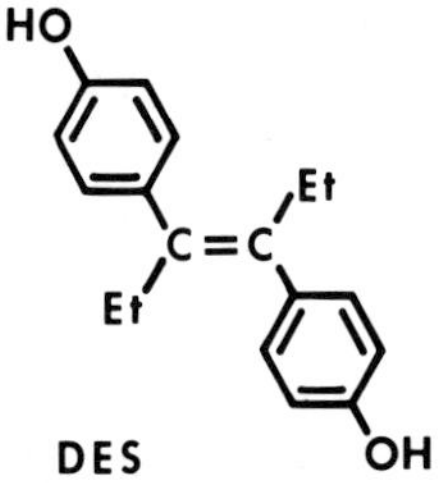

PHENOBARBITONE   **THIOUREA**

Class II **False Negatives** (activation).

Butter Yellow   **Hydrazine**   **HMPA**

DMN   **o – Toluidine**   **Safrole**   **Urethane**

Fig. 6. Animal carcinogens whose negative response in vitro is probably associated with a failure of the in vitro activation system (S-9 mix) to simulate correctly metabolism in vivo

liver. When a compound is tested in vitro, metabolic activation is *simulated* with a sub-fraction of an homogenate of rat liver, the S-9 mix.

For compounds that require several separate steps to achieve their activation it is to be expected that the S-9 mix will not always exactly re-create the enzyme activities and balances of the liver in vivo. For example, a key activation enzyme may be absent from the S-9 mix or particular deactivation enzymes may be over-represented. In such cases the S-9 mix may be incapable of generating the necessary *dynamic balance* of active species needed to inflict the required damage upon DNA: they will therefore appear to be inactive.

This type of false-negative chemical is characterized by giving an erratic or negative response in vitro. Such compounds can or should be able to give a positive response in vitro, but such a response cannot always be reproduced under apparently identical conditions. Possible examples of compounds within this category are shown in Fig. 6. These compounds present the added problem that it would, in most cases, be possible technically to modify the *test system* such that they would be routinely detected as positive, but although this seems to be desirable it implies both that a standard test protocol is not practical and that the required protocol changes can be anticipated for all test compounds, which is unlikely. Figure 7 shows results obtained in the Styles cell transformation assay for a series of derivatives of the carcinogen HMPA. Reproducibly positive or reproducibly negative results can be obtained simply by making changes to the S-9 activation system, thereby illustrating the principles discussed above. HMPA itself is negative in the *Salmonella* assay.

False-Positive Results. The identification of false-positive results presents a greater problem than do false-negative results. This is primarily due to the absence or inadequacy of supportive long-term animal data. Nonetheless, such results are certain to exist and an attempt is made below to delineate from whence they might come.

Class I False Positives (Transport; Fig. 8). The basic reason for anticipating disagreements of this type is that in vitro tests present their DNA in a very exposed environment compared with that of the DNA of mammals. Thus, methyl orange (Fig. 8), a fairly well established non-carcinogen, is positive in the cell transformation assay of Styles. It may be that this compound is non-carcinogenic in vivo because the polar and lipophobic sulphonic acid group imposes a distribution profile on this chemical in a living animal, which prevents the potentially DNA-reactive NMe_2 group from reaching and interacting chemically with DNA.

In an in vitro test such distribution barriers are weakened or absent, thus, the molecule may be forced "unnaturally" into contact with DNA, and when this happens a positive response will be obtained. The basis of this rather diffuse class lies

COMPOUND EXPERIMENT	CLASS + VE CONTROL $\begin{bmatrix} CH_3 \\ \diagdownNP=O \\ CH_3 \diagup \end{bmatrix}_3$ (HMPA)	$\begin{bmatrix} CH_3 \\ \diagdownNP \\ CH_3 \diagup \end{bmatrix}_3$	$\begin{bmatrix} CH_3 \\ \diagdownNP=S \\ CH_3 \diagup \end{bmatrix}_3$	$\begin{bmatrix} ONP=S \end{bmatrix}_3$	$\begin{bmatrix} NP=O \end{bmatrix}_3$	$\begin{array}{c} O \\ \parallel \\ EtO-P-OEt \\ \parallel \\ O \end{array}$ (DEMPA)	CLASS − VE CONTRO $\begin{bmatrix} PhNHP=O \end{bmatrix}_3$
10 μl S−9 MIX 1:9 — 1	+	+	−	−	−	−	−
10 μl S−9 MIX 1:9 — 2	+	+	−	−	−	−	−
50 μl S−9 MIX 1:1 — 3	+	+	+	+	+	+	−
50 μl S−9 MIX 1:1 — 4	+	+	+	+	+	+	−

Fig. 7. In vitro response obtained for a series of potential carcinogens related to the rodent carcinogen hexamethylphosphoramide (HMPA). The results demonstrate that changes to the S-9 mix (activation system) can critically affect the in vitro response obtained (results generated in the Styles cell transformation assay, see Ref. 4)

Class I. False Positives (Transport).

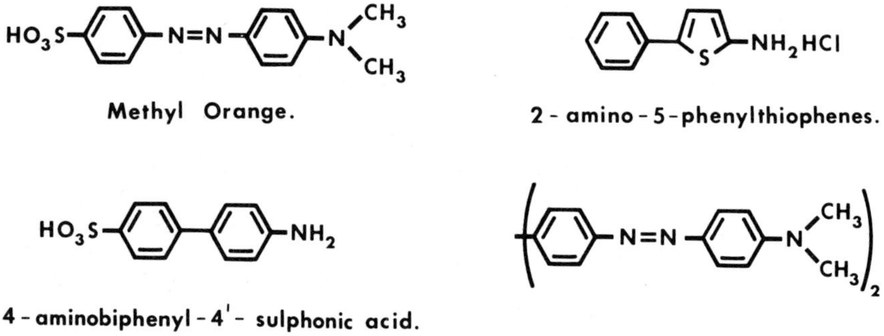

Methyl Orange.

2 - amino - 5 - phenylthiophenes.

4 - aminobiphenyl - 4' - sulphonic acid.

Fig. 8. Chemicals whose non-carcinogenicity (or anticipated non-carcinogenicity) may be associated with specific transport effects in vivo rather than with an absolute inability of the chemical to react with DNA. These compounds may give a positive response in some in vitro assays

in the concept that "a pulmonary carcinogen which never comes into contact with the lungs of a living animal is not a pulmonary carcinogen". Specific animal studies will be required to estimate the importance of this group. Some other possible examples of this class of chemicals are shown in Fig. 8.

Class II False Positive (Reactivity; Fig. 9). This class arises from an extension of the above considerations, that is, that in vitro tests may fail to anticipate correctly the deactivation forces acting on a reactive chemical in vivo. Some possible examples of chemicals within this class are shown in Fig. 9, and the underlying principle for their giving false results is shown diagrammatically in Fig. 10. The reaction of DNA with an electrophilic chemical species is influenced by two main factors:

1. The *inherent reactivity* of the chemical to DNA; this will vary from chemical to chemical, and will depend upon the substitution pattern and steric effects associated with each particular chemical.
2. The *attractiveness* of nuclear DNA to the reactive species as compared with competing nucleophiles (such as water, -SH and -NH$_2$ groups) and competing deactivating enzymes.

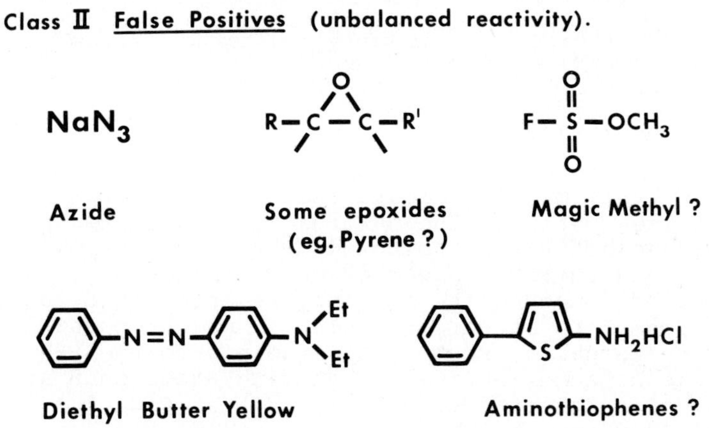

Class II <u>**False Positives**</u> **(unbalanced reactivity).**

NaN$_3$

Azide

Some epoxides (eg. Pyrene ?)

Magic Methyl ?

Diethyl Butter Yellow

Aminothiophenes ?

Fig. 9. Compounds whose positive-response in some in vitro assays may not accurately predict carcinogenicity in vivo. This may be due to a failure of the in vitro assay medium to anticipate correctly the "obstacles" which will be encountered in vivo

If these two factors are related to an animal carcinogenicity study it becomes clear that within a given chemical class of potential carcinogens (such as alkylating agents) there will be a smooth transition, with changes in chemical structure, from complete inactivity to DNA, through optimum reactivity to DNA, and finally to non-reactivity to DNA. The latter stage will be reached when the chemical is *so* reactive to other nucleophiles that it cannot exist for a long enough time to complete the hazardous journey to intranuclear DNA.

This smooth transition in vivo is represented in Fig. 10 by the continuous curve. The dotted extension curve represents activity in vitro. Faced with a diminished number of biological

82

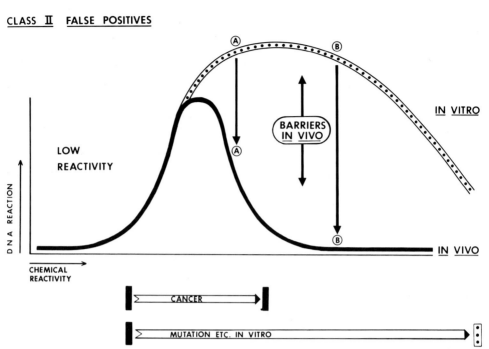

Fig. 10. Illustration of how carcinogenicity may be related to "optimum" chemical reactivity (electrophilicity) and how mutagenicity etc. in vitro may respond to a much larger range of chemical reactivity

hurdles, activity in vitro may outstretch activity in vivo. Therefore, in vitro tests might indicate that both of compounds Ⓐ and Ⓑ are active, yet when the natural in vivo obstacles are imposed upon these activities compound Ⓑ might dissipate its DNA reactivity, and thereby appear as non-carcinogenic, whilst the activity of compound Ⓐ may only be attenuated, and it will therefore appear to be carcinogenic. It may be possible to add a specific nucleophile, such as piperidine, to the S-9 mix which would make a "super-active" alkylating agent such as Magic Methyl (FSO_3Me) (suggested to be point Ⓑ in Fig. 10) appear as negative in vitro whilst leaving as positive a carcinogenic alkylating agent of medium reactivity such as dimethyl sulphate [$(CH_3O)_2SO_2$] (suggested to be point Ⓐ in Fig. 10). In this way conditions in vitro could be regulated to those occurring in vivo by means of titrating the S-9 mix to a given "piperidine figure". This class of result is epitomized by the concept that "an expert pearlfisher who cannot swim underwater is no pearlfisher at all".

It was recently observed that the addition of cysteine to the medium of the Ames assay can profoundly affect the mutagenic potency of chemicals, and this is clearly related to the above considerations. Perhaps the bacterial mutagens to be most concerned about are those which can show activity over a wide range of metabolic conditions. Conversely, chemicals whose mutagenicity is observed in vitro only under carefully regulated conditions may be less likely to act as mutagens in vivo.

What Do Predictivity Figures of ~90% Really Mean? The real and hypo-
thetical considerations outlined above indicate that the *predictivity figure* associated with an in vitro assay will depend upon
the type of chemical that is tested. If long-term animal-testing
facilities are used only to confirm the predictions made by in
vitro assays for chemicals such as dimethylsulphate and sugar,
then these assays will appear to be highly predictive of carcinogenicity. This is because the activity of such compounds
could have been correctly anticipated via chemical and biochemical considerations. At the other extreme, if problem compounds and their structural analogues, such as those discussed
above, are pursued, these tests may well appear to be completely
non-predictive of carcinogenicity (see Fig. 11).

✪ METHYL ORANGE	● CHLOROFORM
✪ AMINOTHIOPHENES	● D.D.T.
✪ BIS-BUTTER YELLOW	● D.E.S.
✪ 4- AB SULPHONIC ACID	● SACCHARIN
✪ MAGIC METHYL	● PHENOBARBITONE
✪ SOME EPOXIDES	● THIOUREA
✪ DIETHYL BUTTER YELLOW	● BUTTER YELLOW
✪ SODIUM AZIDE	● H.M.P.A.
● D.M.N.	● SAFROLE
● URETHANE	● DIELDRIN

● = Carcinogen

✪ = Non-carcinogen

A~100% PREDICTIVE STUDY WOULD BE
EVEN EASIER TO DESIGN.

Fig. 11. Validation to
show in vitro tests
~ 0% predictive

Alternatively, the study of such compounds might confirm the
suggestion that the present *false* predictions of in vitro assays
would disappear if these compounds were to be tested adequately
in vivo. Should this prove true these assays would then be
established as capable of replacing animal studies. Either way,
such studies would be worthwhile.

Carcinogenic Inhibition and Potentiation

The problems which already have been, or predictably could be, encountered with in vitro assays are already well established in the field of animal carcinogenicity. For example, it is well known that the co-administration of certain chemicals (usually competing nucleophiles, specific enzyme "poisons" or free-radical scavengers) with a carcinogen can reduce or abolish the carcinogenicity of the latter. A specific example is afforded by the carcinogenicity of 2-acetylaminofluorene (2-AAF) (Fig. 12) which is dramatically reduced if acetanilide (Fig. 13), a non-carcinogen, is co-administered. This effect has been associated with the ability of acetanilide to poison the $N \rightarrow O$ transacetylase enzyme system which is critical to the metabolic activation of 2-AAF as a carcinogen.

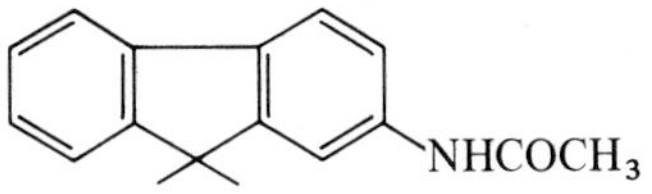

Fig. 12. 2-Acetyl-aminofluorene

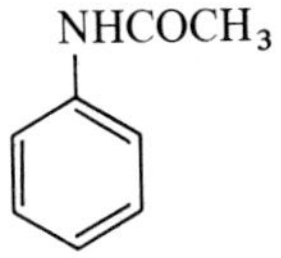

Fig. 13. Acetanilide

The related topic of carcinogenic potentiation, or synergism, will probably be governed by similar laws, although this subject has not yet been studied in detail. An indication that carcinogenic synergism *may* be an important consideration when assessing the hazard from human exposure to chemicals is afforded by the following in vivo/in vitro observations.

The carcinogenic potency of the rat-liver carcinogen butter yellow (Fig. 14) is heavily dependent upon the levels of the deactivating azoreductase enzymes present in the liver of the test animal. These in turn depend on the riboflavin content of the test-animal diet. Thus, when these levels are low, butter yellow appears to be a moderately potent carcinogen, but when they are high it appears to be almost non-carcinogenic. The metabolic interconversions observed for this chemical (Fig. 15) enable the above variations to be explained. In order for butter yellow to react with DNA, the $-NMe_2$ group must be enzymically transformed whilst the remainder of the molecules remains intact. Acting against this *activation* pathway are two *deactivating* pathways, namely, splitting of the molecule via azoreductase enzymes and ring hydroxylation and conjugation of the intact molecule. The net activation of DAB obtained (and thereby the *net* carcinogenicity observed) will depend upon the *balance* of activation and deactivation, a balance which in this case depends upon the riboflavin content of the test-animal diet. It has been observed that the in vitro response given by this chemical can be increased by the addition of the non-mutagen nor-harman (Fig. 16) to the assay medium. It is therefore possible that the latter is inhibiting, either competitively or non-competitively, the ring-hydroxylation enzyme system which deactivates butter yellow, thereby increasing its apparent potency in vitro (Fig. 17). It could equally be anticipated that "diversion" (either competitively or non-competitively) of the

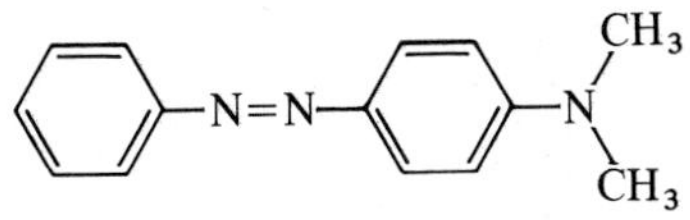

Fig. 14. Butter yellow

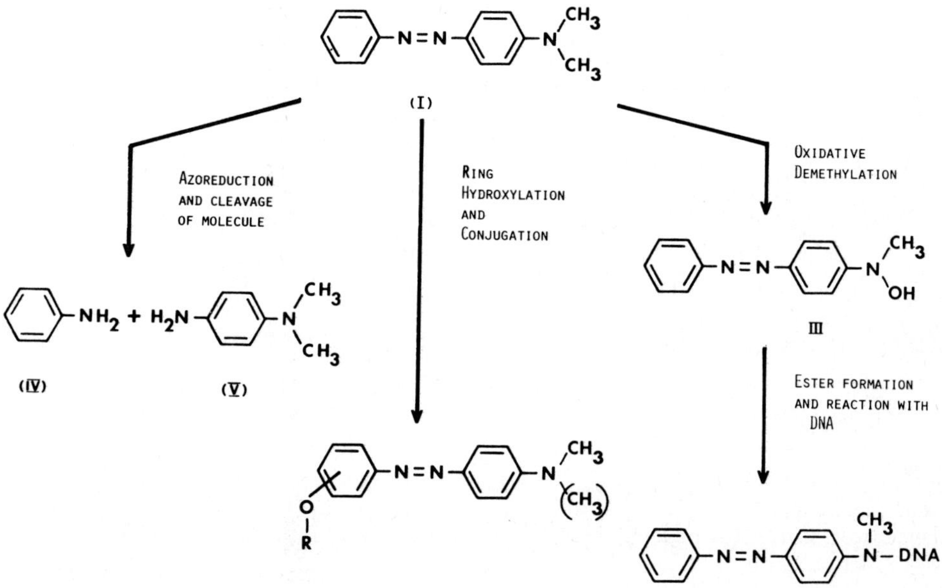

Fig. 15. Metabolism (based on both in vivo and in vitro studies) of 4-(dimethylamino)azobenzene (butter yellow)

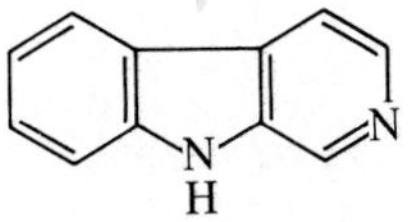

Fig. 16. Norharman

azoreductase enzyme system with a suitable competitive substrate, such as the non-carcinogen azobenzene (Fig. 18), would also increase the net activation of butter yellow (Fig. 19).

Such an effect has been demonstrated in vitro using the Styles cell transformation assay. Figure 20 shows the negative response given by azobenzene (AB) and the positive response given by butter yellow (BY) when tested alone. The third response is that given by a 1:1 mixture of azobenzene and butter yellow (AB + BY) and it shows a 25-fold increase in the potency of butter yellow as a cell-transforming agent in vitro. This apparent demonstration of synergism in vitro should not be translated into synergism in vivo too readily. For example, the only relevant experiment conducted in vivo concerns the co-administration of butter yellow (Fig. 14) and 4,4-dimethylazobenzene (Fig. 21). In this case, which may have been expected to follow the in vitro azobenzene experiment referred to above, a marked protective effect was observed, tumour appearance being delayed as compared with butter yellow. Nonetheless, carcinogenic

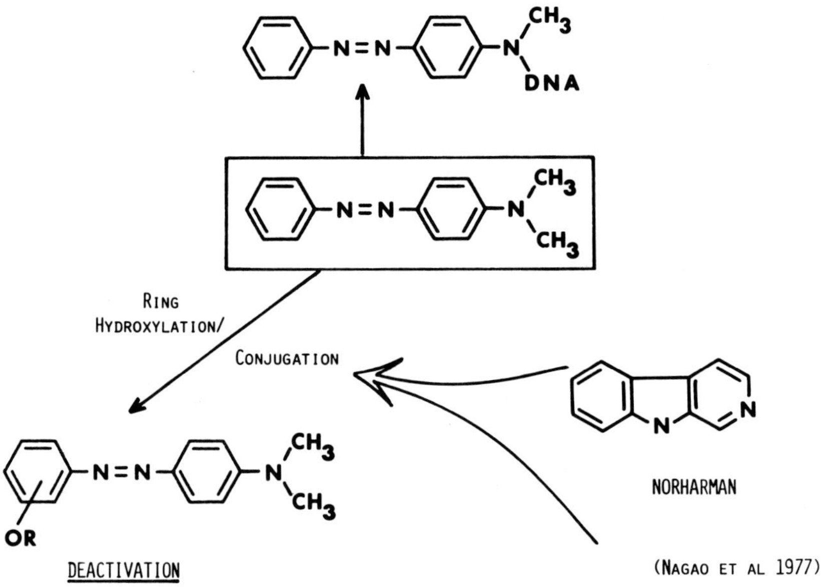

Fig. 17. Illustration of how norharman is suggested to interfere with the detoxification of butter yellow via either competitive or non-competitive interaction with the ring-hydroxylation detoxification enzyme system of the S-9 mix

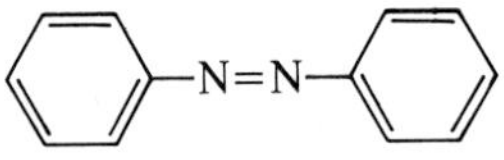

Fig. 18. Azobenzene

potentiation or synergism experiments conducted in vivo are bound to be realized in some cases.

The considerations developed throughout this article have been summarized in Fig. 22. This figure enables the phrase *potential carcinogen* to be accurately defined and suggests that there may be two classes of non-carcinogens recorded in the literature: the first, a group of *absolute* non-carcinogens, and the second, compounds which are *potential* carcinogens but which have so far *failed* to produce a carcinogenic effect in vivo. Chemicals within the latter group could possibly be induced to produce tumours by the appropriate choice of animal species and strain, or diet etc. These arguments cast some doubt on the historical concept of *absolute* carcinogens and non-carcinogens but this should not be abandoned too readily, at least not until an alternative ground-rock can be found upon which to base decisions concerning the potential human hazard presented by exposure to a given chemical.

The above reasoning also leads to the hypothesis that many compounds may be chemically equipped and theoretically able to cause cancer under individually optimized metabolic circumstances,

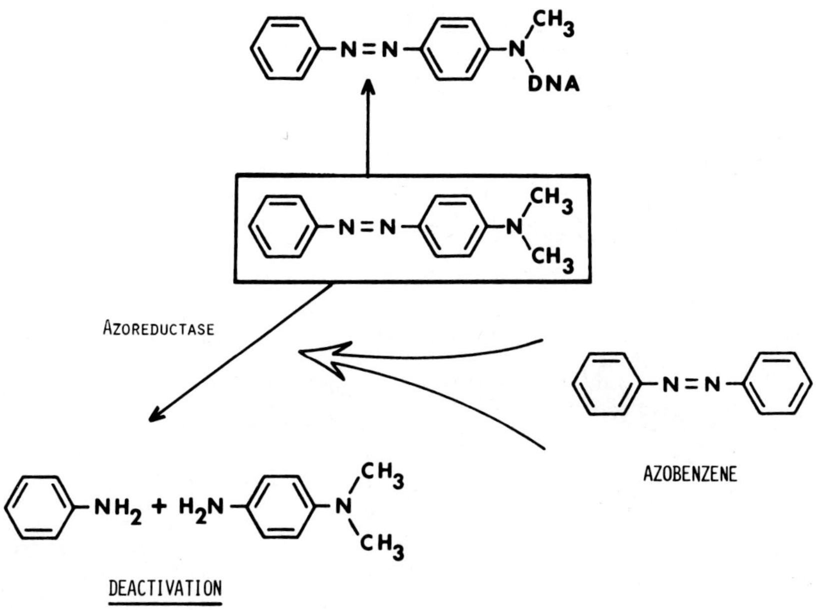

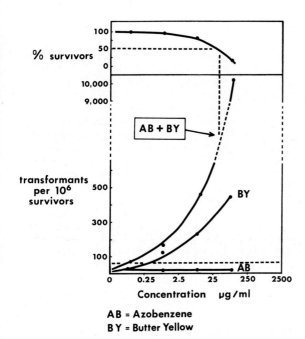

Fig. 19. Illustration of how azobenzene is suggested to interfere with the detoxification of butter yellow via either competitive or non-competitive interaction with the azoreductase detoxification enzyme system of the S-9 mix

AB = Azobenzene
BY = Butter Yellow

Fig. 20. Response given by the non-carcinogen azobenzene (AB), the carcinogen butter yellow (BY) and a 1:1 mixture of azobenzene + butter yellow (AB + BY) in the Styles cell transformation assay (see 1)

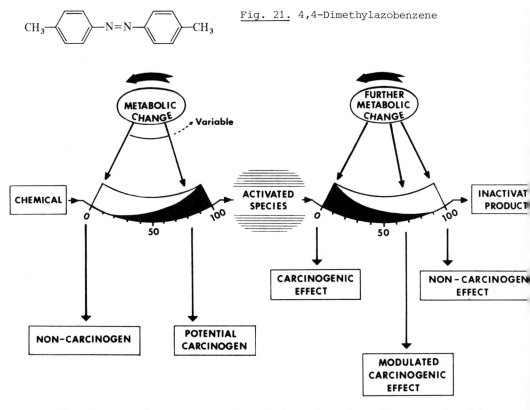

Fig. 21. 4,4-Dimethylazobenzene

Fig. 22. Diagrammatic representation of the moderating effects produced by competitive metabolic pathways on the carcinogenicity of a compound. The starting compound is assumed not to be a direct-acting carcinogen. In such cases the compound would be placed directly in the central box. The position of the indicator in each dial could affect both the in vivo and in vitro response given by a compound. The exact indicator positions will be influenced by the diet, sex, age, species and strain of test animal, and dose levels employed in an in vivo study; the method of induction, preparation and storage of the liver S-9 mix used in an in vitro assay; and the presence of competitive enzyme substrates, both in vivo and in vitro

but only a proportion of these may be capable of inducing tumours under the metabolic conditions of an in vivo study. If this is the case, a dilemma is posed by the fact that in vitro carcinogenicity assays detect the *potential* rather than the *ability* in vivo of a chemical to cause cancer. As the number of compounds in the former category may be significantly larger than those in the latter, some attention should be given to what is inferred from the results of such in vitro assays. In particular, the following question should be answered: are carcinogen-screening programmes designed to protect the majority of a population from exposure to easily demonstrable animal carcinogens, or are they also to be used to protect all metabolically idiosyncratic minorities of a population from each and every possible carcinogen? (The metabolic differences of these sub-groups may be environmentally or genetically determined.) The existence of such sub-groups is probably evidenced by the non-uniform incidence of tumours generally observed when either animals or humans are exposed to chemical carcinogens. The answer to the above question will determine whether the enzyme profile of the S-9 liver fraction used in in vitro assays should be regulated, as far as is possible, to that encountered by a chemical in the liver of an average man, or whether is to be individually optimized, perhaps as a "cocktail" of individually purified enzymes, to give the maximum chance of obtaining a positive response for each compound.

Emphasis has been placed throughout this article on the concept that the *total* available data on a chemical should be considered when assessing its carcinogenicity or potential carcinogenicity. These ideas have been summarized in Fig. 23, which also illustrates the various strategies which can be adopted when attempting to screen large numbers of chemicals for potential human carcinogens. Whatever strategy is adopted, some random screening in vitro of hitherto untested chemicals must be carried out. This is because chemical considerations may not always alert us to the *potential* carcinogenicity of some chemicals.

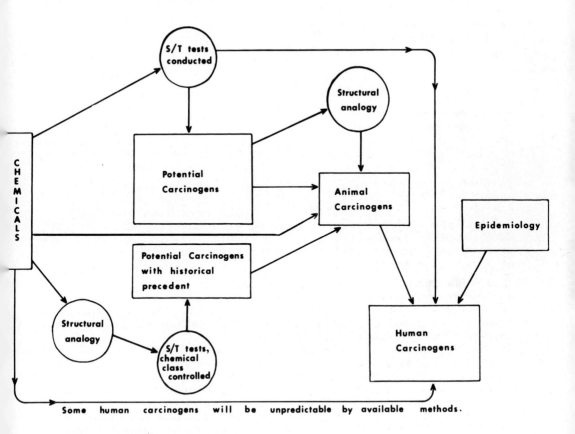

Some human carcinogens will be unpredictable by available methods.

Fig. 23

Secondly, one does not necessarily need an historical precedent
for the carcinogenicity of a given "class" of compounds. For
example, structural considerations indicate that the indoline
derivate (Fig. 24) and the indene derivate (Fig. 25) may possess
carcinogenic potential simply because they are "functionally"
related to the animal carcinogens butter yellow (Fig. 26) and
safrole (Fig. 27), respectively. Such concerns are realized *despite* the fact that, to date, no derivatives of either indoline
(Fig. 28) or indene (Fig. 29) have been established as carcinogens (i.e. strict adherence to *chemical* nomenclature is a trap
to be avoided).

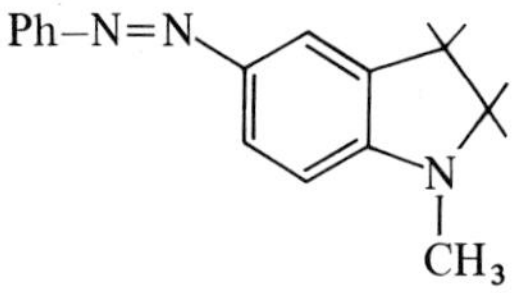

Ph—N=N...

Fig. 24. Indoline-
derivate

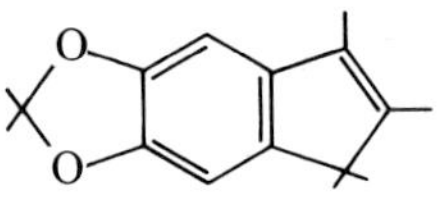

Fig. 25. Indene-
derivate

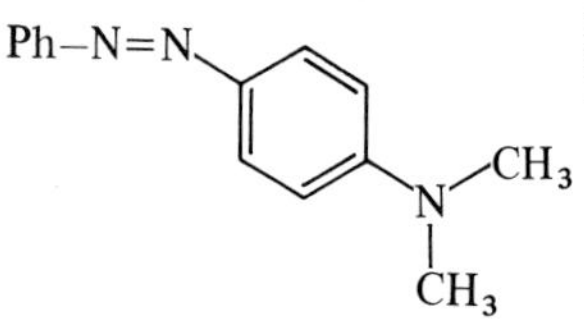

Ph—N=N...

Fig. 26. Butter
yellow

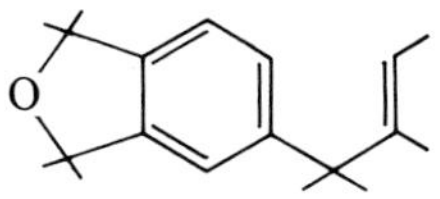

Fig. 27. Safrole

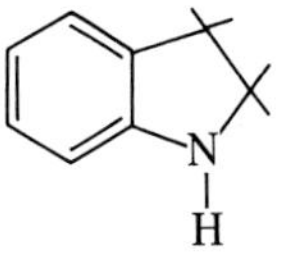

Fig. 28. Indoline

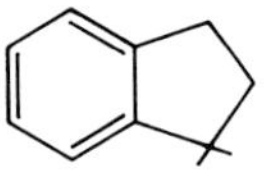

Fig. 29. Indene

In summary, carcinogenic and mutagenic effects are complex
phenomena. This complexity will of necessity be increased by
the need to study such effects in lower organisms and then
extrapolate such results to man. We will never be able to protect *everybody* from every possible genetic hazard, and so a compromise must be reached. This compromise can only be arrived
at after a balanced consideration of the following factors:

1. Likely human exposure to the chemical.
2. The predictions of in vitro carcinogenicity tests.
3. Chemical, biochemical and pharmacokinetic considerations
   which will help to estimate the *likelihood* of expression in
   man of effects observed in vitro.
4. The protective defences (non-critical nucleophiles, detoxification enzymes, immunosurveillance mechanisms etc) of animals
   and man. To swamp these defences in an animal carcinogenicity
   or mutagenicity study, by using very high exposure levels,
   may generate data which will be of academic interest, but of
   little or no value for extrapolating to an average man, with
   intact defences, who is experiencing low levels of exposure
   to that chemical.

To realize the above objectives, specific carcinogenicity studies
are required to evaluate the nature and likely frequency of false
predictions made by in vitro tests (summarized in Tables 1 and 2).
Further, in order that general credibility in short-term tests
should be retained, a *justification* for any new test, and perhaps
some of the recently announced ones, should be clearly given.
It is no longer justifiable to develop a new assay (e.g. a new
strain of *E. coli* or of *S. typhimurium*) and *then* decide whether it
could be useful. Rather, new tests should be sought which fill
a gap left by the currently available tests. A short-term test
which *clearly* and *reliably* detected saccharin or DDT as positive
may be of more immediate value than yet another test which detected, in common with most other tests, benzo(a)pyrene and
aflatoxin B_1 as positive. For example, specific enzyme changes
have recently been associated with exposure of animals to both
saccharin and dieldrin. If pursued, these may form the basis of
a test for the "carcinogenicity" of such agents.

Table 1. Possible genesis of false-negative in vitro predictions

Negative in vitro test results for an animal carcinogen may occur
for one or more of the following reasons:

1. The carcinogenic effect observed may have been mediated via a
   mechanism that did not involve covalent interaction of the
   chemical with the DNA of the host animal. For example,
   a) Hormonal carcinogens (diethylstilboestrol?)
   b) Physical carcinogens (asbestos?)
   c) Inorganic carcinogens (some nickel compounds?)
   d) Epigenetic carcinogens (includes a-c, see ref. 3; saccharin?)
2. The in vitro test system, in particular the S-9 mix, has not been
   optimized for the particular class of compound under study. The
   use of *structurally appropriate positive* control chemicals alerts
   to this situation (see ref. 6)
3. An *inappropriate* in vitro assay is being employed for a particular
   class of compounds (see ref. 6)

Table 2. Possible genesis of false-positive in vitro predictions

Positive in vitro test results for a putative non-carcinogen may
occur for one or more of the following reasons:

1. The chemicals' non-carcinogenic status has been defined in-
   adequately. For example,
   a) Too short a study period or too low a dose level employed.
   b) "Inappropriate" route of administration used.
   c) "Inappropriate" test-animal species used.
   d) Inadequate pathology undertaken.
2. The in vitro test has failed to take account fully of the deactivation processes that operate on active electrophiles in vivo
   (either enzymic or chemical).
3. Whole body chemical transport effects, which may influence access
   of the chemical to DNA in vivo, are not adequately represented in
   the in vitro assay.
4. The in vitro assay is responding positively to a physical or chemical (or physicochemical) property of the chemical which is not
   cancer-related.

92

Acknowledgments. The biological data shown in Figs. 7 and 20 were generated by Jerry Styles using his own cell transformation assay. I also wish to acknowledge the British Journal of Cancer for granting permission to reproduce Figs. 7, 15, 20, and 22 (for all of which they hold the copyright) and ICI, Ltd., for supporting fundamental research.

References

To ease the flow of this article it has not been specifically referenced. Nonetheless, all of the work discussed above, both from our laboratory and from others, has been described and referenced in detail in the following publications:

1. Ashby J, Styles JA, Paton D (1978) In vitro Evaluation of some derivatives of the carcinogen butter yellow: implications for environmental screening. Br J Cancer 38:34-50
2. Ashby J, Styles JA (1978) Comutagenicity, competitive enzyme substrates, and in vitro carcinogenicity assays. Mutat Res 54:105-112
3. Ashby J, Styles JA, Anderson D, Paton D (1978) Saccharin: an epigenetic carcinogen mutagen? Fd Cosmet Toxicol 16:95-103
4. Ashby J, Styles JA, Paton D (1978) Potentially carcinogenic analogues of the carcinogen hexamethylphosphoramide (HMPA). Br J Cancer 38:418-427
5. Ashby J, Anderson D, Styles JA (1978) The potential carcinogenicity of methyl fluorosulphonate (CH_3OSO_2F; Magic Methyl). Mutat Res 51:285-287
6. Ashby J, Purchase IFH (1977) The selection of appropriate chemical class controls for use with short-term tests for potential carcinogenicity. Ann Occup Hyg 20:297-301
7. Ashby J, Styles JA, Anderson D (1977) Selection of an in vitro carcinogenicity test for derivatives of the carcinogen hexamethylphosphoramide. Br J Cancer 36:564-571
8. Ashby J, Styles JA (1978) Does carcinogenic potency correlate with mutagenic potency in the Ames assay? Nature 271:452-455 and subsequent correspondence Nature 274:19-22
9. Ashby, J, Anderson D, Styles JA, Paton D (1978) Thiophene analogues of the carcinogens benzidine and 4-aminobiphenyl: evaluation in vitro. Br J Cancer 38:521-530
10. Purchase IFH, Longstaff E, Ashby J, Styles JA, Anderson D, Lefevre PA, Westwood FR (1978) An evaluation of six short-term tests for detecting organic chemical carcinogens. Br J Cancer 32:873-959 (in particular, Appendix I, 904-923)
11. Crabtree HG (1955) Retardation of azo-carcinogenesis by non-carcinogenic azo-compounds. Br J Cancer 9:310-317
12. Wattenberg LW (1978) Inhibitors of chemical carcinogenesis. Adv Cancer Res 26:197-226
13. Moriya M, Kato K, Shirasu Y (1978) Effects of cysteine and liver metabolic activation system on the activities of mutagenic pesticides. Mutat Res 57:259-263
14. Rosin MP, Stich HF (1978) The inhibitory effect of cysteine on the mutagenic activities of several carcinogenesis. Mutat Res 54/73-81
15. Yamamoto RS, Williams GM, Richardson HL, Weisburger EK, Weisburgher JH (1978) Effects of p-hydroxyacetanilide on liver cancer induction by N-hydroxy-N-2-fluorenylacetamide. Cancer Res 33:454

16. Vesely DL, Levy GS (1978) Saccharin inhibits guanylate cyclase activity —
    possible relationship to carcinogenesis, Biochem Biophys Res Commun
    81:1384
17. Kohli K, Venkitasubramanian TA (1978) Effect of dieldrin toxicity on
    pyridine nucleotides and activities of NADH and NADPH oxidase in rat
    liver. Chem Biol Interact 21:337-341
18. Nagao M, Yahagi T, Kawachi T, Sugimura T, Kosuge T, Tsuji K, Wakabayashi
    K, Mizusaki S, Matsumototo T (1977) Comutagenic action of norharman and
    harman. Proc Jpn Acad 53:95-98

Some Aspects of Bacterial Mutagenicity Testing

J. Ellenberger[1] and G. R. Mohn[2]

In routine mutagenicity testing of environmental chemicals, bacterial systems occupy an important place in test strategies such as those developed by Flamm (1), by Bridges (2), by Bora (3), and by others, and which are in current use in several institutions. The common phases of these tier systems for mutagenicity have been recognized and described by Sobels (4) as (i) primary detection of mutagenic effects in short-term assays, (ii) verification in tests using eukaryotic indicators, (iii) quantification of the effects in animals (in comparison to known mutagens), and (iv) extrapolation to man. Bacterial indicators can and have been used to quantify genetic effects in mammals, for example in the body-fluid test (5) and in host-mediated assays (6-8), but their main role lies in the primary detection of environmental chemicals to be further evaluated for mutagenic and carcinogenic hazards, and several systems in bacteria such as *Escherichia coli* and *Salmonella typhimurium* have been described (see 9 and 10).

As exemplified in comparative studies involving the assay of many chemicals of known carcinogenic effects in bacterial mutation test systems using several auxotrophic strains of *S. typhimurium*, it could be empirically shown that there is a reasonable degree of correlation between carcinogenicity and mutagenicity of chemicals (11-17). Furthermore, attempts are presently being made to directly and quantitatively relate the mutagenic potency of chemicals in bacteria with their carcinogenic potency in mammals (18). The attractive possibility arises to use only a standard set of few bacteria and techniques (e.g., Salmonella) to detect and quantify the potential risk presented by environmental carcinogens and mutagens. Such an important role can be assumed by bacterial systems, however, only after a thorough evaluation of the advantages and limitations and the accurate determination of sensitivity and reliability. An active discussion on the quantitative predictability of effects in mammals from bacterial tests is presently being conducted (19-22). An interlaboratory comparison of results gained in one of the standard systems (Salmonella) showed great variations (23). Possible restrictions due to the complex, multistep nature of the mutation induction process have been pointed out several years ago (24) and this presentation describes a further few examples which in-

[1]Zentrallaboratorium für Mutagenitätsprüfung der Deutschen Forschungsgemeinschaft, Freiburg i.Br./FRG

[2]Department of Radiation Genetics and Chemical Mutagenesis, University of Leiden, Leiden/The Netherlands

dicate that a large overestimation or a large underestimation
of mutagenic potency of chemicals can be reached in bacterial
test systems upon slight modification of test procedure and
which make further comparative studies, improvements, and deve-
lopments necessary.

The physiologic state of the indicator cell seems to play an
important role in detecting mutagenic activity of certain classes
of chemicals. This has been demonstrated, for example, with sodium chromate and related compounds, which shows a strong mutagenic activity in growing *E. coli* cells and only a weak effect if
stationary cells are used (25). With aminoacridines the difference is even more pronounced and growing cells seem to be an
absolute prerequisite for detecting mutagenicity of these compounds (25). Another very striking example is given by caffeine,
a compound which exerts obviously very specific effects, being
mutagenic only in certain back mutation systems (26).

Differences in the method of performing a test may also lead to
large differences in sensitivity toward chemicals, as shown by
the fact that the bacterial strain *E. coli lys*$_{60}$ is not mutagenized
by ethyl methanesulfonate (EMS, a potent mutagen) in the spot
test (27) — this strain reverts readily with both base-pair substitution-inducing agents (methyl methanesulfonate, nitroso-
guanidine) and frameshift-inducing agents (acriflavine, pro-
flavine) — but in liquid test there is a very pronounced dose-
dependent mutagenic effect with EMS (28). Analogous results
were obtained with compounds requiring metabolic activation, the
dialkylnitrosamines, which are not mutagenic in the standard
plate test (11) but are active in modified plate tests (12,29)
or in liquid tests (25,30,31). On the other hand, some compounds
such as polycyclic hydrocarbons are active in plate tests but
seem to be inactive in liquid suspension tests (Bartsch, personal
observation cited in 32).

The influence of pH on mutagenicity is usually not taken into
consideration in standard testing protocols unless it is clear
that the formation of active chemical species is strongly pH
dependent (as in the mutagenicity of nitrite and of sulfite).
Recent results with the compound procarbazine (Natulan), a drug
of cytostatic activity, have unexpectedly shown that the pH
has a very strong effect on the mutagenic activity of this compound toward *E. coli* strain 343/113; a decrease in pH below 7
strongly increases the mutagenic activity of the compound. This
is probably due to the differences in charge and solubility of
the acidic and neutral or basic form. These differences may influence the rate of penetration of procarbazine into bacteria
(33).

The influence of light in some cases in performing bacterial
experiments is also of great importance, as shown in very early
studies on the photodynamic activity of dyes (34), and it has
been shown that simple irradiation of plates containing bacteria
and acriflavine with white light has a photodynamic, mutagenic
effect (24). Recent studies (35) confirm the ease with which
mutagenic effects can be inadvertently obtained, e.g., by ir-

radiating solutions of 8-methoxypsoralen and neutral red with white light. The different mutational spectra induced in light and in dark conditions are, furthermore, probably indicative of different modes of action.

A further possibility of enhancing the sensitivity of tester strains is, for example, to make use of comutagenic additives. The enhancing effect of nonmutagenic acridines on the mutagenic activity of ethyl methanesulfonate in *E. coli* was demonstrated several years ago (28). In these investigations the acridine derivative 6,9-diamino-2-ethoxyacridine (Rivanol) enhances the frequency of EMS-induced arg^+ and gal^+ mutations in strain *E. coli* 343/113. This effect could be due to an interaction with DNA, making it more susceptible to mutation by EMS; alternatively, 6,9-diamino-2-ethoxyacridine could interfere with the repair of EMS-induced premutations. Further compounds with comutagenic effects are harman and norharman, and riboflavin as reported in these proceedings (36), and it might be of interest to investigate the comutagenic properties of compounds known as strong protein alkylators, such as iodoacetamide.

In conclusion, it appears that slight changes in the testing procedure can result in great variation of genetic response. In routine testing of compounds of unknown mode of action, the exclusive use of a single standard protocol (e.g., the plate test) is likely to lead to underestimating of the mutagenic activity of some compounds (e.g., procarbazine, hydrazine sulfate, some nitrosamines, some metal salts).

Manipulation of the genetic background of tester strains can greatly influence the spontaneous and chemically induced mutability of certain genes. Examples of mutability changes after introduction of different repair deficiencies in the multipurpose strain *E. coli* 343/113 are various. Results with 9-aminoacridine, for example (33), show that the compound exerts moderate genetic effects (induction of frameshifts in the nad^+ back mutation system) in the standard spot test and that these effects are not increased upon introduction of plasmid pKM101. Introduction of the *dam*-4 mutation, however, which suppresses the cell's ability to methylate adenine residues after DNA replication and, therefore, restricts the ability to recognize parental from daughter DNA strands, has a very pronounced effect in enhancing the mutagenicity of 9-aminoacridine; *dam*-4 also enhances the mutagenic effect of EMS and of methylphenyl-nitrosamine (MPNA), a carcinogen which requires mammalian metabolic activation and which is not detected in standard plate tests (37). Introduction of pKM101 on the other hand, has different effects; whereas the mutagenic activity of MPNA and 9-aminoacridine is not markedly affected (33), compounds such as different alkylating agents, nitroheterocycles, and mito-mycin C are much more mutagenic when pKM101 is present in the cells (33).

Finally, another modification of the genetic background of tester strains which has a drastic influence on mutagen sensitivity is the introduction of excision repair deficiencies such as *uvrA* or *uvrB*. While the mutagenic activities of chemicals such as mitomycin C and malonaldehyde are suppressed or strongly reduced in excision repair-deficient strains (38,39) several classes of compounds exhibit very enhanced mutagenicity in *uvrA* or *uvrB* backgrounds. These include alkylating agents as well as frameshift inducers (40,41) and chemicals of weak mutagenicity can be easily detected, as demonstrated by the recent findings that 8-methoxypsoralen in the dark is more mutagenic in a *uvrB* derivative of *E. coli* K12 (35). The fact that no effect of *uvrB* on 8-methoxypsoralen activity was found in the *lac z* strain of *E. coli* K12 (42) again demonstrates the possible selective activity of chemicals upon different genes or gene loci.

These examples show that manipulation of the capacity of the indicator strains to metabolize and repair DNA damage can profoundly alter the observed mutational response toward certain classes of chemical mutagens. The most sensitive conditions (such as a combination of DNA repair deficiencies) certainly are most appropriate for detecting potential mutagens, but they will be of only limited value for quantifying genetic effects of chemicals or for extrapolation to mammalian cells, as long as the nature of the intracellular processes leading to mutagenic events remain largely unknown, especially in mammalian cells. Recent experimental evidence suggests that mutation induction pathways in mammalian cells might proceed through some different repair steps than in bacteria (for review see 43).

Back mutation systems have been repeatedly used for the determination of molecular mechanisms which lead to induction of mutations and have served to distinguish several classes of point mutations such as base-pair substitutions and frameshifts in bacteria such as *E. coli* (44), *S. typhimurium* (41), and *Serratia marcescens* (24). A large part of induced mutations arise by misrepair rather than mispairing (45). Therefore, the uncritical use of repair-deficient strains in mutagenicity tests will lead to misunderstanding and perhaps misinterpretation of what happens in normal repair-proficient bacteria. The reason is that deficiency of a given repair system probably forces premutagenic alterations into a different pathway and leads to additional or different observed mutants. This is probably the reason why 4-nitroquinoline-1-oxide was shown to induce mainly frameshifts in repair-deficient *Salmonella* (46) and base-pair substitutions in repair-proficient *E. coli* and *Neurospora* (47). This is also demonstrated in tests including the substance 1,1,1-trichloropropane-2,3-oxide (TCPO), an alkylating epoxide, and *S. typhimurium* strains (unpublished data). TCPO is slightly active without metabolic activation by mammalian enzymes in the base substitution-sensitive strain TA 1535. The mutagenicity is extremely enhanced in its resistance factor-bearing derivative, TA 100. While TCPO has been not detected as mutagen in the frameshift-sensitive strains, TA 1537 and TA 1538, a weak but significant dose-dependent and reproducible positive effect could be shown in strain TA 98, a derivative of TA 1538 bearing the plasmid pKM101.

It has also been shown, however, that even in wild-type genetic
background strains such as *E. coli* 343/113 even strong base-pair
substitution or strong frameshift-detecting systems do not allow
an absolute distinction between those two types of premutagenic
alterations. This is demonstrated by the fact that the arg^+ back
mutation system which seems to be strongly sensitive for base-
pair substitution-inducing agents is also sensitive to the mutagenic activity of 9-aminoacridine (25) and by the fact that
the frameshift mutation system nad^+ is also sensitive to the
mutagenic activity of alkylating compounds such as 1-chloro-
cyclohexene-1 and others (unpublished data).

Even in forward mutation systems where one might expect that
the gene can be attacked by different classes of chemical mutagens there is still some specificity present which is probably
due to differential expression of induced mutations and differential phenotypic lags, as shown in the cyclophosphamide
results (48). While cyclophosphamide is nonmutagenic in the gal^+
forward mutation system of *E. coli* 343/113 after biotransformation through extracts of mouse liver this substance shows a
dose-dependent mutagenic effect in the arg^+ back mutation system
of the same bacterial strain.

A potentially useful system with probably very decreased mutagen
specificity is the induction of the vegetative growth of prophage
in lysogenic bacteria (49). This test system was described
several years ago and has also been shown to be sensitive to
several different classes of substances (50-54). It was recently reactivated as the *inductest* with the possibility of including
mammalian biotransformation with it (55). The use of lysogenic
strains, however, in routine mutagenicity testing experiments is
somewhat restricted because of the induction of vegetative growth
of prophage which leads to increasing killing of the cells as
compared with the wild-type non-prophage-bearing strain (35).

In conclusion, we have shown examples which demonstrate that
mutation tests based on repair-deficient indicators may not give
results that are representative of those to be expected in wild-
type populations. In some systems, such as those detecting forward mutations and possibly lysogenic induction, mutagen specificity is greatly reduced because of the increased number of
available target sites; these systems should be given preference
if informations on generalized gene sensitivity to mutagens are
to be obtained.

With studies of bioactivation using mammalian metabolizing systems, a relatively simple situation exists if the major mammalian
metabolites of a given compound are known and can be isolated
and tested. In an attempt to determine which of the known mammalian metabolites of cyclophosphamide is responsible for the
mutagenic (and probably carcinogenic) properties of the compound,
several synthetic metabolites were tested for their mutagenicity
in *E. coli* 343/113 (56). The results show large differences in
the direct mutagenicity of the various cyclophosphamide metabolites. Most of the metabolites are mutagenic per se (4-hydroxy-
cyclophosphamide, carboxyphosphamide, 4-ketocyclophosphamide,

phosphoramide mustard, and nornitrogen mustard). In contrast, acrolein (known as a cytotoxic compound) did not exhibit any mutagenic activity (either with or without liver homogenates). These results indicate that mutagenic metabolites arise early in the cyclophosphamide metabolic pathway and that this mutagenicity is retained through several degradation steps.

Satisfactory results are also obtained when mammalian organ homogenates are used which are known to activate mainly the compound, such as using liver microsomes in checking the mutagenic activity of dimethylnitrosamine. Problems arise when the mutagenic activity of a compound is assayed in organ homogenates in which the compound is not activated. This is demonstrated in the case of cycasin, a natural product which needs activation via a β-glucosidase before liberating the alkylating moiety methylazoxymethanol (36). This step is carried out by the bacterial microflora of the intestine and does not take place in the mammalian liver. This is why cycasin cannot be demonstrated in a mammalian-microsome test whereas it is easily shown as mutagen in the host-mediated assay (57). A further clear demonstration of compound activated outside mammalian liver has been reported by Batzinger et al. (58), who found that the non-mutagenic compound 4-isothiocyano-4'-nitrophenylamine is not activated by mammalian liver preparations, but by a representative member of the enteric bacterial flora, and would have been missed using a routine standard S-9 assay.

In summary, it appears that for the important task of primary identification of chemical mutagens and carcinogens one single bacterial test procedure is not sufficient to effectively detect all possible genetic alterations and use should be made of several different kinds of test systems including those which register both forward and back mutations. It seems also clear that the repair capacity of the tester strains has an important influence on sensitivity for various mutagenic chemicals. In addition it appears that the kinds of mutations detected can be altered appreciably by such changes in repair capacity. Therefore, primary areas of investigation will include the more precise elucidation of pharmacologic and pharmacokinetic properties of foreign compounds in mammalian systems and possibly the elaboration of new test systems in microbes which reduce mutagen specificity by greatly enhancing the number of investigated genes, and which possibly assay for genetic effects so far not thoroughly investigated, such as lysogenic induction of prophage, induction of gene or genetic duplications of part of the genome, induction of displacements of inserted sequence elements within different genes of bacteria (for review see 59). Induction of the so-called *inserted sequence elements* is a phenomenon related to induction of prophage and possibly a future research area in chemical mutagenesis and carcinogensis.

References

1. Flamm WG (1974) A tier system approach to mutagen testing. Mutat Res 26:329-333
2. Bridges BA (1974) The three-tier approach to mutagenicity screening and the concept of radiation-equivalent dose. Mutat Res 26:335-340
3. Bora KC (1976) A hierarchical approach to mutagenicity testing and regulatory control of environmental chemicals. Mutat Res 41:73-82
4. Sobels FH (1977) Some problems associated with the testing for environmental mutagens and a perspective for studies in "comparative mutagenesis". Mutat Res 46:245-260
5. Legator MS, Pullin TG, Connor TH (1977) The isolation and detection of mutagenic substances in body fluid and tissues of animals and body fluid of human subjects. In: Kilbey BJ et al. (eds) Handbook of Mutagenicity Test Procedures. Elsevier, Amsterdam, pp 149-159
6. Mohn GR (1977) Actual status of mutagenicity testing with the host-mediated assay. Arch Toxicol 38:109-133
7. Maier P, Feldman DB, Ficsor G (1978) Host-mediated assay in Rhesus monkey (*Macaca mulatta*): Mutagenicity of mitomycin C. Mutat Res 57:91-95
8. Wheeler LA, Carter JH, Soderberg FB, Goldman P (1975) Association of Salmonella mutants with germfree rats: Site specific model to detect carcinogens as mutagens. Proc Natl Acad Sci USA 72:4607-4611
9. Kilbey BJ, Legator M, Nichols W, Ramel C (eds) Handbook of Mutagenicity Test Procedures. Elsevier, Amsterdam (1977)
10. Hollaender A (ed) Chemical Mutagens. Principles and Methods for their Detection, Vol 1. Plenum Press, New York (1971)
11. McCann J, Choi E, Yamasaki E, Ames BN (1975) Detection of carcinogens as mutagens in the Salmonella/microsome test: Assay of 300 chemicals. Proc Natl Acad Sci USA 72:5135:5139
12. McCann J, Ames BN (1976) Detection of carcinogens as mutagens in the Salmonella/microsome test: Assay of 300 chemicals: Discussion. Proc Natl Acad Sci USA 73:950-954
13. Andrews AW, Thibault LH, Lijinsky W (1978) The relationship between carcinogenicity and mutagenicity of some polynuclear hydrocarbons. Mutat Res 51:311-318
14. Andrews AW, Thibault LH, Lijinsky W (1978) The relationship between mutagenicity and carcinogenicity of some nitrosamines. Mutat Res 51:319-326
15. Zeiger E, Sheldon AT (1978) The mutagenicity of heterocyclic N-nitrosamines for *Salmonella typhimurium*. Mutat Res 57:1-10
16. Rao TK, Young JA, Lijinsky W, Epler JL (1979) Mutagenicity of aliphatic nitrosamines in *Salmonella typhimurium*. Mutat Res 66:1-7
17. Bartsch H, Camus A, Malaveille C (1976) Comparative mutagenicity of N-nitrosamines in a semi-solid and in a liquid incubation system in the presence of rat and human tissue fractions. Mutat Res 37:149-162
18. Meselson M, Russell K (1977) Comparisons of carcinogenic and mutagenic potency. In: Hiatt HH, Watson JD, Winsten JA (eds) Origins of Human Cancer, Book C. Cold Spring Harbor Laboratory, pp 1473-1481
19. Ashby J, Styles JA (1978) Does carcinogenic potency correlate with mutagenic potency in the Ames assay? Nature 271:452-455
20. Ames BN, Hooper K (1978) Does carcinogenic potency correlate with mutagenic potency in the Ames assay? Nature 274:19-20
21. Ashby J, Styles JA (1978) Factors influencing mutagenic potency in vitro. Nature 274:20-22
22. McGregor DB (1978) Cotton rat anomaly. Nature 274:21
23. Rosenkranz HS (These proceedings)

24. Mohn G (1971) Microorganisms as test systems for mutagenicity. Arch Toxikol 28:93-104
25. Mohn GR, Ellenberger J (1977) The use of *Escherichia coli* K12/343/113 (λ) as a multi-purpose indicator strain in various mutagenicity testing procedures. In: Kilbey BJ et al. (eds) Handbook of Mutagenicity Test Procedures. Elsevier, Amsterdam, pp 95-118
26. Clarke CH, Wade MJ (1975) Evidence that caffeine, 8-methoxypsoralen and steroidal diamines are frameshift mutagens for *E. coli* K-12. Mutat Res 28:123-125
27. Mohn G, Ellenberger J, McGregor D (1974) Development of mutagenicity tests using *Escherichia coli* K-12 as indicator organism. Mutat Res 25:187-196
28. Mohn G, Ellenberger J, McGregor D, Merker H-J (1975) Mutagenicity studies in microorganisms in vitro, with extracts of mammalian organs, and with the host-mediated assay. Mutat Res 29:221-233
29. Nakajima T, Iwahara S (1973) Mutagenicity of dimethylnitrosamine in the metabolic process by rat liver microsomes. Mutat Res 18:121-127
30. Frantz CN, Malling HV (1975) The quantitative microsomal mutagenesis assay method. Mutat Res 31:365-380
31. Green MHL, Muriel WJ (1975) Use of repair-deficient *E. coli* strains and liver microsomes to characterize mutagenesis by dimethylnitrosamine. Chem Biol Interact 11:63-65
32. Ames BN, McCann J, Yamasaki E (1975) Methods for detecting carcinogens and mutagens with the Salmonella/mammalian-microsome mutagenicity test. Mutat Res 31:347-364
33. Mohn GR (To be published)
34. Kaplan RW (1949) Mutations by photodynamic action in *Bacterium prodigiosum*. Nature 163:573-574
35. Ellenberger J (To be published)
36. Matsushima T, Sugimura T (These proceedings)
37. Drevon C, Kuroki T, Montesano R (1977) Microsome-mediated mutagenesis of a Chinese hamster cell line by various chemicals. In: Scott D, Bridges BA, Sobels FH (eds) Progress in Genetic Toxicology. Elsevier, Amsterdam, pp 207-213
38. Kondo S (1973) Evidence that mutations are induced by errors in repair and replication. Genetics Suppl 73:109-122
39. Mukai FH, Goldstein BD (1976) Mutagenicity of malonaldehyde, a decomposition product of peroxidized polyunsaturated fatty acids. Science 191:868-869
40. Bridges BA, Mottershead RP, Rothwell MA, Green MHL (1972) Repair-deficient bacterial strains suitable for mutagenicity screening: Tests with the fungicide captan. Chem Biol Interact 5:77-84
41. Ames BN (1971) The detection of chemical mutagens with enteric bacteria. In: Hollaender A (ed) Chemical Mutagens. Principles and Methods for their Detection, Vol. 1. Plenum, New York, pp 267-282
42. Bridges BA, Mottershead RP (1977) Frameshift mutagenesis in bacteria by 8-methoxypsoralen (methoxalen) in the dark. Mutat Res 44:305-312
43. Hart RW, Hall KY, Daniel FB (1978) DNA repair and mutagenesis in mammalian cells. Photochem Photobiol 28:131-155
44. Yanofsky C (1971) Mutagenesis studies with *Escherichia coli* mutants with known amino acid (and base-pair) changes. In: Hollaender A (ed) Chemical Mutagens. Principles and Methods for their Detection, Vol 1. Plenum, New York, pp 283-287
45. Bridges BA (1977) Recent advances in basic mutation research. Mutat Res 44:149-164

46. Ames BN, Lee FD, Durston WE (1973) An improved bacterial test system for the detection and classification of mutagens and carcinogens. Proc Natl Acad Sci USA 70:782-786
47. Ong T-M, Matter BE, De Serres FJ (1975) Genetic characterization of adenine-3 mutants induced by 4-nitroquinoline 1-oxide and 4-hydroxyamino-quinoline 1-oxide in *Neurospora crassa*. Cancer Res 35:291-295
48. Ellenberger J, Mohn G (1975) Mutagenic activity of cyclophosphamide, ifosfamide, and trofosfamide in different genes of *Escherichia coli* and *Salmonella typhimurium* after biotransformation through extracts of rodent liver. Arch Toxicol 33:225-240
49. Lwoff A (1953) Lysogeny. Bacteriol Rev 17:269-337
50. Epstein SS, Saporoschetz IB (1968) On the association between lysogeny and carcinogenicity in nitroquinolines and related compounds. Experientia 24:1245-1248
51. Fleck W (1968) Eine neue mikrobiologische screening-Methode für die Suche nach potentiellen Carcinostatica und Virostatica mit Wirkung im Nuclein-säure-Stoffwechsel. Z Allgem Mikrobiol 8:139-144
52. Heinemann B (1971) Prophage induction in lysogenic bacteria as a method of detecting potential mutagenic, carcinogenic, carcinostatic, and teratogenic agents. In: Hollaender A (ed) Chemical Mutagens. Principles and Methods for their Detection, Vol 1. Plenum, New York, pp 235-266
53. Ikeda Y, Iijima T (1965) Simplified methods for selecting mutagenic and phage inducing agents from microbial products. J Gen Appl Microbiol 11:129-135
54. Kondo S, Ichikawa H, Iwo K, Kato T (1970) Base-change mutagenesis and prophage induction in strains of *Escherichia coli* with different DNA re-pair capacities. Genetics 66:187-217
55. Moreau P, Bailone A, Devoret R (1976) Prophage λ induction in *Escherichia coli* K12 *envA uvrB*: A highly sensitive test for potential carcinogens. Proc Natl Acad Sci USA 73:3700-3704
56. Ellenberger J, Mohn GR (1977) Mutagenic activity of major mammalian metab-olites of cyclosphamide toward several genes of *Escherichia coli*. J Toxicol Environ Health 3:637-650
57. Gabridge MG, Denunzio A, Legator MS (1969) Cycasin: Detection of associ-ated mutagenic activity in vivo. Science 163:689-691
58. Batzinger RP, Bueding E, Reddy BS, Weisburger JH (1978) Formation of a mutagenic drug metabolite by intestinal microorganisms. Cancer Res 38:608-612
59. Starlinger P (1977) DNA rearrangements in procaryotes. Annu Rev Genetics 11:103-126

Mutagenicity of Closely Related Carcinogenic and Noncarcinogenic Compounds Using Various Metabolizing Systems and Target Cells

H. R. GLATT[1], H. SCHWIND[1], L. M. SCHECHTMAN[2], S. BEARD[2], R. E. KOURI[2], F. ZAJDELA[3], A. CROISY[4], F. PERIN[4], P. C. JACQUIGNON[4], and F. OESCH[1]

Summary

A total of 49 heteropolycyclic compounds belonging to structurally homogenous series was investigated for bacterial mutagenicity in the Ames test. The same batches of compounds were tested for carcinogenicity by injection into subcutaneous tissue of mice; 22 test compounds were carcinogenic, some strongly, others weakly. With the exception of one weak carcinogen, all these compounds were mutagenic. However, 15 of 27 noncarcinogens (56%) were also mutagenic. Moreover, noncarcinogenic, weakly carcinogenic, and strongly carcinogenic mutagens showed very similar mutagenic potencies.

To investigate the reasons for the many apparently false positives in the Ames test and for the complete lack of quantitative correlation, two groups of isomers were selected for further investigation. The first group of isomers consisted of the noncarcinogenic nonmutagen 2-fluoro-7-methyl-6H-[1]benzothiopyrano-[4,3-b]quinoline (2-F-MBTQ), the noncarcinogenic mutagen 3-F-MBTQ, and the carcinogenic mutagen 4-F-MBTQ. The second group of isomers consisted of 7-methylbenzo(c)acridine and 12-methylbenzo-(a)acridine. Both were mutagenic, but whereas 7-methylbenzo(c)-acridine produced tumors essentially in all (522 of 523) animals surviving the minimal latency time of the experiment, no indication of carcinogenicity was found with 12-methylbenzo(a)acridine, although it was tested in many experiments using various strains and various routes of application with totally 554 animals.

Modifications of the mammalian activating system in the mutagenicity test, such as the use of tissue preparations from mice treated with enzyme inducers, or the addition of cofactors for conjugating, potentially inactivating enzymes, had very similar effects on the mutagenicity of carcinogenic and noncarcinogenic isomers. Carcinogenic and noncarcinogenic isomers also did not

[1]Section of Biochemical Pharmacology, Institute of Pharmacology, University of Mainz, Obere Zahlbacher Straße 67, D-6500 Mainz

[2]Department of Biochemical Oncology, Microbiological Associates, Bethesda, Maryland 20016/USA

[3]Unité de Physiologie Cellulaire, Institut National de la Santé et de la Recherche Médicale, F-91405 Orsay/France

[4]Institut de Chimie des Substances Naturelles du CNRS, F-91190 Gif sur Yvette/France

differ in their enzyme-inducing ability. All five MBTQs and methylbenzoacridines were mutagenic to mammalian (Balb 3T3) cells.
In these cells carcinogens were more potent mutagens than the
noncarcinogenic isomers, but the quantitative difference in
mutagenicity was much smaller than the minimal estimate of the
difference in carcinogenicity.

The elucidation of the reasons for such discrepancies is important for the interpretation of data obtained in short-term tests
for carcinogenicity.

Introduction

A high reliability is essential for a short test for carcinogenicity. It is obtained by empirical evaluation and by understanding the biological basis of the test. For the microsome/
Salmonella test developed by Ames' group (1), very high correlations with carcinogenicity were found by several groups (2-4).
These studies were essentially empirical and did not analyze
the reason for the correlation or noncorrelation. We may sub-
divide these reasons in three classes.

Artifical Reasons. The first evaluation is strongly interrelated
with the development of a test. The test is optimized and criteria for a positive result are defined using certain known
carcinogens and possibly also certain noncarcinogens. Considering the usually large number of reasonable variables — Ashby and
Styles (5) have recently listed 14 main variables for the Ames
test — the inclusion in the evaluation of the test of the same
compounds which had been used for the development of the test
or an insufficiently defined test program may be significant
sources for an artifical correlation. A second important group
of artifical factors arises from the use of literature data for
carcinogenicity. These data were obtained using different species,
routes of application, and dosage schedules. Different batches
of test compound which therefore very likely contained different
impurities were used for carcinogenicity and mutagenicity. Frequently carcinogenicity data obtained in different laboratories
and by different methods disagree and the significance of the
results for the classification of a compound as a carcinogen or
noncarcinogen has to be decided subjectively. It has also to be
noted that noncarcinogenicity can not be proven; experiments
can only show that a compound produces less than a certain number of tumors in a certain system. Thus, carcinogenicity always
implies a quantitative aspect, but only an extremely crude comparison of the carcinogenic potency of various compounds is
possible when literature data are used.

Technical Reasons. A second group of factors disturbing the correlation are real, but not fundamental, differences between the
two systems. They include pharmacokinetic differences between
the two systems, such as the existence of permeability barriers
in one system but not in the other.

Fundamental Reasons. The two fundamental reasons for noncorrelation
are that the metabolism of a compound is critically different
in the two systems and that different metabolites are responsible for the two different endpoints.

For a rational analysis of whether a given system is fundamentally representative of or fundamentally different from another
system, it is desirable to exclude the artificial and to reduce
the technical reasons for correlation and noncorrelation. In
the present study we therefore investigated struturally homogeneous compounds in order to minimize the pharmacokinetic
differences. We studied the correlation between mutagenicity
in the Ames assay and carcinogenicity of 49 tetra- and penta-
cycles with heteroatoms; 44 of them were tested for carcinogenicity under identical conditions; for the other five compounds
very similar methods were used. The same batches were used for
the mutagenicity experiments. A standard protocol for the mutagenicity tests was devised in advance. Furthermore, the mutagenicity tests were performed without knowledge of the carcinogenicity results.

Much to our surprise we found marked differences between whole
animal carcinogenicity and mammalian-enzyme-mediated mutagenicity.
Therefore we selected compounds where carcinogenicity and mutagenicity data correlated and isomers with a lack of such a correlation. Using these isomers we tried to find the reasons for
the noncorrelation.

Screening of Chemical Homogeneous Compounds for Mutagenicity and Carcinogenicity

Test Compounds. A total of 49 tetra- and pentacyclic compounds
with heteroatoms was investigated. They were originally synthesized in order to investigate the effect of a modification
of the K-region in the benzoacridine, benzocarbazole, and ben-
zopyridocarbazole parent compounds. A carbon at the K-region was
replaced by sulphur or oxygen. Furthermore, fluoro and trifluoromethyl substituents were introduced at various distances
in the benzene ring next to the modified K-region. The fluoro
substituent has the same size as hydrogen, but is strongly elec-
tronegative and therefore impedes electrophilic substitution
reactions such as metabolic oxidation in its neighborhood.
Furthermore, the fluorine shows mesomerism with the aromatic
ring system, which results in a strong directing effect for substitution reactions. The trifluoromethyl group is electron withdrawing but it does not show mesomerism. Compared with hydrogen
or fluorine it is also larger. This may sterically affect interactions with enzymes or with target molecules for carcinogenesis
or mutagenesis. The synthesis of the test compounds is described
in references 6-12.

Carcinogenicity Experiments. In the standard carcinogenicity test,
28 mice of the strain XVIInc/Z (14 males and 14 females) received
three subcutaneous injections of 0.6 mg test compound (dissolved
in olive oil) at monthly intervals. The animals received the
first treatment when they were 3-4 months old and they were

sacrificed when they had tumors or when they were 700-800 days
old. During the experiment they were tested weekly by palpation,
after sacrifice they were autopsied, and, in unclear cases,
examined histologically. Differences in this standard protocol
(different number of animals; in the case of one compound different mouse strains) and additional carcinogenicity experiments
are mentioned together with the results in Table 1. It should
be noted that the strain XVIInc/Z shows an extremely low incidence of spontaneous tumors and a high sensitivity of the subcutaneous tissue to carcinogenesis by polycyclic aromatic
hydrocarbons. In a survey of 2500 control animals older than
20 months and of 24,000 control animals older than 15 months,
no single subcutaneous tumor was observed. Therefore, even one
subcutaneous tumor in a group of treated animals is statistically highly significant. All tumors induced after subcutaneous
application of the test compounds were fibrosarcomas. The incidence of other tumors was not statistically significantly different from controls (0% mammary tumors, 2.7% hepatomas, 2.6%
leukemias).

Of the 49 compounds tested five produced tumors in > 80% of the
treated animals, nine in 20%-80%, eight were weakly carcinogenic (<20% tumor incidence), and 27 compounds were inactive.
Thus, the carcinogenic potency of the tested compounds covered
a whole spectrum from strong carcinogens to apparently inactive
compounds.

Some of the test compounds were also tested with other mouse
strains, other dosage schedules or with other modes of application (Table 1). No discrepancies were observed between the
results of these different tests compared with those obtained
with the standard subcutaneous test in XVIInc/Z mice. This indicates that this test has some representative character for
the carcinogenicity of this class of compounds, at least as long
as mice are used. Carcinogenicity in other species has not been
studied, but such experiments are now in progress.

Bacterial Mutagenicity. The mutagenicity experiments were performed
essentially as described by Ames et al. (1). The person doing
the experiments was not aware of the carcinogenicity data. A
standard testing program was defined in advance. The *Salmonella
typhimurium* strains TA 1535, TA 1537, TA 98, and TA 100
(0.5 - 1.0 × 10^8 bacteria/plate) were used. The compounds were
tested at doses of 1, 3, 10, 30, and 100 µg/plate. Those doses
were chosen after an estimation of the toxicity of some of these
heteropolycyclic compounds. In case of weak effects, other concentrations around the optimal dose were often included in re-
peat experiments. The compounds were tested in the presence
and in the absence of a mammalian metabolizing system. This was
fresh liver S-9 mix [= postmitochondrial fraction plus NADPH-
generating system (1)] from Aroclor-1254-treated adult male
Sprague-Dawley rats which were killed on the day of the experiment. Only one dose of postmitochondrial fraction (equivalent
to 50 mg liver) per plate was used for the screening. As we observed in later studies this amount was sometimes not optimal.
Some compounds showed severalfold stronger mutagenic effects at

Table 1. Carcinogenicity and mutagenicity of 49 heteropolycycles. Carcinogenicity was tested by thrice subcutaneous injections of 0.6 mg test compound in XVIInc/Z mice (14 males and 14 females). All tumors induced
were fibrosarcomas. Further carcinogenicity experiments are mentioned in the last column. Mutagenicity was
investigated in the Ames test (1) in the presence and absence of liver S-9 mix from Aroclor-1254-treated rats.
Only two compounds showed direct mutagenicity (marked by an asterisk). A mutagenicity index (MI) is defined
as the number of revertants over spontaneous revertants per nmol from TA 100 plus twice this number from
TA 98 plus four times this number from TA 1537. Three polycyclic hydrocarbons, the last compounds on the list,
were used as positive controls in the mutagenicity experiments

Test compound	Mutagenicity Revertants/nmol			MI	Carcinogenicity XVIInc/Z mice with tumors (%)	Other carcinogenicity experiments
	TA 98	TA 100	TA 1537			
BTQ	0.06	0.37	0.08	0.83	0	
2-Fluoro-BTQ	0	1.4*	0	1.40*	0	
3-Fluoro-BTQ	0.57	0.4 (0.9*)	0.29	2.7 (0.9*)	0	
4-Fluoro-BTQ	0.15	1.0	0.03	1.42	28	
3-Trifluoromethyl-BTQ	0	0	0	0	0	Only 14 mice were used.
4-Trifluoromethyl-BTQ	0	0.84	0	0.84	0	
BPQ	0.18	1.9	0.25	3.26	0	
7-Methyl-BTQ (MBTQ)	0.18	0.27	0.13	1.15	57	
2-Fluoro-MBTQ	0	0	0	0	0	
3-Fluoro-MBTQ	1.2	0.57	0	2.97	0	
4-Fluoro-MBTQ	0.27	0.39	0.08	1.25	85	
3-Trifluoromethyl-MBTQ	0	0	0	0	0	
4-Trifluoromethyl-MBTQ	0	0	0	0	0	
7-Methyl-BPQ	0.30	0.63	0.30	2.43	0	
BTI	0.45	1.3	0.12	2.68	0	Also no tumors in 20 XVIInc/Z mice which received 10 subcutaneous doses of 0.6 mg.
2-Fluoro-BTI	0.31	0.55	0.10	1.57	7	
3-Fluoro-BTI	0.42	0.39	0.27	2.23	0	
4-Fluoro-BTI	0.29	0.38	0.07	1.24	15	
2-Fluoro-6,11-dihydro-BTI	0.81	0.41	0.17	2.41	7	

Table 1 (continued)

Compound					%	
3-Fluoro-6,11-dihydro-BTI	0	0	0	0	0	
4-Fluoro-6,11-dihydro-BTI	0.05	0.16	0.03	0.38	7	
2-Fluoro-BgBTI	0.47	0.76	0	1.70	0	
3-Fluoro-BgBTI	0.14	0.48	0	0.76	15	
4-Fluoro-BgBTI	0.31	0.68	0	1.30	7	
3-Trifluoromethyl-BgBTI	0	0	0	0	0	Only 14 mice were used.
4-Trifluoromethyl-BgBTI	0	0	0	0	0	
2-Fluoro-6,13-dihydro-BgBTI	0	0.55	0.11	0.99	15	Also no tumors in 20 XVIInc/Z mice which received 10 subcutaneous doses of 0.6 mg.
3-Fluoro-6,13-dihydro-BgBTI	0	0.43	0	0.43	0	
4-Fluoro-6,13-dihydro-BgBTI	0	0.40	0.14	1.04	0	
3-Trifluoromethyl-6,13-dihydro-BgBTI	0	0	0	0	0	
4-Trifluoromethyl-6,13-dihydro-BgBTI	0	0	0	0	0	
2-Fluoro-BeBTI	0.27	1.12	0	1.66	21	
3-Fluoro-BeBTI	2.07	1.91	0	6.05	50	
4-Fluoro-BeBTI	0.63	2.48	0	3.11	57	
3-Trifluoromethyl-BeBTI	0	0	0	0	0	
6,13-Dihydro-BeBTI	0.17	1.01	0	1.35	78	
2-Fluoro-6,13-dihydro-BeBTI	0.21	0.49	0	0.91	0	Also no tumors in 21 XVIInc/Z mice which received 60 epicutaneous doses of 50 µg.
3-Fluoro-6,13-dihydro-BeBTI	0.41	1.60	0	2.52	65	
4-Fluoro-6,13-dihydro-BeBTI	0.19	1.36	0	1.74	93	
3-Trifluoromethyl-6,13-dihydro-BeBTI	0	0	0	0	0	
4-Trifluoromethyl-6,13-dihydro-BeBTI	0	0	0	0	0	
13H-Benzo[g]-pyrido[2,3-a]-carbazole	0	0	0	0	15	Epithelioma in the stomach after intragastral application (17).
	0.58	3.4	0.38	6.08	100	
13H-Benzo[g]-pyrido[5,6-a]-carbazole	0.55	6.4	0.15	8.10	56	Epithelioma in the stomach after intragastral application (17).
13H-Benzo[e]-isochromano[4,3-b]indole-5-one	0.24	1.8	0.16	3.00	—	Tumors in 96% of C3H mice and in 100% of Swiss mice treated by 3 subcutaneous injections of 0.6 mg (18).

Table 1 (continued)

13H-Benzo[h]-pyrido[2,3-a]-carbazole	0.62	1.1	0.38	3.24	60	
13H-Benzo[a]-pyrido[2,3-i]-carbazole	0.63	2.6	0.63	5.75	0	Also not carcinogenic after subcutaneous application to 15 C57bl mice(19).
12-Methylbenzo[a]acridine	0.09	0.99	0.14	1.73	0 other	Not carcinogenic in many other experiments (cf. Table 3).
7-Methylbenzo[c]acridine	0.35	3.40	0.15	4.70	100	Also strongly carcinogenic in many other experiments (cf. Table 4).
3-Methylcholanthrene	3.15	17.43	0.47	25.6	–	
7,12-Dimethylbenz[a]anthracene	0.88	6.79	0.31	9.79	100	After a single dose of 100 μg.
Benzo(a)pyrene	13.1	34.3	4.5	78.5	65	After a single dose of 150 μg.

BTQ, 6H-[1]benzothiopyrano[4,3-b]quinoline; BPQ, 6H-[1]benzopyrano[4,3-b]quinoline; MBTQ, 7-methyl-BTQ; BTI, [1]benzothiopyrano[4,3-b]indole; BeBTI, benzo[e]-BTI; BgBTI, benzo[g]BTI.

lower doses, others were more active with more postmitochondrial fraction[5]. Thus, the rank order of the mutagenic potency of various compounds depends on the dose of postmitchondrial fraction. This was not unexpected and probably a large number of reasonable test variations exist which could increase the mutagenic effects of some compounds, but not of others. In spite of these problems intrinsically connected with screening, we tried to quantitate roughly the mutagenic potency by the introduction of a mutagenicity index (MI) which we defined as the maximal mutagenic effect (number of revertant colonies above spontaneous revertants) per nanomole with TA 100 plus twice this effect with TA 98 plus four times this effect with TA 1537 (no mutagenicity was observed to TA 1535 with any test compound). The factors for TA 98 and TA 1537 were introduced since the numbers of spontaneous and of the average-mutagen-induced reversions are lower for these strains than for TA 100. To improve quantitative reproducibility, only experiments in which blank (solvent) and positive controls gave the normal number of colonies were used for this study. Furthermore, all compounds were tested at least twice.

The results of the mutagenicity study are shown in Table 1. Of the 49 tested heteropolycyclic compounds, 36 were mutagenic. Only two compounds (the second and the third compounds in Table 1) were directly mutagenic. The others required activation by the S-9 mix. All 36 mutagens could be detected by the strain TA 100 (Table 2), 31 also reverted TA 98, and 22 were mutagenic with TA 1537. In contrast, no single compound showed mutagenicity with TA 1535. The mutagenic potencies of the heteropolycyclic compounds were relatively low compared with the positive controls 7,12-dimethylbenz[a]anthracene, benzo[a]pyrene, and 3-methylcholanthrene (Table 1).

Comparison of Mutagenicity and Carcinogenicity Results. The higher mutagenicity of the tested polycyclic aromatic hydrocarbons fits well their high carcinogenicity in this system. A single subcutaneous injection of 10 µg or 100 µg 7,12-dimethylbenz[a]anthracene caused subcutaneous tumors in 56% and 100%, respectively, of the treated XVIInc/Z mice. After a single subcutaneous dose of 150 µg benzo[a]pyrene, subcutaneous tumors were found in 69% of the treated mice.

When mutagenicity and carcinogenicity of the heteropolycyclics are compared (Table 2), we find that all compounds which produced tumors were also detected as mutagens, with the exception of one weak carcinogen (95% correlation). However, only 13 of 27 (48%) noncarcinogens were also nonmutagenic. This means that the probability for a nonmutagen to be also a noncarcinogen was 92%, whereas only 61% of the mutagens were carcinogenic. As also seen from Table 2, noncarcinogenic mutagens showed mutagenic potencies

---

[5]In the more detailed studies of five selected compounds described later in this manuscript, permutations of varying concentrations of test compounds as well as varying concentrations of activating systems have been tested.

Table 2. Comparison of mutagenic, carcinogenic, and structural properties of 49 heterocycles, using the data of Table 1

Class of compounds	Number of compounds	Mutagenic (%)	Mean MI $\pm$ SD of mutagens	Carcinogenic (%)
All tested heterocycles	49	73	2.4 ± 1.8	45
Noncarcinogens	27	56	2.1 ± 1.4	–
Carcinogens	22	95	2.6 ± 2.0	–
Tumor incidence <20%	8	88	1.2 ± 0.6	–
Tumor incidence 20%-80%	9	100	3.2 ± 2.4	–
Tumor incidence >80%	5	100	3.4 ± 2.0	–
Nonmutagens	13	–	–	8
Mutagens	36	–	–	61
Mutagenic with TA 100	36	–	–	61
Mutagenic with TA 98	31	–	–	65
Mutagenic with TA 1537	22	–	–	59
Mutagenic with TA 1535	0	–	–	–
Mutagenic with 3 strains	20	–	–	60
Compounds with CF_3 substituent	12	8	0.84	8
Compounds without CF_3 substituent	37	95	2.4 ± 1.8	57

indistinguishable from those of the carcinogens. Furthermore, the detection of a mutagen by all three sensitive strains did not improve the predictability of tumor production, nor did we observe that one of the strains was superior in distinguishing between mutagens which produced tumors and mutagens which were inactive in the carcinogenicity test.

When structures and biologic activities of the test compounds were compared, it was conspicuous that introduction of a trifluoromethyl substituent at the benzo ring next to the modified K-region strongly inactivated the compounds with respect to carcinogenicity as well as mutagenicity (Table 2). Of the 12 compounds possessing a trifluoromethyl group, only one was carcinogenic and only one was mutagenic. Both activities were very weak. In contrast, practically all (95%) compounds without a trifluoromethyl group were mutagenic. Within this latter group of 37 compounds, therefore, mutagenicity data were useless to distinguish between carcinogens (57% of the compounds) and noncarcinogens (43%). The observation that a relatively small alteration, introduction of a trifluoromethyl substituent (instead of a fluoro substituent and also compared with the mother compounds without substitutes), removed carcinogenic and mutagenic activities in a whole group of compounds suggests the possibility that clinically or industrially useful chemicals with a carcinogenic or mutagenic potential may be rendered harmless by relatively small chemical modifications which may be possible to introduce without destroying the desired therapeutic or technical properties of the compound in question.

Examination of Possible Sources of Noncorrelation Between Mutagenicity in the Ames Test and Carcinogenicity

Insufficient Carcinogenicity Studies. The simplest explanation for the large number of apparently false positives in the Ames test is that these compounds were just not investigated sufficiently for carcinogenicity. Indeed, it cannot be excluded that these compounds would have shown carcinogenic activity in larger experiments, in other species, or with a different mode of application. However, the similar mutagenic potency of carcinogenic and apparently noncarcinogenic mutagens suggests that this is not a main reason for the noncorrelation. A qualitative correlation without at least a partial quantitative correlation is hardly believable. The structural homogeneity of the test compounds makes it very unlikely that small differences are strongly potentiated by pharmacokinetic differences such as solubility or penetration.

Selection of Test Compounds for More Detailed Investigations. For further analysis we selected two groups of test compounds. The structures of these compounds are shown in Fig. 1. The first group consists of the 2-, 3-, and 4-fluoro isomers of 7-methyl-6H-[1]-benzothiopyrano[4,3-b]quinoline (MBTQ). The first isomer was neither mutagenic (Fig. 2) nor carcinogenic (Table 1). The second was mutagenic (Fig. 2) and strongly carcinogenic; it produced tumors in 85% (Table 1) of the treated animals with a mean

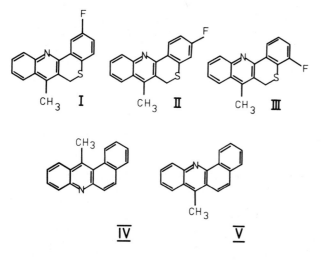

Fig. 1. Structures of 2-fluoro-7-methyl-6H-[1]-benzothiopyrano[4,3-b]-quinoline (*I*); 3-fluoro-7-methyl-6H-[1]benzothiopyrano[4,3-b]quinoline (*II*); 4-fluoro-7-methyl-6H-[1]benzothiopyrano[4,3-]quinoline (*III*); 12-methylbenzo[a]acridine (*IV*); and 7-methylbenzo[c]-acridine (*V*)

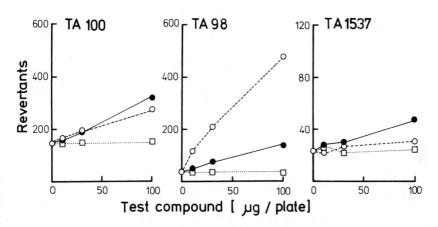

Fig. 2. Mutagenicity of 2-fluoro-MBTQ (□), 3-fluoro-MBTQ (O), and 4-fluoro-MBTQ (●) with various *S. typhimurium* strains using for activation liver S-9 mix (equivalent to 50 mg liver/plate) from Aroclor-1254-treated rats. Values are means of two plates; the standard deviations were normally smaller than 10% of the mean

latency of 182 days (159-414 days). 7-Methylbenzo[c]acridine and 12-methylbenzo[a]acridine are the second group. They were investigated very thoroughly for carcinogenicity (Tables 3 and 4) using various strains of mice and various modes of application. 7-Methylbenzo[c]acridine was tested with a total of 632 animals. All but one of the 523 animals which survived longer than the minimal latency time in the respective experiment developed tumors at the application site. The mean latency times were very similar after different modes of application (about 140 days). 12-Methylbenzo[a]acridine was tested with 585 animals. No tumors at the application site were observed in any of these animals. It is especially noteworthy that 320 of them survived the first

Table 3. Carcinogenicity experiments with 7-methylbenzo[c]acridine. The experiments were performed between 1950 and 1976. The better survival in the later experiments (nos. 20-26) than in the earlier experiments is due to better housing conditions and to the use of SPF animals. The many identical experiments with XVIInc/Z mice were performed to regularly check the reproducibility of our stock with a reference compound with respect to tumor incidence and latency period. The animals received the first treatment when they were 3-4 months old. Latency and survival times are defined beginning with the first treatment

Experiment number[a]	Animals (number, mouse strain)	Treatment	Tumors
1	10 XVII	Painting with 0.3% solution in acetone twice weekly till dead.	Eight of nine animals surviving longer than 90 days developed epitheliomas at the application site. Mean latency period: 141 days.
2-16	299 XVIInc/Z (15 independent experiments)	3 Subcutaneous injections of 0.5-0.6 mg at monthly intervals.	All 242 animals surviving the minimal latency period developed fibrosarcomas at the application site.
17	20 XVIInc/Z (10 ♂ + 10 ♀)	Same as in experiment 1.	All 12 animals surviving the minimal latency period (105 days) developed epitheliomas. Mean latency period: 146 days.
18	21 C3H Radium (11 ♂ + 10 ♀)	Same as in experiment 1.	All 13 animals surviving minimal latency period (112 days) developed epitheliomas. Mean latency period: 136 days.
19	40 XVIInc/Z (21 ♂ + 19 ♀)	24 Intragastral applications of 0.5 mg at weekly intervals.	All 22 animals surviving the treatment developed tumors.

Table 3 (continued)

20-26	89	XVIInc/7 (63 ♂ + 14 ♀)	Same as in experiment 2.	All 235 animals surviving the minimal latency period developed fibrosarcomas. Mean latency period with XVIInc/7 mice: 140 days.
	28	C57bl Carshalton (14 ♂ + 14 ♀)		
	28	C3H Carshalton (14 ♂ + 14 ♀)		
	27	Swiss Carshalton (14 ♂ + 13 ♀)		
	28	XVIInc/z (14 ♂ + 14 ♀)		
	21	Swiss Carshalton (13 ♂ + 8 ♀)		
	21	XVIInc/z (14 ♂ + 7 ♀)		

[a]Experiment 1: ref. 22; experiments 2-26: this study

Table 4. Carcinogenicity experiments with 12-methylbenzo[a]acridine. For explanation see Table 3.

Experiment number[a]	Animals (number, mouse strains)	Treatment	Tumors
1	10 XVII	Painting with 0.3% solution in acetone twice weekly till dead.	No tumors; 6 animals survived longer than 90 days (143-323 days).
2	10 XVII	3 Subcutaneous injections of 0.5-0.6 mg at monthly intervals.	No tumors; 7 animals survived longer than 90 days (95-537 days).
3-16	278 XVIInc/Z	Same as in experiment 2.	No tumors at the injection site; frequencies of other tumors not different from control animals; 103 animals survived longer than 500 days.
17	42 XVIInc/Z (20 ♂ + 22 ♀)	Same as in experiment 1.	No epidermal tumors; frequencies of other tumors not different from control animals; 18 animals survived longer than 450 days.
18	35 XVIInc/Z (21 ♂ + 22 ♀)	30 Intragastral applications of 0.6 mg at weekly intervals.	No tumors were observed in stomach, intestines and liver; frequencies of other tumors not different from control animals; 19 animals survived longer than 400 days.
19-22	82 XVIInc/Z (40 ♂ + 42 ♀)	Same as in experiment 2.	No tumors at the injection site; frequencies of other tumors not different from control animals; 135 animals survived 602 days.
	28 C57bl Carshalton (14 ♂ + 14 ♀)		
	27 C3H Carshalton (♂)		

Table 4 (continued)

28	Swiss Carshalton (♂)		
23	XVIInc/Z (21 ♂ + 14 ♀)	12 Subcutaneous injections of 0.6 mg at intervals of 15-20 days.	No subcutaneous tumors; frequencies of other tumors not different from controls; 29 animals survived 582 days.
24	XVIInc/Z (7 ♂ + 7 ♀)	Same as in experiment 2.	No subcutaneous tumors; frequency of other tumors not different from controls; 13 animals survived 627 days.

[a]Experiments 1 and 2: ref. 22; experiments 3-24: this study

treatment, which was performed at an age of 3-4 months, by more than 450 days. This is more than three times the mean latency time after which tumors were observed with the carcinogenic isomer 7-methylbenzo[c]acridine. In spite of this very large difference in carcinogenicity, both compounds were mutagenic with various *Salmonella* strains (Fig. 3). Their mutagenic potency as indicated by the mutagenicity index (MI) differed by a factor smaller than 3 (Table 1).

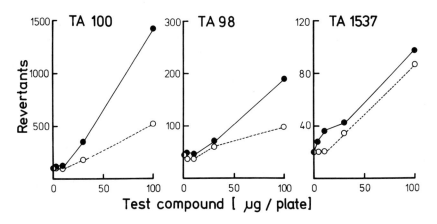

Test compound [μg / plate]

Fig. 3. Mutagenicity of 12-methylbenzo[a]acridine (O) and 7-methylbenzo[c]-acridine (●) with various *S. typhimurium* strains using activation for S-9 mix (equivalent to 50 mg liver/plate) from Aroclor-1254-treated rats. Values are means of two plates; the standard deviations were normally smaller than 10% of the mean

The Role of Monooxygenases and Enzyme Induction in the Ames Test. For the preceding screening part of this study, S-9 mix from liver homogenate of Aroclor-1254-treated rats was used because this activation is proposed by Ames et al. (1) and is used by most laboratories for routine investigations. Since we had studied carcinogenicity in XVIInc/Z mice, we used homogenate from this mouse strain for the subsequent experiments on mechanisms of metabolic activation and inactivation. Because it was not possible to get sufficient, pure, and locally defined material from the target tissue, i.e., subcutaneous mesenchymal tissue possibly with local enzyme induction by the test compound, we used liver homogenate. Liver most likely contains all the drug-metabolizing enzymes present in fibroblasts, but in different proportions, and it may possess additional enzymes not present in fibroblasts.

When metabolic variations were studied, suboptimal doses of mutagen were used to avoid the possibility that an increased concentration of reactive metabolites would decrease the observable mutagenic effect by toxicity instead of increasing it. However, optimal amounts of postmitochondrial fraction were used in the activating system. The optimal amounts were different for different mutagens. Interestingly, however, within the groups of

isomers they were identical (Figs. 4 and 5 and other data),
suggesting similar mechanisms for activation of carcinogenic
and noncarcinogenic isomers. Using Aroclor-1254-treated mice and
50-100 µg test compound, 50 µl postmitochondrial fraction [S-9
fraction prepared as described by Ames et al. (1)] were optimal
for the fluoro-MBTQ series (data not shown), 100 µl for the
methylbenzoacridine series (Fig. 4), and 200 µl for the fluoro-6,
13-dihydro-benzo[e]-[1]benzothiopyrano[4,3-b]indoles, compounds
of a series not discussed in this paper. When S-9 mix from control livers was used for activation, larger doses of postmitochondrial fraction were required for maximal mutagenic effects
and these maximal effects were lower than with Aroclor S-9 mix
with both the fluoro-MBTQ (data not shown) and the methylbenzoacridine series (Fig. 4). The postmitochondrial fractions were
able to activate these test compounds only when a NADPH-generating system was present, indicating that monooxygenases were required for activation. Induction by 3-methylcholanthrene inten-
sified the activation similar to induction by Aroclor 1254, indicating that cytochrome P-448 dependent monooxygenases were
mainly responsible for the activation. This was observed for the
fluoro-MBTQ (data not shown) and methylbenzoacridine series
(compare Fig. 4 with Fig. 5). No difference was observed between
carcinogenic and noncarcinogenic isomers. Since carcinogenic
but not noncarcinogenic isomers might have induced the enzymes
required for activation, we treated mice with the test compounds
and used S-9 mix from these animals for activation of the same
compounds. This experiment was performed only with the methylbenzoacridines, since the fluoro-MBTQs were available only in
small quantities. As seen from Fig. 5, neither the carcinogenic
nor the apparently noncarcinogenic of the mutagenic methylbenzoacridines induced the activating enzymes. However, in a more
sensitive system, mammalian cells in culture, it was demonstrated
that both compounds and also the fluoro-MBTQs are monooxygenase
inducers, probably of the 3-methylcholanthrene type. However,
much larger doses than of polycyclic aromatic hydrocarbons were
required for monooxygenase induction (Fig. 6). Whether or not
the compounds induced their own activation in the carcinogenicity
experiment, enzyme induction could not explain the difference
in carcinogenicity, since the inducing effects of carcinogenic
and noncarcinogenic isomers could not be distinguished.

Effect of Cofactors for Conjugation Reactions in the Ames Test. The most
fundamental function of drug metabolism is to render lipophilic
foreign compounds sufficiently hydrophilic for their excretion.
Typically, excretability of lipophilic compounds is achieved by
introduction of a chemical function ("phase I reaction") which
allows conjugation with a hydrophilic moiety ("phase II reaction"). Phase I reactions thus necessarily tend to increase the
reactivity of a compound. Therefore, it is not surprising that
the majority of reactive metabolites are phase I reaction products, whereas highly reactive conjugation products are exceptions. Since reactive intermediates with identical reactive
groups but which are otherwise nonidentical may be metabolized
at different rates by enzymes, differences in carcinogenicity
of chemically similar compounds may be caused not only by differences in the formation but also by differences in the inac-

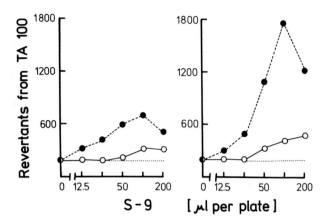

Fig. 4. Activation of 12-methylbenzo[a]cridine (*left*) and 7-methylbenzo[c]
acridine (*right*) by liver S-9 mix from control (O) and Aroclor-1254-treated
(●) XVIInc/Z mice. Treated animals received a single intraperitoneal injection of Aroclor 1254 (500 mg/kg, diluted 1:5 with sunflower oil) 6 days
before sacrifice. The liver was homogenized in three volumes 150 mM KCl-10 mM
Na phosphate pH 7.4. The homogenate was centrifuged at 9000 *g* for 10 min.
Various amounts of the resulting supernatant (S-9, postmitochondrial fraction) were used for the preparation of the S-9 mix (1). The figures show the
numbers of revertant colonies in the presence of 50 μg of test compounds.
The number of spontaneous revertants is indicated by a *dotted line*. Values
are means of three parallel plates; the standard deviation was normally
smaller than 10% of the mean

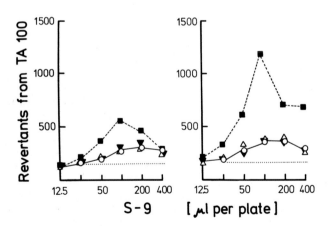

Fig. 5. Activation of 12-methylbenzo[a]acridine (*left*) and 7-methylbenzo[c]-
acridine (*right*) by liver S-9 mix from control (O), 3-methylcholanthrene-(■),
12-methylbenzo[a]acridine-(Δ), and 7-methylbenzo[c]acridine-treated (▼)
XVIInc/Z mice. Treated animals received a single intraperitoneal injection
(60 mg/kg dissolved in 0.2 ml sunflower oil) 40 h before sacrifice. Experiments were performed as described in Fig. 4

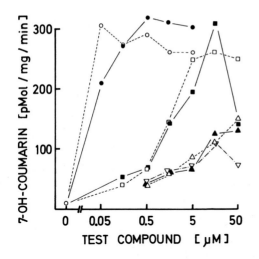

Fig. 6. Induction of ethoxycoumarin O-deethylase activity in Reuber H-4-II-E cells. The cells were seeded at a density of 20,000/cm^2 in Eagle's minimum essential medium containing 10% fetal calf serum. After 2 days the medium was changed and the inducer dissolved in acetone was added. The acetone concentration was 0.17% on all plates. Cells were harvested after 16 h and washed several times. The ethoxycoumarin O-deethylase activity was determined essentially as described by Ullrich and Weber (13), but by using unbroken cells instead of microsomes

tivation of reactive metabolites. However, in the Ames test cofactors for conjugation reactions are present only at low concentrations. This can increase the lifespan of reactive intermediates and favors further phase I metabolism which can lead to otherwise rare metabolites. Both effects increase the sensitivity of the test but also remove differences which are introduced in vivo by conjugating enzymes.

Therefore, we studied the effect of addition of cofactors for conjugation reactions upon the mutagenicity of carcinogenic and noncarcinogenic isomers. For these experiments we used the standard Ames test (1), but we included a preincubation for 30 min at 37°C. We checked that monooxygenase [with 7-ethoxycoumarin as substrate (13)] glutathione S-transferase [with 2,4-dinitrochlorobenzene as substrate (14)], epoxide hydratase [with benzo(a)pyrene 4,5-oxide as substrate (15)], and UDP-glucuronyltransferase [determined by continuous fluorimetric observation of conjugation of 1-naphthol (Stasiecki et al., unpublished work)] activities did not significantly change during this preincubation. Table 5 shows the effects of the various cofactors upon the mutagenicity of 3- and 4-fluoro-MBQT. The data for 2-fluoro-MBTQ are not shown because it remained nonmutagenic under all conditions. The cofactors for UDP-glucuronyltransferases, sulfotransferases, and acetyltransferases did not significantly alter the mutagenicity of the MBQTs. Glutathione markedly decreased it, but the effect upon the carcinogenic and the noncarcinogenic isomers were quantitatively similar. Cysteine as model for nonenzymic conjugation with glutathione only had a marginal effect with 3-fluoro-MBQT.

Although not identical, the results observed with the methylbenzoacridines were generally similar to those with the MBQTs (Table 6). Cofactors for sulfo- and acetyltransferases had no effect. UDP-glucuronic acid increased the mutagenicity of both compounds. Possible mechanisms are the formation of mutagenic conjugates or the removal of competitive substrates for the activating enzyme. In contrast to UDP-glucuronic acid, glutathione

Table 5. Effect of cofactors for conjugating enzymes on the mutagenicity of fluoro-MBTQs. Mutagenicity was tested as described by Ames et al. (1) with 50 µg test compound, the strain TA 98, and 50 µl liver postmitochondrial fraction from Aroclor-1254-treated XVIInc/Z mice, but performing a 30-min preincubation at 37°C before addition of the top agar and using dialyzed S-9, 10 mM MgSO$_4$ (required for the generation of PAPS from ATP) and the respective cofactors for conjugation reactions

Modification	His[+] induced by 3-F-MBTQ	His[+] induced by 4-F-MBTQ
Standard S-9 mix	900 ± 80	190 ± 17
+ 1.5 mM Glutathione	510 ± 30[a]	105 ± 27[a]
+ 15 mM Glutathione	270 ± 20[a]	46 ± 25[a]
+ 8 mM ATP	1010 ± 80	196 ± 12
+ 6 mM UDP-glucuronic acid	910 ± 50	221 ± 28
+ 0.25 mM Acetyl-CoA	1050 ± 70	224 ± 35

[a] $P < 0.01$ (*t*-test)

Table 6. Effect of enzyme inhibition and of cofactors for conjugation reactions on the mutagenicity of methylbenzoacridines. Mutagenicity was tested as described by Ames et al. (1) with 50 µg test compound, the strain TA 100, and 100 µl liver postmitochondrial fraction from Aroclor-1254-treated XVIInc/Z mice, but performing a 30-min preincubation at 37°C before addition of the top agar and using dialyzed S-9, 10 mM MgSO$_4$ (required for the generation of PAPS from ATP) and cofactors for conjugation reactions. TCPO (1,1,1-trichloropropene 2,3-oxide) was used as an inhibitor of epoxide hydratase (20, 21)

Modification	His[+] induced by 12-methyl-benzo-[a]acridine	His[+] induced by 7-methylbenzo-[c]acridine
Standard S-9 mix	516 ± 22	1600 ± 180
+ 0.3 mM TCPO	445 ± 26	1410 ± 180
+ 15 mM Glutathione	104 ± 25[a]	990 ± 90[a]
+ 15 mM Cysteine	402 ± 24[a]	1560 ± 70
+ 15 mM ATP	458 ± 99	1500 ± 190
+ 15 mM UDP-glucuronic acid	735 ± 76[a]	1830 ± 140
+ 0.75 mM Acetyl-CoA	520 ± 25	1610 ± 160
− NADPH generating system	2 ± 6[a]	5 ± 10[a]

[a] $P < 0.01$ (*t*-test)

decreased the mutagenicity. The effect was stronger with the non-carcinogenic isomer. But although this effect could contribute to the difference in carcinogenicity, it could not explain it completely, since the mutagenicity of the two isomers in the presence of glutathione differed by a factor of only 10, whereas the carcinogenic potency of the carcinogenic compared with the apparently noncarcinogenic isomer differs by a factor of more than 100 (cf. Tables 3 and 4).

Mutagenicity in Mammalian Cells. Since metabolic activation and inactivation were very similar for carcinogenic and noncarcinogenic isomers and quantitative differences in these processes could not explain the differences in carcinogenicity, we investigated the possibility that mutagenesis in bacteria and in mammalian cells is very different. Differences could be created, for example, by differences in the protein content of chromosomes or by differences in repair mechanisms or capacity. Since the compounds had produced fibrosarcomas in mice, the mammalian mutagenicity experiments were performed with a mouse fibroblast cell line (Balb 3T3 Cl. A31-1). Mutation to ouabain resistance was studied as described by Schechtman and Kouri (16). The results are shown in Tables 7 and 8. In contrast to the bacteria, exogenous activation by an S-9 mix was not required. All bacterial mutagens were mutagenic with fibroblasts. Besides, 2-fluoro-MBQT was also slightly mutagenic. In contrast to the bacterial test, the carcinogen 4-fluoro-MBQT was clearly more strongly mutagenic than the noncarcinogen 3-fluoro-MBQT. Considering the lower doses at which 4-fluoro-MBQT could be tested due to its higher toxicity, and assuming a linear dose-mutagenicity relationship, it was about ten times more mutagenic than 3-fluoro-MBTQ. This factor correlates with the *minimal* difference in carcinogenic potency between 3-fluoro-MBTQ (tumor induction in 0 of 28 treated animals) and 4-fluoro-BMTQ (fibrosarcomas in 24 of 28 treated animals). However, in the methylbenzoacridine pair, where a difference in carcinogenic potency of a factor more than 100 (Tables 3 and 4) was established, the carcinogenic isomer was again more strongly mutagenic to mammalian cells but only by a factor of about 10 (Table 8).

Table 7. Mutation of Balb 3T3 cells to ouabain resistance by fluoro-MBTQs. Cells in suspension were exposed to the test compound for 2 h in the presence or absence of liver S-9 mix from Aroclor-1254-treated rats as described (16). After an expression time of 6-8 days, cells were replated and exposed to the selecting agent ouabain (1 mM) for 4 weeks; MF, mutation frequency

Test compound (µg/ml)	S-9 mix	Dishes with mutations/ total dishes	MF (10^{-5})
Acetone control	+, O	1/136	0.009
12.5 Benzo(a)pyrene	+	13/15	3.03
3	+	2/14	0.19
10	+	1/13	0.06
30 2-Fluoro-MBTQ	+	0/10	< 0.1
30	Boiled	0/15	< 0.08
30	O	1/15	0.18
3	+	0/14	< 0.07
10	+	1/15	0.08
30 3-Fluoro-MBTQ	+	5/13	0.59
30	Boiled	7/15	0.67
30	O	3/15	0.33
1	+	2/15	0.23
3	+	5/15	0.45
10 4-Fluoro-MBTQ	+	12/13	1.83
10	Boiled	9/13	1.25
10	O	5/14	1.37

Table 8. Mutation of Balb 3T3 cells to ouabain resistance by methylbenzoacridines. Cells in suspension were exposed to the test compound for 2 h
in the presence or absence of liver S-9 mix from Aroclor-1254-treated rats
as described (16). After an expression time of 8 days, cells were replated
and mutants determined using 1 mM ouabain in the culture medium; MF,
mutation frequency

Test compound (µg/ml)		S-9 mix	Dishes with mutations/ total dishes	MF (10^{-5})
Acetone control		+, O	1/136	0.009
3		+	0/15	< 0.8
10		+	1/15	0.8
30	12-Methylbenzo(a)acridine	+	1/15	1.1
30		Boiled	0/15	< 0.4
30		O	2/15	2.2
3		+	1/15	0.3
10		+	8/15	4.0
30	7-Methylbenzo(c)acridine	+	3/15	10
30		Boiled	11/15	12
30		O	5/15	9

Discussion

Correlation between mutagenicity in the Ames test and carcinogenicity in mice after subcutaneous application was studied
qualitatively and quantitatively with 49 structurally homogeneous
compounds, with the aim of determining the reasons for noncorrelation. This was mainly done by comparing correlating and non-
correlating isomers with respect to metabolic activation, inactivation, and enzyme induction. Tests were also performed using
mammalian cells instead of bacteria as indicators for mutagenicity.

Qualitative Correlation. A total of 95% of the carcinogens were mutagenic in bacteria. However, an unexpectedly high number (56%)
of the apparently noncarcinogenic isomers were mutagenic in the
Ames test. All five compounds tested were mutagenic in mammalian
cells, although only two of them were carcinogenic and four were
mutagenic in bacteria. Thus, both mutagenicity tests if used
for the prediction of carcinogenicity apparently tended to give
false-positive results.

Quantitative Correlation. Noncarcinogenicity is not an absolute
term; it signifies that a compound at a certain dose and in a
certain number of animals did not significantly increase the
tumor frequency. Similar considerations apply to nonmutagenicity.
Thus, any correlation study should take into account these quantitative aspects. However, carcinogenicity can be tested in
various animals, using different dosage schedules or modes of
application. Also bacterial or mammalian mutagenicity tests can
be performed in many ways. Results obtained under different

conditions can not be compared quantitatively and different tests may show different relative potencies of different compounds. In spite of these grave problems we tried to describe our results quantitatively. To improve comparability, we tested all the compounds under principally the same conditions for carcinogenicity and for mutagenicity, and we used the same batches of compounds for both tests. The effect of a specific test method on the relative potency of carcinogenicity or mutagenicity is expected to be much smaller than usual, due to the structural homogeneity of the test compounds. In spite of this experimental design we could not observe any correlation between the potency of the bacterial mutagens and their carcinogenicity. Also we could not find any sufficient explanations for this lack of correlation. Carcinogenic and noncarcinogenic isomers had similar requirements for metabolic activation and no differences in the inactivation mechanisms were observed between them. Mammalian cell mutagenicity partially distinguished between carcinogens and noncarcinogens: Carcinogens were much stronger mutagens than their noncarcinogenic isomers. This finding requires confirmation with a large number of test compounds and by mutation at other loci. However, the mutagenicity of noncarcinogens in this system will remain a problem. Therefore, we are now investigating whether cell transformation which can be performed with the Balb 3T3 cells used for this study (16) is a better indication for whole animal carcinogenicity.

Thus, with the 49 heteropolycyclic compounds tested, no short test was able to predict the observed carcinogenic potencies with a sufficient certainty. This, of course, does not prove either that the usual animal carcinogenicity studies with high doses of test compounds are good at predicting carcinogenicity in man under his exposure conditions.

Acknowledgments. This work was supported by the Deutsche Forschungsgemeinschaft and by funds provided in part by the International Cancer Research Data Bank Programme of the National Cancer Institute, National Institutes of Health, USA, under contract NO1-CO-65341 with the International Union Against Cancer. We thank Dr. B. Ames for *S. typhimurium* strains, Dr. J. Gielen for Reuber cells, Dr. T. Kakunaga for Balb 3T3 cells, and Dr. C. Clegg for critically reading the manuscript.

References

1. Ames BN, McCann J, Yamasaki E (1975) Methods for detecting carcinogens and mutagens with the Salmonella/mammalian-microsome mutagenicity test. Mutat Res 31:347-364
2. McCann J, Choi E, Yamasaki E, Ames BN (1975) Detection of carcinogens as mutagens in the Salmonella/microsome test: assay of 300 chemicals. Proc Natl Acad Sci USA 72:5135-5139
3. Sugimura T, Sato S, Nagao M, Yahagi T, Matsushima T, Seino Y, Takenchi M, Kawachi T: Overlapping of carcinogens and mutagens. In: Magee PN, Takayama S, Sugimura T, Matsushima T (eds) Fundamentals in cancer prevention. University Tokyo Press, Tokyo, pp 191-215
4. Anderson D, Styles JA (1978) The bacterial mutation test. Br J Cancer 37:924-930

5. Ashby J, Styles JA (1978) Factors influencing mutagenic potency in vitro. Nature 274:20-22
6. Croisy A, Jacquignon P, Fravolini A (1974) Sur quelques analogues fluorés des [1]benzothiopyrano[4,3-b]-indoles et des 6H[1]benzothiopyrano[4,3-b]-quinoléines. J Heter Chem 11:113-118
7. Buu-Hoi NP, Martani A, Croisy A, Jacquignon P, Perin F (1966) Carcinogenic nitrogen compounds. Part LII. [1]Benzothiopyrano[4,3-b]indoles, [1]benzopyrano[4,3-b]indoles, and related pseudo-azulenes. J Chem Soc [C]:1787-1789
8. Jacquignon P, Fravolini A, Feron A, Croisy A (1974) Dérivés trifluoro-méthylés des [1]benzothiopyrano[4,3-b]indoles et des 6H-[1]benzothio-pyrano[4,3-b]quinoléines. Experientia 30:452-455
9. Jacquignon P, Croisy A, Ricci A, Balucani D (1973) Synthése et prop-riétés de 6H-[1]benzopyrano[4,3-b]quinoléines et de 6H-[1]benzothio-pyrano[4,3-b]quinoléines. Collect Czech Chem Comm 38:3862-3871
10. Buu Hoi NP, Perin F, Jacquignon P (1962) Carcinogenic nitrogen compounds. Part XXXII. The synthesis of new highly active benzopyridocarbazoles. J Chem Soc 146-150
11. Buu Hoi NP, Perin F, Jacquignon P (1960) Carcinogenic nitrogen compounds. Part XXVIII. Azadibenzofluorenes and related compounds. J Chem Soc [Perkin I]:4500-4503
12. Postovskii Y, Lundin BN (1940) Chemistry of carcinogenic substances. I. Synthesis of 9-azacholanthrene and certain ms-alkyl derivatives of 1,2- and 3,4-benzacridine. J Gen Chem USSR 10:71-76
13. Ullrich V, Weber P (1972) The O-dealkylation of 7-ethoxycoumarin by liver microsomes. A direct fluorimetric test. Hoppe Seylers Z Physiol Chem 353:1171-1177
14. Habig WH, Pabst MJ, Jacoby WB (1974) Glutathione S-transferases: the first enzymatic step in mercapturic acid formation. J Biol Chem 49:7130-7139
15. Schmassmann HU, Glatt HR, Oesch F (1976) A rapid assay for epoxide hydratase activity with benzo(a)pyrene 4,5-(K-region-)oxide as substrate. Anal Biochem 74:94-104
16. Schechtman LM, Kouri RE (1977) Control of benzo(a)pyrene induced mammalian cell cytotoxicity, mutagenesis and transformation by exogenous enzyme fractions. In: Scott D, Bridges BA, Sobels FH (eds) Progress in genetic toxicology. Elsevier, Amsterdam, pp 307-316
17. Lacassagne A, Buu-Hoi NP, Zajdela F, Jacquignon P, Perin F (1963) Re-lations entre structure moléculaire et activité cancérogéne chez les benzopyridocarbazoles et les composés polycycliques analogues. CR Acad Sci (Paris) 257:818-822
18. Lacassagne A, Buu-Hoi NP, Zajdela F, Jacquignon P, Mangane M (1967) 5-Oxo-5H-benzo(e)isochromeno-[4,3-b]indole, a new type of highly sarco-magenic lactone. Science 158:387-388
19. Lacassagne A, Buu-Hoi NP, Zajdela F, Perin-Roussel O, Jacquignon P, Perin F, Hoeffinger J-P (1970) Activité sarcomogène chez deux nouveaux types d'hétérocycles: les benzocarbolines et les thiénopyridocarbazoles. CR Acad Sci (Paris) 271:1474-1479
20. Oesch F (1973) Mammalian epoxide hydrases: inducible enzymes catalys-ing the inactivation of carcinogenic and cytotoxic metabolites derived from aromatic and olefinic compounds. Xenobiotica 3:305-340
21. Glatt HR, Oesch F, Frigerio A, Garattini S (1975) Epoxides metaboli-cally produced from some known carcinogens and from some clinically used drugs. I. Differences in mutagenicity. Int J Cancer 16:787-797
22. Lacassagne A, Buu-Hoi NP, Daudel R, Zajdela F (1956) The relation between carcinogenic activity and the physical and chemical properties of angular benzacridines. Adv Cancer Res 4:315-369

Possibilities for an Adequate Stepwise Carcinogenicity Testing Procedure

D. STEINHOFF[1]

The difference between the cost of a short-term test, e.g., the *Salmonella* test according to Ames, and that of an officially recognized carcinogenicity experiment is very great. The main reason for performing short-term tests is, after all, to keep expenditure to the minimum. But the use of short-term tests ceases to be inexpensive as soon as one tries to improve by a few percent the agreement of the results with those which are given by long-term tests by greatly increasing the number and diversity of the experiments performed. Where in vivo carcinogenicity studies are concerned, one is accustomed to think in completely different terms. In this case the feeding of the test compound to two species of animals at three different concentrations, with 100 animals per dose and, practically speaking, all-embracing histological examinations of all the animals, is regarded by some as the very least that should be demanded. Therefore a carcinogenicity study is generally expected to cost "several hundred thousand dollars". That testing of such comprehensiveness is seldom possible while compounds are in the early stages of their development is self-evident. Hence there will generally be a considerable lapse of time between the arrival of the results of the short-term test and that of the results of the carcinogenicity study. In most cases much money will be spent on the technical development of the product during the interval —money which could be lost if the compound turns out to be carcinogenic.

I regard this state of affairs as unfortunate and consider that it would be better to approach the goal in some steps that are adequate to the particular circumstances. I therefore shall review the potentialities of carcinogenicity testing on "whole animals" with a view to determining whether it is possible to bridge the great gap between short-term tests and the customary — and costly — carcinogenicity studies.

Inhalation

On the whole it would appear that an inhalation test is the best method by which to investigate all substances that are absorbed by humans mainly through the respiratory organs. The difficulties, however, are readily apparent. Inhalation carcinogenicity tests have so far been performed on only a limited scale owing to their

[1]Bayer AG, Institut für Toxikologie, Friedrich-Ebert-Straße 217, 5600 Wuppertal-Elberfeld/FRG

high cost and to the need for extensive safety precautions to
protect personnel.

Other problems arise from the very nature of such tests, however.
It is true that in many instances no other test provides conditions which are more similar to those under which humans may
be exposed to the substance in question. Yet there are important
differences. Unlike man, the animals used in the majority of
experiments, i.e., rodents, breathe through the nose obliga-
torily and their nasal cavity is quite different from that of
man with regard to its filtering effect and absorption (1).

Oral Application

The method generally recommended for routine carcinogenicity
testing is oral application to rats or mice. Altogether, this
method appears to be the one with the fewest problems, as well
as directly or indirectly corresponding to the actual exposure
of humans in a very large number of cases.

There are, though, at least two not inconsiderable difficulties:

1. Application with the food, which is the normal technique,
   contaminates the room and thus — if the substance is carcinogenic — places the personnel at risk, unless very costly
   safety precautions are taken (2).
2. Results may be falsified by poor absorption or by reactions
   between highly active compounds and the contents of the
   stomach and intestines.

Room contamination by the test substance in food given in the
normal way can be considerably reduced by stomach tube application five times a week. This procedure is also very costly,
however, and only practicable if very experienced staff is
available. Apart from this, the room may still be contaminated
by any portion of the substance which is not absorbed.

Cutaneous Application

Cutaneous application to mice is a method which in many cases
simulates the exposure of humans. At a rate of five applications
a week it is not inexpensive either. It must be added that, depending on the solubility and absorption conditions, it is possible for considerable quantities of the applied substances to
run off the skin and to contaminate the room, with the result
that extensive safety precautions have to be taken. It must be
pointed out, finally, that the ability of the shaved skin of a
mouse and that of the human skin to absorb a particular substance
are not necessarily equal. It is also possible that the carcinogenic effects of substances with high vapour pressures may not
be comprehended. Last not least, difficulties will be encountered
in recognizing systemic carcinogenic effects.

Implantation in the Lung and Intratracheal Application

The use of a single implantation is of some importance, especially where the lung is concerned. After narcotization of the animal, a pellet consisting of the test compound together with a carrier material (generally beeswax-tricapryline or cholesterol) is implanted in a bronchus (3) or directly in the lung tissue (4) by means of an operation. The method has considerable disadvantages, one of which is the fact that the highest dose applicable to a rodent by means of a single intra-bronchial pellet implantation is about 2 mg of the test compound. If no carcinogenicity is seen, one cannot be certain that the dose has been high enough, especially as pellets do not always stay exactly at the implantation sites. On the other hand, though the total dose is low, the local dose may be excessive, with the result that the target cells are killed and thus prevented from undergoing cancerification. The implantation of pellets directly in the lung parenchyma sometimes causes considerable traumatic damage, which may influence the tumorification through secondary tissue reactions.

By virtue of its technical simplicity, intratracheal application is often performed in rats or golden hamsters to determine possible carcinogenic effects on the respiratory tract.

This method permits accurate dosage. Relatively high doses can be applied. Even daily applications over a long time are possible without substantial mechanical damage to the respiratory tract. Intratracheally applied substances are distributed very uniformly throughout the entire lung. A very important advantage of intratracheal application is that it avoids nasal respiration, which is obligatory for rodents. It is therefore possible that a method which is not at first sight similar to the exposure of humans may produce conditions which are similar in fact.

Intraperitoneal Application

Intraperitoneal application can often be used as an alternative to intravenous application, which in many cases is difficult to continue over the entire lifespan of the animals. Absorbable substances rapidly find their way from the abdominal cavity to all parts of the body. This method, unlike intravenous injection, also permits the recognition of possible local carcinogenic effects. The method is also suitable for compounds which are otherwise difficult to apply. For example, the intraperitoneal implantation of pieces of rubber in rats leads to the formation of local sarcomas no less than does the implantation of ivory, platinum, gold, silver etc. (5). This does not imply that the method is of no value, but that such manipulations would not be entirely without risk in humans (6).

It must be pointed out, however, that such experimentally produced local tumours following the intraperitoneal application of a test compound must be carefully analyzed according to the parameters of the dose (or form and size) of the material applied, the latency period, the frequency of the application, and the biological behaviour. The fact that a simple test of this nature generally enables such an analysis to be performed highly satisfactorily can be illustrated with reference to the testing of a coarsely crystalline substance of low solubility in comparison with asbestos: when 1 × 50 mg or 1 × 10 mg of chrysotile per rat were administered intraperitoneally, practically all rats developed a local malignant tumour within 620 days after the beginning of the experiment; but the test compound, administered at the rate of 34 × 25 mg (= 850 mg/rat), has so far (i.e., after 620 days, counting from the beginning of the experiment) caused no tumour of this kind (Fig. 1)

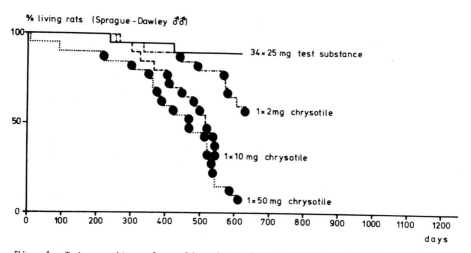

Fig. 1. Intraperitoneal application of a fibrous test substance in comparison to asbestos. Test substance: a coarsely crystalline fibrous substance of low solubility (34 × 25 mg/rat within 547 days). Positive control substance: chrysotile (1 × 2; 1 × 10 or 1 × 50 mg/rat). Within 620 days nearly all chrysotile-treated rats developed a local i.p. tumour (●). The test compound has so far caused no tumours of this kind. The experiment will be continued

In common with intraperitoneal application, intramuscular, intrapleural or subcutaneous application does not generally correspond to the conditions under which humans are exposed to substances. Yet each of these methods has important advantages. Subcutaneous application is the one most commonly used and for this reason I will now consider it in some detail.

Subcutaneous Application

The advantages of testing a substance by subcutaneous application to rats are as follows: The test is relatively simple to perform and it is not too expensive. In most cases contamination

of the laboratory with carcinogens can be avoided without difficulty. Local and systemic carcinogenic effects can be easily
distinguished. The test is sensitive.

For all of these reasons subcutaneous application is a very useful method, particularly in the early stages of testing. In
particular the high sensitivity of this method makes it extremely useful for initial testing of compounds, since, if
properly performed, the method rarely gives false-negative results. The main objection, therefore, to subcutaneous application is that it gives too many false-positive results —not of
a general nature, but only with respect to a local carcinogenic
effect in the sensitive subcutaneous tissue. Before considering
this objection I would like to review the major potential results of subcutaneous testing:

1. No carcinogenicity is apparent despite the fact that the
   highest applicable or tolerated doses have been given
   (4,4'-diaminodiphenylmethane in Figs. 2 and 3). In such a
   case it is fairly certain that the tested compound has no
   carcinogenic effect in the rat, or, at the most, a very slight
   one. This conclusion may be drawn not only because the subcutaneous tissue is highly sensitive but also because practically no other method enables larger total doses to be absorbed by the body.
2. A systemic carcinogenic effect is observed (benzidine in
   Figs. 2 and 3; Fig. 4). This is a strong indication that the
   compound will also have a systematic carcinogenic effect in
   humans. If a relatively equal amount of the compound enters
   the circulation of the rat when other methods of application
   are used, a similar carcinogenic effect can be expected.
3. A strong local carcinogenic effect is seen (Fig. 5). In other
   words malignant tumours appear at the injection site in practically all the rats after only a relatively small total
   dose has been applied and within a short time. A result of
   this sort makes it highly probable that a primarily local
   carcinogenic effect will be produced, not only in rats when
   other methods of application are used, but also in humans.
   After inhalation, for example, the substances in question
   may be expected to induce, above all, tumours of the naso-
   pharyngeal cavity or lung.
4. In the treated animals, as compared with those of the control
   group, there is a significant increase in the occurrence of
   local sarcomas at the injection site. The effect is not,
   however, entirely convincing. It may be, for example, that
   the required total dose is very high, that the survival times
   are not significantly reduced or are, indeed, extended,
   despite the increased occurrence of local tumours, or that
   the tumour rate exceeds that of the controls to a small extent only, or that the local tumours appeared after strong
   local irritation by the test substance. Interpretation of
   the result is difficult in this case. The method has given a
   result which is not unequivocal, but other methods frequently
   do the same.

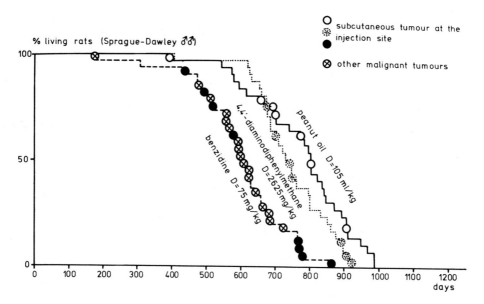

Fig. 2. Subcutaneous injection of 4,4'-diaminodiphenylmethane (in peanut oil) in comparison to benzidine (in peanut oil) (positive control) and to peanut oil alone (negative control) (25 male rats per group). 4,4'-Diamino-diphenylmethane: 1×25 mg/kg/week; total dose = 2625 mg/kg. Benzidine: 1×0.93 mg/kg/week; total dose = 75 mg/kg. Peanut oil: 1×1 ml/kg/week; total dose = 105 ml/kg.

In the male Sprague-Dawley rat treatment with peanut oil caused 7 subcutan-eous tumours at the injection site. With regard to such tumours this strain is very sensitive. In spite of this, 4,4'-diaminodiphenylmethane (in peanut oil) in the highest tolerated doses induced no additional subcutaneous tumours; there were 7 such tumours as was the case with peanut oil alone. On the other hand, benzidine at much lower doses induced, in a shorter time, 8 subcutaneous tumours and 17 other tumours not seen in the peanut oil or 4,4'-diaminodiphenylmethane group (mainly tumours of the auditory canal)

The three most plausible interpretations are as follows:

1. A slight carcinogenic effect must indeed be attributed to the test substance.
2. The sensitive subcutaneous tissue indicates, though not dis-tinctly, a carcinogenic effect which is difficult to detect in rats by other methods (Fig. 6).
3. A false, though weak, positive effect has been produced.

False-positive results are therefore possible. The great ma-jority of these, however, are *weak*. Nevertheless, the use of suitable control groups, coupled with the experience of the experimenter, will keep the number of false-positive results very small or even to zero.

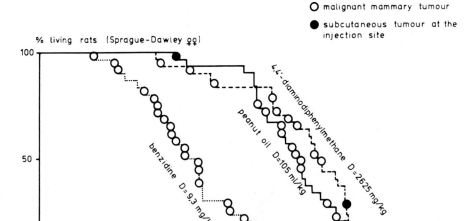

Fig. 3. Subcutaneous injection of 4,4'-diaminodiphenylmethane (in peanut oil) in comparison to benzidine (in peanut oil) (positive control) and to peanut oil alone (negative control) (25 female rats per group). 4,4'-Di-aminodiphenylmethane: 1×25 mg/kg/week; total dose = 2625 mg/kg. Benzidine: 1×0.93 mg/kg/week; total dose = 9.3 mg/kg. Peanut oil: 1×1 ml/kg/week; total dose = 105 ml/kg.

The female Sprague-Dawley rat is sensitive to the induction of mammary carcinomas. In this case treatment with peanut oil caused 1 subcutaneous tumour at the injection site and 12 mammary carcinomas. In the group treated with the highest tolerated doses of 4,4'-diaminodiphenylmethane (in peanut oil) there were 3 subcutaneous tumours at the injection site and 9 mammary carcinomas. On the other hand, the very low total dose of 9.3 mg benzidine/kg induced 23 malignant mammary tumours in a much shorter time

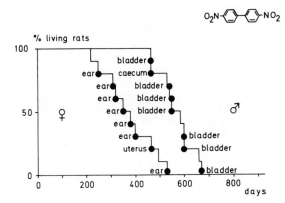

Fig. 4. Systemic carcinogenic effect of 4,4'-dinitrobiphenyl after subcutaneous application to Wistar rats. Dosage: 25-100 mg/kg/week; total dose = 750 mg/kg. In male rats the substance induced mainly bladder tumours (malignant) (●), in female rats mainly tumours of the auditory canal (malignant) (●)

134

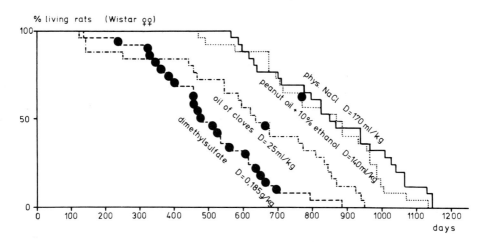

● subcutaneous tumour at the
   injection site

Fig. 5. The subcutaneous injection of dimethylsulfate in peanut oil (once
a week; total dose = 185 mg/kg) led in nearly all rats to the induction of
malignant subcutaneous tumours at the injection site. In contrast, the
highly irritant oil of cloves, in spite of the high total dose of 25 ml/kg,
caused only one such tumour out of 25 rats. The same result was obtained
after subcutaneous injection of a mixture of peanut oil + 10% ethanol up
to a total dose of 140 ml/kg. No subcutaneous tumours appeared after similar
treatment (5 ml/kg/week) with physiological saline solution up to a total
dose of 170 ml/kg

Furthermore, substantial subcutaneous implantations, like intraperitoneal implantations, may induce local sarcomas in rats.
It is still a question whether sarcomas produced under these
circumstances are relevant to humans, but there is some evidence
to suggest that they might be (6). Interpretation of such experimental results poses no special difficulty for the experienced worker.

Nevertheless, the occurrence of such non-specific cancer induction has brought the subcutaneous test into disrepute among a
fair number of cancer research workers. But a test which has
proved sensitive as an indicator of chemical carcinogens can
hardly be invalidated by the fact that it also responds to certain, and to some extent extreme, non-chemical stimulations,
which, incidentally, can hardly lead to false conclusions if
the results are correctly interpreted.

Druckrey and Van Duuren came to have a good opinion of the subcutaneous test in the light of their very extensive experimental
experience (7,8). Recently Tomatis, who compared the results
of experiments carried out by a variety of methods, came to a
similar conclusion (9).

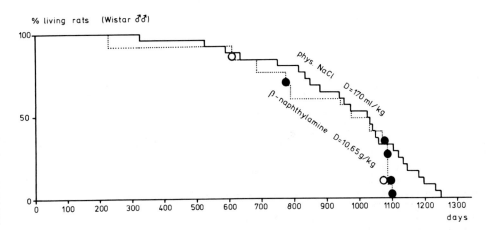

Fig. 6. The carcinogenic effect of β-naphthylamine is difficult to detect in rats. After weekly subcutaneous injections of β-naphthylamine (in physiol. NaCl solution) and a total dose of 10.65 g/kg, 50% of the treated rats developed malignant tumours as compared with 26% in the control group. This figure shows for the male rats the appearance of 2 liver tumours and 5 subcutaneous tumours at the injection site, tumours not seen in the control group

On the other hand, the method of subcutaneous application has been rejected as irrelevant by several authors, particularly Grasso, because the formation of subcutaneous tumours can be influenced in several ways (10-14). But it is true of all test methods that the induction of tumours by carcinogens, and also the spontaneous tumour rate of the experimental animals, can be inhibited or promoted by a large number of factors which can be manipulated in many different ways. Apart from this it should be repeated that some increase in the number of subcutaneous sarcomas, as compared with that found in the controls, represents only one of four possible results (see above). We have seen already that the three other possible results raise no comparable problems.

It seems to me, however, that a method which in a case of doubt gives a false, weakly positive result rather than a false-negative result is particularly suitable for the early stages of testing.

Comparative Evaluation of the Various Tests

It is clear, then, that every test has advantages and disadvantages. The greater the variety of the tests performed, the better the prospect of obtaining a picture of the potential risk to man. Of the large number of possible in vivo tests, about ten deserve particular attention. Of these there are three whose

conditions largely correspond to those that occur when humans
are exposed to substances, namely oral application, cutaneous
application and inhalation. All three have also disadvantages.
On the other hand, three other methods, though they do not correspond to the conditions of humans, have important technical
advantages, that is to say intratracheal, intraperitoneal and
subcutaneous application.

For the following reasons the latter three methods are particularly suitable for testing at the early stages of development:

1. At this stage it is not always certain how humans will be
   exposed to the substance in question.
2. Very expensive tests are seldom justified when a substance
   is still at the early stages of development.
3. The methods are so sensitive that false, weakly positive
   results are more probable than false-negative results. But
   interpretation of the results poses no special difficulty
   for the experienced worker.
4. They permit relatively safe handling of substances about whose
   carcinogenic propensities very little is yet known.
5. They enable the results of short-term tests to be checked
   without too much expenditure. For this reason these tests
   recommend themselves for bridging the gap between short-term
   tests and full-scale carcinogenicity studies.

Proposals for Step-By-Step Carcinogenicity Testing

Therefore it would appear that sensible, cost-saving step-by-step
carcinogenicity testing of laboratory products, technical products, and of possible development products etc., could be performed as follows (Fig. 7)

A suitable short-term test should be the first step. As long as
the uncertainties regarding the interpretation of the results
of short-term tests cannot be disposed of, a subcutaneous or
intratracheal or an intraperitoneal test forming a second step
should be performed as soon as possible, at least for the more
important substances.

The subcutaneous (or i.t.- or i.p.-) test need not be very expensive. It would be sufficient to apply a dose which is in
the vicinity of the maximum tolerated dose but also avoiding
local incompatibility reactions, and, as a second dose, an
amount representing one tenth, for example, of the maximum tolerated dose. Both dose groups and the corresponding control
group should comprise about 25 male and 25 female rats each. A
second control group should comprise an equal number of rats
which would not be treated in any way. Treatment at weekly
intervals would be sufficient. The scope of the histological
examinations would depend on the macroscopic findings.

Though the subcutaneous test is relatively simple, its proper
performance and evaluation demands — like that of all other
carcinogenicity tests — the knowledge of an experienced experimenter.

Proposals for step-by-step carcinogenicity testing

Fig. 7. Proposal for a testing procedure (see text)

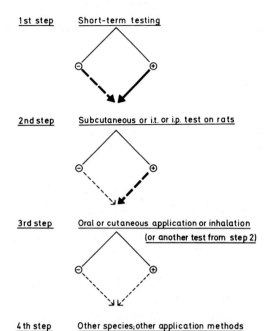

1st step   Short-term testing

2nd step   Subcutaneous or i.t. or i.p. test on rats

3rd step   Oral or cutaneous application or inhalation
             (or another test from step 2)

4th step   Other species; other application methods

Once one has performed short-term testing and a carcinogenicity test by the subcutaneous or intraperitoneal or intratracheal method much information will be available as a basis for further testing or even enough information to make further testing superfluous in many cases. (Especially if two or even three of the latter methods have been used.) At any rate a subcutaneous or intraperitoneal or intratracheal test appears suitable to bridge the gap between a short-term test and a very expensive carcinogenicity study on the classical pattern. One should take advantage of this opportunity.

References

1. Wynder EL, Hoffmann D (1967) Tobacco and tobacco smoke. Academic Press, New York, London
2. Sansone EB, Losikoff AM, Pendleton RA (1977) Potential hazards from feeding test chemicals in carcinogen bioassay research. Toxicol Appl Pharmacol 39:435-450
3. Laskin S, Kuschner M, Drew RT (1970) Studies in pulmonary carcinogenesis. In: Hanna MG, Nettesheim P, Gilberg JR (eds) Inhalation carcinogenesis. US Atomic Energy Commission, Symposium Series 18, pp 321-351
4. UICC Technical Report Series, Vol 25 (1976) Lung Cancer. Wynder EL, Hecht S (eds). UICC, Geneva, pp 81-130
5. Druckrey H, Schmähl D, Mecke R, Jr (1956) Cancerogene Wirkung von Gummi nach Implantation an Ratten. Z Krebsforsch 61:55-64

6. Ott G (1970) Fremdkörpersarkome. Springer, Berlin, Heidelberg, New York
7. Druckrey H, Preussmann R, Ivankovic S, So BT, Schmidt CH, Bucheler J (1966) Zur Erzeugung subcutaner Sarkome an Ratten. Z Krebsforsch 68:87-102
8. Van Duuren BL, Langseth L, Orris L, Teebor G, Nelson N, Kuschner M (1966) Carcinogenicity of epoxides, lactones, and peroxy compounds. IV. Tumor response in epithelial and connective tissue in mice and rats. J Natl Cancer Inst 37:825-838
9. Tomatis L (1977) Comment on methodology and interpretation of results. J Natl Cancer Inst 59:1341
10. Grasso P, Golberg L (1966) Subcutaneous sarcoma as an index of carcinogenic potency. Fd Cosmet Toxicol 4:297-320
11. Grasso P, Gangolli SD, Golberg L, Hooson J (1971) Physicochemical and other factors determining local sarcoma production by food additives. Fd Cosmet Toxicol 9:463-478
12. Gangolli SD, Grasso P, Golberg L, Hooson J (1972) Protein binding by food colourings in relation to the production of subcutaneous sarcoma. Fd Cosmet Toxicol 10:449-462
13. Hooson J, Grasso P, Gangolli SD (1973) Injection site tumours and preceding pathological changes in rats treated subcutaneously with surfactants and carcinogens. Br J Cancer 27:230-244
14. Grasso P (1976) Review of tests for carcinogenicity and their significance to man. Clin Toxicol 9:745-760

Section II

Correlations Between in Vitro
and in Vivo Results –
Investigations Using Different Test Systems

Validity of Test Systems Used in the Detection of Mutagenic and Carcinogenic Properties of Chemical Substances

D. Müller[1]

Abstract

Firstly, the results of comparative investigations with 14 mutagenic or carcinogenic substances in seven different mutagenicity test systems are presented. Two test systems were used for the detection of point mutations: (a) *Salmonella*/mammalian microsome mutagenicity test, i.e., the Ames test (AT); and (b) the point mutation test with mouse lymphoma cells (L5178Y), in vitro, and in the host-mediated assay (MLC). In addition, four cytogenetic test systems were used: (a) chromosome studies of the bone marrow of the Chinese hamster; (b) the nucleus anomaly test in the bone marrow of the Chinese hamster, (NAT); (c) chromosome studies in spermatogonia of mice (Spg); and (d) chromosome studies in spermatocytes of mice (Spct). Finally, the dominant lethal test was carried out in male mice. Two substances, vincristine and 5-fluorouracil, were AT-negative; vincristine produced positive cytogenetic results (NAT and Spct), but was MLC-negative; 5-fluorouracil was MLC-positive and NAT-positive. Twelve substances were AT-positive. Thiotepa, triaziquone, adriamycin, ethyl methanesulphonate, MNNG, and daunomycin showed positive results both in the cytogenetic investigations and in the dominant lethal test, as well as in the MLC. N-propylmethanesulphonate and isopropylmethanesulphonate, benzpyrene and *p*-dimethylaminoazobenzene caused structural chromosomal aberrations and/or dominant lethals, but were MLC-negative. N-nitrosodiethylamine and 20-methylcholanthrene induced neither structural aberrations nor point mutations.

Certain fundamental aspects are discussed that have to be considered in assessing the value and the importance of short-term test systems in relation to mammalian systems. In this context, mutation is postulated to be a causal pathogenic principle of cancer, and the induction of cancer by chemical agents is expounded with the aid of a model. The possibility of arriving at a quantitative estimate of the risk associated with chemical mutagens is considered. The significance of dose-effect relations is examined. It is explained that in evaluating experimental results a distinction has to be drawn between two reactions that determine the result, namely, the reaction of the genetic material and the physiologic reaction of the species. The physiologic parameters that influence the relation between dose and exposure are enumerated, and possibilities of determining this relation discussed.

[1]Ciba-Geigy AG, CH-4002 Basel/Switzerland

Some views on the selection of appropriate tests from the currently available in vitro and in vivo systems and on the sequence of application of test systems and groups of test systems are presented and reasons given for these suggestions are offered concerning aspects on which emphasis should be placed in developing and establishing the validity of new test systems.

Until a few years ago, no evidence could be presented to prove that the carcinogenic effect of environmental influences comes about by way of mutation. In other words, the causal pathogenesis of cancer was unknown. If one considers the cancer theories of the recent past, one finds among them a "radiation theory," a "chemical cancer theory," and finally the very correct observation that chemical measures or exposure to radiation play only an instrumental part in carcinogenesis. We know now that this concept was already very close to the truth. Exposure to radiation and chemical measures alike are instruments capable of inducing mutations and thereby exempting the cell from its constraint toward normal growth.

The view that carcinogenic effects are mediated by mutations has been proved correct by various findings. Cleaver (1) demonstrated that cells from patients with xeroderma pigmentosum had a defect in their DNA-repair capactiy, recognizable after the induction of DNA damage by ultraviolet irradiation. Setlow and Regan (2) showed the same effect after DNA destruction by the carcinogen N-acetoxy-2-acetylaminofluorine. The decisive evidence was finally presented by Ames et al. (3), whose test system made it possible to demonstrate the mutagenic properties of the active form of many chemical carcinogens.

The discovery in recent years that chemical carcinogens are to be found in various clases of chemical substances in everyday use for a multitude of purposes brought with it the realization that the systematic investigation of environmental chemicals is not an extravagant demand, but a rational precaution. The success of this comprehensive investigation, however, depends to a great extent on the quality and the applicability of the available systems, which is precisely the subject under consideration here today.

It is desirable that laboratories whose task it is to test chemical substances for potentially mutagenic or carcinogenic properties should also perform comparative investigations with known mutagenic or carcinogenic substances in a battery of test systems, and in so doing contribute to the evaluation of the usefulness of these systems. It is in this sense that the studies I now wish to report upon are intended. In them, 14 mutagenic or carcinogenic substances were examined in seven mutagenicity test systems. The test systems used were:

1. *The Salmonella/mammalian microsome mutagenicity test*, with and without microsomal activation, *i.e., the Ames test*. This test was carried out with the five strains TA 92, TA 98, TA 100, TA 1535, and TA 1537. Where known results were reproduced, the experiments were limited to the strains indicated in the original publications.

2. *The point mutation assay with mouse lymphoma cells (L5178Y)*, which was developed by Fischer together with Calabresi, Chu, Lee, and Momparler, in particular (4-6). The experiments were performed both in vitro and in the host-mediated assay system.

3. *Cytogenetic studies in the bone marrow of the Chinese hamster (CYS)*. The doses used corresponded to 1/12, 1/6, and 1/3 of the LD_{50} and were administered twice, on two consecutive days. The animals were killed 6 h after the second dose. Four animals from each of the treated groups and four controls were examined, and 100 metaphases from each animal inspected.

4. *The nucleus anomaly test (NAT)*. A description of this test was last given at the EEMS meeting in Edinburgh by Langauer and Müller (7). It differs fundamentally from the micronucleus test in that besides polychromatic erythrocytes the developmental stages of the leukopoietic system are examined, and in the erythropoietic system the other developmental stages as well as the polychromatic erythrocytes. In addition, the animals are killed not 6, but 24 h after the administration of the last dose. This system has proved twice four, or eight times as sensitive as the micronucleus test. Six Chinese hamsters per group were studied and 1000 cells from each animal analyzed. The doses administered corresponded to those used in the cytogenetic studies in the bone marrow.

5. *Studies of spermatogonia from mice (Spg)*. The animals received five doses on five consecutive days and were killed one day after the last dose. As a rule, the doses given were 1/24, 1/12, and 1/6 of the LD_{50}. Six mice from each group were examined and 100 metaphases from each mouse evaluated.

6. *Studies of spermatocytes I and II from mice (Spct)*. The doses administered were generally 1/12, 1/6, and 1/3 of the LD_{50}, and these were given 12, 10, 9, 7, and 3 days before sacrifice. The cells studied in metaphase had thus been exposed in all the preceding prophase stages. Six animals from each group, and 100 metaphase I and 100 metaphase II figures from each animal were examined.

7. *The dominant lethal test in the male mouse (DLT)*. In general, doses equivalent to 1/9 and 1/3 of the LD_{50} were used. The animals received one dose, and then followed eight mating periods of one week each. The treated groups and the controls consisted of 20 males each, and in each of the mating periods 40 females were used per group.

The results are presented in Table 1. In connection with the dominant lethal test, GON stands for spermatogoniogenesis, CYT for spermatocytogenesis, and ZOON for spermatohistogenesis.

Looking first at the carcinogen *N-nitrosodiethylamine*, according to Malling (8) and Malling and Frantz (9) this compound requires metabolic activation before it produces carcinogenic or mutagenic effects. Accordingly, positive results in the Ames test were only observed after activation. In the mammalian systems it caused neither point mutations nor structural aberrations.

Table 1. Comparative investigations with 14 known mutagenic or carcinogenic substances in a battery of test systems

Test substance	Mode of application	Ames test without/with activation		Test with mouse lymphoma cells		Test systems in vivo					DLT	
				in vitro	in vivo	CYS	NAT	Spg	Spct	GON	CYT	ZOON
N-Nitrosodiethyl-amine	PO	O	++	O		O	O	O	O	O	O	O
20-Methyl-cholanthrene	PO	O	+++	−		O	O	O	O	O	O	O
Benzo[α]pyrene	PO	O	+++	O		O	(+)	O	O	O	O	O
Paradimethyl-aminoazobenzene	PO	O	+++	O		O	(+)	O	O	O	O	O
Paradimethyl-aminoazobenzene	IP	−				−	−	−	−	O	O	O
MNNG	PO	+++			+++ (SC)	O	(+)	O	O	O	O	O
MNNG	IP	+++	−	O		−	+++	−	−	+	O	O
N-Propylmethane-sulphonate (PMS)	PO	+++	−	O		O	O	O	(+)	O	O	O
N-Propylmethane-sulphonate (PMS)	IP					−	−	−	−	+	++	+++
Isopropylmethane-sulphonate (iPMS)	PO	O	+++	O		O	O	O	O	O	O	O
Isopropylmethane-sulphonate (iPMS)	IP					−	−	O	O	O	O	O
Ethyl methane-sulphonate (EMS)	IP	+++	−	++	+++ (SC)	(+)	+++	O	O	O	O	O

Table 1 (continued)

Thiotepa	IP	++	-	+	(+) (IV)	+++	+++	+	+	0	+++	+++
Triaziquone	PO	++	-	+	+	+++	++	0	(+)	0	++	++
Adriamycin	SC	+++	-	0	(+)	+++	+++	+++	+++	0	0	0
Daunomycin	IP	++	-	0	(+) (IV)	0	+	0	(+)	0	0	0
Vincristine	IP	0	0	0	0 (IV)	0	++	0	+	0	0	0
5-Fluorouracil	PO	0	0	+	(+) (SC)	0	+	0	0	0	0	0

The carcinogen *methylcholanthrene* requires activation to induce
mutagenic effects on *Salmonella typhimurium*. It displayed no activity either in the point mutation test with mouse lymphoma
cells or in any of the other systems.

As McCann et al. (10) had already demonstrated, the carcinogen
benzo(a)pyrene only induces mutagenic effect in *S. typhimurium* after
activation. It proved negative in the tests with mouse lymphoma
cells. Rüdiger and his group showed in 1976 (11) that the compound has to be converted by intracellular metabolism to the
epoxide before mutagenicity occurs. They demonstrated sister-
chromatid exchanges after exposure to benzo(a)pyrene. Basler
and Röhrborn (12) found structural aberrations in metaphase II
oocytes of the mouse and in the bone marrow cells of the Chinese
hamster. We were unable to reproduce the cytogenetic findings in
the bone marrow, but we did observe a weak, yet significant effect in the nucleus anomaly test.

The carcinogen *paradimethylaminoazobenzene* has to be activated before
it produces an effect on *S. typhimurium*. It is negative in the
test system with the mouse lymphoma cells. In the nucleus anomaly
test it displayed a weak, but significant degree of activity.

The mutagenic activity of the carcinogen *MNNG* has already been
demonstrated in microbial systems and on plants. It produced
mutagenic effects on *S. typhimurium* with activation, but only
affected mouse lymphoma cells in the host-mediated assay. In
the nucleus anomaly test it had a weak, but significant effect.
In the dominant lethal test we did not observe the effects on
postmitotic stages reported by Ehling et al. (13) and Parkin et
al. (14), but we did find an effect on spermatogoniogenesis.

n-Propylmethanesulphonate, which is positive in the Ames test without activation, was inactive on mouse lymphoma cells. After oral
administration, only weak positive effects on the spermatocytes
were detectable. The results observed after intraperitoneal
administration agreed with the findings of Ehling et al. (15),
but corresponding cytogenic studies have not yet been performed.

Isopropylmethanesulphonate required activation in the Ames test.
All the other assays, including the dominant lethal test in NMRI
mice, gave negative results. Ehling et al. (15), on the other
hand, found the compound active in (101 × C3H) mice, except with
regard to spermatogoniogenesis.

Ethyl methanesulphonate was mutagenic without activation in the
Ames test and positive in the test systems with mouse lymphoma
cells. Cytogenetic studies of bone marrow and the nucleus anomaly test both yielded positive results. In contrast to the
findings reported by Ehling et al. (13) and Lavappa and Yerganian
(16) but in agreement with those of Cattanach and Williams (17)
and Ray et al. (18), we did not detect indications of dominant
lethal effects and translocations in postmeiotic cells in our
investigations in NMRI mice treated with 125 mg/kg.

Thiotepa proved positive in the Ames test without activation and in the test with mouse lymphoma cells in vivo also. All the other assays gave positive results, save that the cytogenetic findings in spermatogonia could not be confirmed in the dominant lethal test.

Triaziquone was positive in the Ames test without activation and already positive in vitro with mouse lymphoma cells. Positive results were also obtained in all the other test systems, but no effect on spermatogoniogenesis was demonstrable either in the cytogenetic studies or in the dominant lethal test.

Adriamycin is positive without activation in the Ames test. When tested on mouse lymphoma cells, it was only in the host-mediated assay that weakly positive effects were observed. Vig (19,20) has on several occasions reported positive cytogenetic findings after treatment in vitro. The cytogenetic in vivo studies all gave clearly positive results, while the results of the dominant lethal test were negative.

The carcinogen *daunomycin* had positive effects on *S. typhimurium* without activation, but only in the host-mediated assay on mouse lymphoma cells. According to Vig et al. (21), it attacks the prereplicative chromosomes. Gebhart (22) observed chromosome breaks in vitro. In vivo only a slight, though significant activity was detectable in the nucleus anomaly test and on spermatocytes.

The spindle-poison *vincristine* was positive in the Ames test and — as was to be expected — negative when tested on mouse lymphoma cells. Significant effects were observed, on the other hand, in the nucleus anomaly test and on metaphase spermatocytes.

The antimetabolite *5-fluorouracil* was negative in the Ames test. It caused point mutations in mammalian cells, however, and gave positive results in the nucleus anomaly test. Abdulnur (23) attributed its lack of activity in vitro to the absence of the enol tautomer mispairing. The positive in vitro findings with mouse lymphoma cells indicate that these cells provide the nenessary conditions for this mispairing in vitro.

Let us now consider these results in relation to one another (Fig. 1). Of the 14 substances studied, 12 were positive in the Ames test. Among them were two carcinogens that caused neither point mutations nor structural aberrations in the mammalian systems. Of the remaining ten, at least five are known carcinogens, and these substances induced structural chromosomal aberrations or dominant lethals, or both, while three of them also led to point mutations in mammalian cells. The majority of the tested substances producing chromosomal aberrations and dominant lethals, i.e., six of the ten, also gave rise to point mutations in mammalian cells. The two substances that proved negative in the Ames test induced structural aberrations and one of them also caused point mutations in mouse lymphoma cells.

148

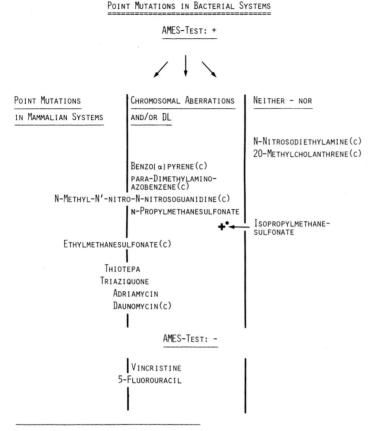

Fig. 1. Relative
mutagenic effects
of 14 substances
in various test
systems

*ACCORDING TO THE FINDINGS OF OTHER AUTHORS
C = CARCINOGEN

I should like straight away to express my own opinion about the
usefulness of the test systems applied here and must call attention in advance to the fact that the composition of this
battery of tests, which was put together at the beginning of
the experiment, no longer entirely coincides with our present
views.

1. *The Ames test.* There is no doubt whatever about the great value
of this test system. The metabolite mixture used in this test
system is prepared from microsomal fractions from the liver of
the mouse or the rat. It is presumed that the enzyme pattern
formed after induction in the liver of these two species corresponds in its action, to a large extent at least, to that of
the primate and in particular the human liver. To test this assumption, we investigated the activity of the S-9 fraction in
mice, Chinese hamsters, rats, mini-pigs, dogs, baboons, and
rhesus monkeys, with and without activation. The substances
studied were benzpyrene, cyclophosphamide, diethylnitrosamine,
β-naphthylamaine, and dimethylaminoazobenzene (Table 2). The two
primates already show an enzyme pattern in the noninduced liver

Table 2. The activity of the S-9 liver fractions of various species in the Ames test [Müller et al., 1978 (24)]

		BP	CPA	DENA	β-NA	DMAB	Activity
Mouse	o	+	(+)	(+)	+	+	4.3
	*	++	++	+	++	++	15.0
Chinese hamster	o	+	+	+	+	(+)	2.1
	*	+	+	++	+	++	5.7
Rat	o	(+)	−	−	+	(+)	3.9
	*	+	+	++	++	++	12.0
Mini-pig	o	−	−	−	+	+	6.1
	*	++	++	+	++	+	24.0
Dog (beagle)	o	−	+	+	++	(+)	3.1
	*	+	++	++	++	+	4.5
Baboon	o	+	+	+	++	+	7.4
	*	++	+	+	++	+	14.0
Rhesus monkey	o	oo	oo	o	oo	o	14.0
	*	++	++	+	++	+	17.0

BP: benzo(a)pyrene, CPA: cyclophosphamide, DENA: diethylnitrosamine, β-NA: β-naphthylamine, DMAB: 4-amino-2,3-dimethylazobenzene. Activity: ethylmorphine demethylase activity expressed as nmol formaldehyde per mg protein per min. o=non-induced, *=induced

that is only demonstrable in the other species after induction. In the mouse and the rat, however, the enzyme pattern found after induction with Aroclor corresponded to that observed in the noninduced primate liver (24).

2. *The point mutation test with mouse lymphoma cells in vitro and in vivo.* We consider this test especially appropriate when the risk associated with a compound that gives positive results in, say, the Ames test, but its usefulness has to be further assessed.

3 and 4. *Chromosomal studies in bone marrow and the nucleus anomaly test.* In all cases in which chromosomal examinations gave positive results, those of the nucleus anomaly test were also positive. On the other hand, positive results were obtained in the nucleus anomaly test in six cases in which the results of the chromosomal studies were negative. The nucleus anomaly test is more sensitive than chromosomal analysis of the bone marrow, and we therefore regard it as an especially valuable test system. Chromosomal examinations can be dispensed with if the nucleus anomaly test is performed and in this way capacity for the application of other test systems can be gained.

5-7. Chromosomal studies on spermatogonia and spermatocytes and the dominant lethal test. The results of these present investigations and experience with other substances have shown that the cytogenetic studies give more reliable results than the dominant lethal test. Performance of the dominant lethal test could accordingly be limited to the spermatohistogenesis phase, i.e., the phase from the end of spermatocyte II until the development of spermatozoa in the cauda epididymidis.

I should like to express my own views concerning the usefulness of some other test systems that were not employed in this study, but first let me mention a few fundamental aspects that have to be considered in appraising the value and the importance of mutagenicity test systems, notably mammalian systems.

Can we also infer, on the basis of the established causal connection, that every system capable of detecting mutagenic characteristics is at the same time capable of detecting carcinogenic properties?

It is easier to come to grips with this subject if one visualizes the mode of development of cancer induced by chemical agents. We know of some theories of carcinogenesis in which it is premised that chemical mutagenesis is the primary event. I should like to abide by Knudson's concept (25), because, with certain modifications, the model he proposed is accepted, and it seems to me particularly well suited to illustrate the circumstances and the course of events (Fig. 2).

According to this model, the development of cancer is conditional upon two mutational events. An initial mutagenic event in a somatic cell leads to a mutation, which predestines the cell for a second initiation event. It is the second event only that induces a transformation, and a cell is created that has all the prerequisites for proliferation and growth into a malignant tumor. That, however, is in turn certainly dependent on a large number of factors. Let us revert to mutation. Two mutagenic events, converging in time and matching in character, are thus the prerequisite for the occurrence of a transformation. A second possibility is that the first event is an inherited characteristic and in the individual case only one event, namely, the second, is necessary to induce transformation. That an individual already carrying a mutation of this nature is exposed to a greater risk is due especially to the fact that the mutated cell is present in a germinal line clone and constitutes the origin of a differential cell type. One example of this is the hereditary retinoblastoma in man.

The foregoing remarks have been intended to show that the risk of an individual's developing cancer depends on various prerequisites: (a) whether a mutation predisposing to cancer has already been acquired prezygotically, (b) the degree of exposure to environmental mutagens, and (c) whether genetic factors that may positively or negatively influence the development of a tumor are present. What is of decisive importance for the population at large, however, is the number of mutation-inducing events.

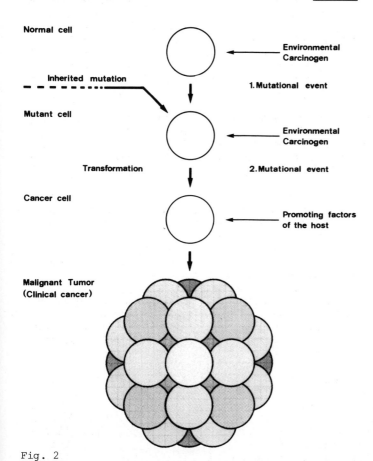

Status of the cell   **Modifiers**

Normal cell   Environmental Carcinogen

Inherited mutation   1. Mutational event

Mutant cell   Environmental Carcinogen

Transformation   2. Mutational event

Cancer cell   Promoting factors of the host

Malignant Tumor
(Clinical cancer)

Fig. 2

As long as it cannot be demonstrated conclusively that mutations can also represent genomic alterations — induced by a certain type or types of substance — that do not entail transformations of the cell, we must go on the assumption that every mutagenic substance can increase the probability of the development of cancer. The presentation of this model is also intended to call attention to the necessity of paying particular heed to exposure of the germinal epithelia to environmental mutagens. The answer to the question of whether mutagenicity test systems can also serve to demonstrate carcinogenic properties is therefore "yes," although with certain reservations.

In radiation genetics there is a direct, linear relation between exposure and effect. In chemical mutagenesis, on the other hand, the effect of a chemical substance is evidently influenced by a number of factors, and these are also species-specific. This raises two questions that I should like to examine now: (a) How far is it possible to extrapolate from the results of a single experiment? (b) Is it possible to consider results as being applicable to other species, in effect, to man, or are such findings only to be regarded as indications? The following remarks are intended to illustrate the difficulties that can arise when an attempt is made to draw inferences from dose-effect relations. If we succeed in constructing a curve of this nature (Fig. 3), we project a line through intersections at dose-levels A and B which intersects X-axis at point D_1. Granting that we are in general only able to depict sections of such a curvilinear course, and assuming that effects in the dose-range between B and C are depictable, then it becomes clear that an extrapolation would have to pass through D_2, which is patently an error.

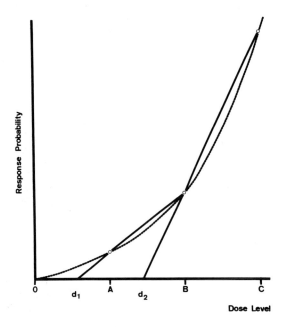

Fig. 3. Linear extrapolations from a convex dose-response curve. Use of dose levels between A and B results in a threshold of D_1 and of doses between B and C in a threshold of D_2. [After Brown, 1976 (34)]

On the other hand, we have been able to observe that known mutagens may cause no visible mutagenic effects in one system or another; in such cases an effect may be present but concealed. Observations of this sort make it compulsory to apply several systems in order to estimate the magnitude of a risk.

The rationale of Bridges' three-tier system (26) is that the first steps in a qualitative test are followed by another, or several others, after which it becomes possible to arrive at a quantitative estimate of risk versus benefit. The mutagenic agents most thoroughly examined with regard to the third step in this system are ionizing radiations. In the investigations of their effects, an increasingly refined technique of quantitatively estimating the risk was introduced. As far as concerns chemical mutagens, however, we do not yet have at our disposal any well-developed and universally applicable technique for the quantitative estimation of risks. The requirements implicit in the three-tier system can, consequently, so far only be met with difficulty.

Lee (27) formulated the following very convincing rule: in so far as it appears desirable to extrapolate from an animal organism to man on Bridges' third plane, the question that has to be put is not simply, "Can this substance be mutagenic in man?", but "Can the mutagenic response observed in the species used in the experiment be correlated quantitatively with the corresponding reaction in man?".

If we wish to answer this question, the following aspect has to be considered. The reaction of the genetic material must not be confused with the physiologic reaction. A distinction has to be made between comparative mutagenesis and comparative physiology. Granting that there can be great variations in metabolism among the species, it is nonetheless true that the genetic mechanism has remained one of the best conserved elements in biology in the course of evolution. Hence, it is reasonable to expect the reaction of the genetic material to show far greater similarities from one species to another than, for example, the metabolism of some chemical substance or other.

The diagram in Fig. 4 will clarify these relationships. If we wish to separate comparative physiology and comparative mutagenesis, we must make a distinction between dose and exposure. In radiobiology, the rad, the standard unit of energy absorbed at the site of action, provides a clear definition. In chemical mutagenetics we have no such definition at our disposal. What we find referred to in the literature as "dose" is, in reality, nothing other than the exposure to which the entire organism is subjected.

Kolbye (28) describes the causation of human cancer as being a three-dimensional problem, which, however, is all too often regarded as a two-dimensional result of dose and reaction. It is equally correct that we should consider the manifestation of a mutagenic effect to be due to the convergence of additional factors in the third dimension.

The relation between dose and exposure is subject to the influence of a number of parameters: absorption kinetics, distribution and elimination, biotransformation outside the target cell, the permeability of the membrane system, and biotransformation within the target cell. The dose is not to be regarded as a factor having a predictable influence on the results observed, in so far as the results are also subject to the influence of various physiologic functions; that is to say, it cannot be assumed that there is a linear relation between the dose of a substance and the concentration of the active form reaching the genome. Hence, neither do we have any foreseeable relation between dose and exposure, nor can it be taken for granted that — beyond certain orders of magnitude, at least — there is a linear relation between dose and exposure. Any relation between dose and effect found in one species is therefore

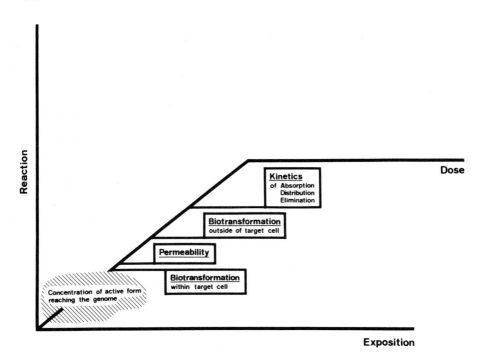

Fig. 4. Factors influencing relationship between dosage and exposure, i.e., the concentration of active form reaching the genome

not necessarily valid for another species, nor must the same relation apply for two different cell types.

It is consequently important that we should strive to determine the relation between these two factors, dose and exposure, at least within certain limits. For the reasons mentioned, it appears that it will be necessary to do so individually for each mutagenic substance.

The technique of molecular dosimetry (27,29,30) that has been developed over the past few years will undoubtedly prove to be a valuable aid in finding the answer to these questions. "Molecular dosimetry" means the measurement of the number of chemical changes occuring at the "genetically significant target," after the administration of a given dose. Since, in the majority of cases, the "genetically significant target" is DNA, DNA can, according to Lee (27) and Aaron (29), be taken as the "selected target molecule"; alkylated DNA would be the "selected reaction product." Strictly speaking, however, these propositions require some qualification, for the "selected target molecule" need not be DNA. Sega and Owens (31) have lately furnished a most convincing demonstration of the fact that when ethyl methanesulphonate is used the decisive reaction consists in the ethylation of the cysteine sulphydryl groups of the spermatid protamines. This blocks the formation of disulphide bridges and prevents chromatin condensation, leading to modifications of the chromatin structure and possibly to the appearance of chromosome breaks.

As far as dosimetry is concerned we would like to state the following: After the effective molecular dose for a particular genetic test system has been determined it could consequently be possible to correlate the mutagenic effect with the number of chemical changes in the genetically significant target. We shall be hearing more about this technique later today from Mohn and co-workers (32).

In connection with Knudson's model, I mentioned the significance of mutagenic events that can be acquired by the individual through genetic transmission. This makes it easy to understand why among all the cell types represented in the multicellular mammalian organism the germinal cell merits particular attention in regard to mutagenic damage.

Appropriate investigations have revealed distinct differences in the sensitivity of the various developmental stages to mutagens; the source of these lies in the differing functional state of DNA in the respective degree of spiralization or in the histone or protamine content. These differences in the sensitivity of the development stages necessitate very careful investigation and critical evaluation of the results.

In this connection attention has to be called to the possibility of detecting mutagenic effects of chemical substances via the induction of the DNA-repair mechanism. A comparison of the doses required to induce dominant lethal mutations or reciprocal translocations with those required to induce the DNA-repair mechanism in mouse germinal cells demonstrates the sensitivity of this technique. Table 3 is based on data published by Sega (30). On the right are the dosages needed to induce DNA-repair mechanisms; on the left the dosages needed to induce dominant lethal mutations or reciprocal translocations; MMS: 50 mg/kg in contrast to 5 mg/kg; EMS: 50 mg/kg in contrast to 10 mg/kg; PMS: 400 mg/kg in contrast to 50 mg/kg; iPMS: 50 mg/kg in contrast to 10 mg/kg.

Table 3. Doses required for the induction of dominant lethal mutation or reciprocal translocations and for the induction of the DNA-repair mechanism in the germinal cells of the mouse

Substance	Induction of dominant lethal mutations[*] or reciprocal translocations[+] (mg/kg)		Induction on DNA-repair mechanism (mg/kg)
MMS	~ 50[*]	Ehling et al. (13)	5
EMS	~150[*]	Generoso et al. (1974)	10
	~ 50[+]	Generoso et al. (1974)	
PMS	~400[*]	Ehling et al. (15)	50
iPMS	~ 50	Ehling et al. (15)	10

After Sega (30)

156

Let me revert to the selected test systems.

In this simplified scheme presented in Fig. 5, the chronologic displacement of the various test systems or groups of test systems in relation to one another is meant to indicate the sequence in which these tests can be applied. At any given time, the continuation of the investigations will depend on what results have been found in the previous studies and on the importance of the substance in question. Every unnecessary investigation takes up capacity that could be better used for other substances due to be studied.

In the first step, two important systems should be supplemented, if need be, by the mitotic recombination test with *S. cerevisiae*. The cell transformation test should be accorded the same status as the Ames test. The prerequisite for this test is a laboratory meeting all the requirements for cell culture. This test system is described in full by Styles (33).

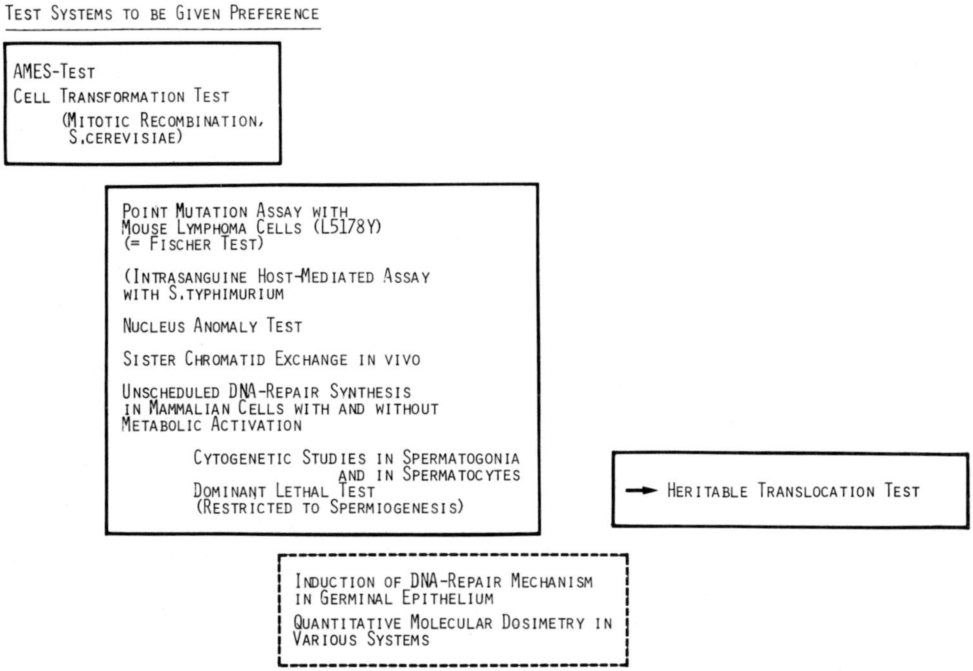

Test Systems to be Given Preference

```
┌─────────────────────────────────────┐
│ AMES-Test                           │
│ Cell Transformation Test            │
│      (Mitotic Recombination,        │
│       S.cerevisiae)                 │
└─────────────────────────────────────┘
```

```
┌──────────────────────────────────────────┐
│ Point Mutation Assay with                 │
│ Mouse Lymphoma Cells (L5178Y)             │
│ (= Fischer Test)                          │
│                                           │
│ (Intrasanguine Host-Mediated Assay        │
│ with S.typhimurium                        │
│                                           │
│ Nucleus Anomaly Test                      │
│                                           │
│ Sister Chromatid Exchange in vivo         │
│                                           │
│ Unscheduled DNA-Repair Synthesis          │
│ in Mammalian Cells with and without       │
│ Metabolic Activation                      │
│                                           │
│      Cytogenetic Studies in Spermatogonia │
│                     and in Spermatocytes  │
│      Dominant Lethal Test                 │        ──▶ Heritable Translocation Test
│      (Restricted to Spermiogenesis)       │
└──────────────────────────────────────────┘
```

```
┌ ─ ─ ─ ─ ─ ─ ─ ─ ─ ─ ─ ─ ─ ─ ─ ─ ─ ─ ─ ┐
  Induction of DNA-Repair Mechanism
  in Germinal Epithelium
  Quantitative Molecular Dosimetry in
  Various Systems
└ ─ ─ ─ ─ ─ ─ ─ ─ ─ ─ ─ ─ ─ ─ ─ ─ ─ ─ ─ ┘
```

Fig. 5. Test systems to be given preference

The test battery is first supplemented by the intrasanguine host-mediated assay with *S. typhimurium*, which should be performed at this time in special cases. Arni (34) describes this test system.

Also added are the systems based on sister chromatid exchange in the bone marrow of the Chinese hamster, and unscheduled DNA-repair synthesis in mammalian cells with and without metabolic activation. The use of the heritable translocation test is only appropriate if the previous investigations in germinal epithelia have yielded positive results.

The importance of the induction of DNA-repair mechanism in germinal epithelium and the quantitative molecular dosimetry systems has already been pointed out. The establishment of these systems should therefore at least be indicated in passing in this scheme.

I have discussed the reliability of short-term tests for the detection of mutagenic and carcinogenic properties of chemical substances. I have refrained from describing individual test systems in detail, and have instead endeavored to explain the conditions that determine the value of the various systems. I wanted to make clear that mutagenicity and carcinogenicity testing must consist in the application of not one single system, or even a few haphazardly chosen systems, but only of a careful selection of systems adapted to one another. My intention was to illustrate the fact that in evaluating any test system two aspects have first to be considered independently of each other: (a) the sensitivity of the genome and the degree of which mutagenic effects can be demonstrated on this target object, and (b) the exposure of the target object in the system in which it is embedded. Many of the systems employed today will be replaced in the course of the next few years by new ones we shall develop.

In 1976, when the short-term test had been newly developed, DeSerres (35) prophesied a period of transition, which, he opined, would be an "extremely difficult period." He was referring to the results that would emerge from the new short-term test and the conclusions that would be drawn from these results. This period of transition will not draw to a close until the development of useful new test systems has ceased. Our task is therefore clearly set.

In his preface to the "Genetics of Human Cancer" Frank J. Rauscher (36) wrote: "The study of cancer genetics has come of age." He meant that the time had come when the causal pathogenetic mechanisms of cancer could be fully fathomed. I should like to go one step further and say that our knowledge has now reached a state that puts us in the position to develop effective methods of self-defence against the risk of cancer.

References

1. Cleaver JE (1969) Xeroderma pigmentosum: a human disease in which an initial stage of DNA repair if defective. Proc Natl Acad Sci USA 63:428-435
2. Setlow RB, Regan JD (1972) Defective repair of N-acetoxy-2-acetylaminofluorene-induced lesions in the DNA of xeroderma pigmentosum cells. Biochem Biophys Res Commun 46:1019-1024

158

3. Ames BN, Durston WE, Yamasaki E, Lee FD (1973) Carcinogens are mutagens: a simple test system combining liver homogenates for activation and bacteria for detection. Proc Natl Acad Sci USA 70:2281-2285
4. Momparler RL, Chu MY, Fischer GA (1968) Studies on a new mechanism of resistance of L5178Y murine leukemia cells to cytosine arabinoside. Biochim Biophys Acta 161:481-493
5. Fischer GA (1973) The host-mediated mammalian cell assay. Agents Actions 3:93-98
6. Fischer GA, Lee SY, Calabresi P (1974) Detection of chemical mutagens using a host-mediated assay (L5178Y) mutagenesis system. Mutat Res 26:501-511
7. Langauer M, Müller D (1978) The nucleus anomaly test as a sensitive method of detecting mutagenic effects on somatic cells. Abstract of paper presented at the 2nd International Conference on Environmental Mutagens, July 11-15, 1977, Edinburgh (Great Britain). Mutat Res 53:216-217
8. Malling HV (1966) Mutagenicity of two potent carcinogens, dimethylnitrosamine and diethylnitrosamine in Neurospora crassa. Mutat Res 3:537
9. Malling HV, Frantz CN (1974) Metabolic activation of dimethylnitrosamine and diethylnitrosamine to mutagens. Mutat Res 25:179-186
10. McCann J, Choi E, Yamasaki E, Ames BN (1975) Detection of carcinogens as mutagens in the Salmonella/microsome test: assay of 300 chemicals. Proc Natl Acad Sci USA 72:5135-5139
11. Rüdiger HW, Kohl F, Mangels W, Von Wichert P, Bartram CR, Wöhler W, Passarge E (1976) Benzpyrene induces sister chromatid exchanges in cultured human lymphocytes. Nature 262:290-292
12. Basler A, Röhrborn G (1976) Chromosome aberrations in oocytes of NMRI mice and bone marrow cells of Chinese hamsters induced with 3,4-benzpyrene. Mutat Res 38:327-332
13. Ehling UH, Cumming RB, Malling HV (1968) Induction of dominant lethal mutations by alkylating agents in male mice. Mutat Res 5:417-428
14. Parkin R, Waynforth HB, Magee PN (1973) The activity of some nitroso compounds in the mouse dominant-lethal mutation assay. I. Activity of N-nitroso-N-methylurea, N-methyl-N-nitroso-N'-nitroguanidine and N-nitrosomorpholine. Mutat Res 21:155-161
15. Ehling UH, Doherty DG, Malling HV (1972) Differential spermatogenic response of mice to the induction of dominant-lethal mutations by n-propyl methanesulfonate and isopropyl methanesulfonate. Mutat Res 15:175-184
16. Lavappa KS, Yerganian G (1969) Viable chromosomal translocations induced by ethyl methanesulfonate in the Armenian hamster, Cricetulus migratorius. Genetics 61:35
17. Cattanach BM, Williams CE (1971) A search for chromosome aberrations induced in mouse spermatogonia by chemical mutagens. Mutat Res 13:371-375
18. Ray VA, Holden HE, Salsburg DS, Ellis JH, Jr, Just LJ, Hyneck ML (1974) Comparative studies of ethyl methanesulfonate-induced mutations with host-mediated, dominant lethal, and cytogenetic assays. Toxicol Appl Pharmacol 30:107-116
19. Vig BK (1971) Chromosome aberrations induced in human leukocytes by the antileukemic antibiotic adriamycin. Cancer Res 31:32-38
20. Vig BK (1973) Synergism between deoxyribose cytidine and adriamycin in causing chromosome aberrations in human leukocytes. Mutat Res 21:163-170
21. Vig BK, Kontras SB, Aubele A (1969) Sensitivity of the G_1 phase of the mitotic cycle to chromosome aberrations induced by daunomycin. Mutat Res 7:91-97

22. Gebhart E (1970) The treatment of human chromosomes in vitro: results. In: Vogel F, Röhrborn G (eds) Chemical mutagenesis in mammals and man. Springer, Berlin, Heidelberg, New York, pp 367-382
23. Abdulnur S (1976) Why is 5-fluorouracil a mutagen? J Theor Biol 53:165-175
24. Müller D, Nelles J, Deparade E, Arni P (1978) Studies of the activity of S9-liver fractions from various species in the Ames test. Presentation at the Annual General Meeting of the European Environmental Mutagen Society, July 10-13,1978, Dublin
25. Knudson AG, Jr (1977) Genetic and environmental interactions in the origin of human cancer. In: Mulvihill JJ, Miller RW, Fraumeni JF, Jr (eds) Genetics of human cancer. Raven Press, New York (Progress in Cancer Research and Therapy, Vol 3, pp 391-399)
26. Bridges BA (1974) The three-tier approach to mutagenicity screening and the concept of radiation-equivalent dose. Mutat Res 26:335-340
27. Lee WR (1976) Molecular dosimetry of chemical mutagens. Determination of molecular dose to the germ line. Mutat Res 38:311-316
28. Kolbye AC, Jr (1976) Cancer in humans: exposures and responses in a real world. Oncology 33:90-100
29. Aaron CS (1976) Molecular dosimetry of chemical mutagens. Selection of appropriate target molecules for determining molecular dose to the germ line. Mutat Res 38:303-310
30. Sega GA (1976) Molecular dosimetry of chemical mutagens. Measurement of molecular dose and DNA repair in mammalian germ cells. Mutat Res 38:317-326
31. Sega GA, Owens JG (1978) Ethylation of DNA and protamine by ethyl methanesulfonate in the germ cells of male mice and the relevancy of these molecular targets to the induction of dominant lethals. Mutat Res 52:87-106
32. Mohn GR, Van Zeeland AA, Glickman BW, Natarajan AT, Aaron CS, Quantitative molecular dosimetry of ethylmethyl sulfonate (EMS) in several genetic test systems. Presentation at this meeting
33. Styles JA, Studies on the detection of carcinogens using a mammalian cell transformation assay with liver-homogenate activation. Presentation at this meeting
34. Arni P, The microbial host-mediated assay in comparison with in vitro systems: problems of evaluation, predictive value, and practical application. Presentation at this meeting
35. De Serres FJ (1976) Perspective in a period of transition. Mutat Res 38:355-358
36. Rauscher FJ (1977) Forewood. In: Mulvihill JJ, Miller RW, Fraumeni JF, Jr (eds) Genetics of human cancer. Raven Press, New York (Progress in Cancer Research and Therapy, Vol 3)
37. Brown CC (1976) Mathematical aspects of dose-response studies in carcinogenesis —The concept of thresholds. Oncology 33:62-65

Quantitative Molecular Dosimetry of Ethyl Methanesulfonate (EMS) in Several Genetic Test Systems

G. R. Mohn[1], A. A. van Zeeland[1], A. G. A. C. Knaap[1,2], B. W. Glickman[3], A. T. Natarajan[1], M. Brendel[4], F. J. de Serres[5], and C. S. Aaron[1,6]

The increasing use of several different organisms (1, 2) to detect, verify, quantify, and extrapolate the potential mutagenic and carcinogenic effects of environmental chemicals (3) makes a critical evaluation of their sensitivity and reliability necessary. Of special interest is the determination to what extent the response to chemical mutagens is influenced by intrinsic cellular factors, such as chromosome structure and DNA content per cell, and also by metabolic and physiologic differences between test organisms or within strains of the same species (4). A quantitative comparison of the induced genetic effects first requires a precise determination of the actual dose at the target molecule, say, DNA. The reason for individual dose measurements in the different indicator organisms is that one cannot, a priori, assume that identical exposure concentrations of a chemical applied to the system will lead to identical dose at the DNA level. Instead, one expects that penetration and metabolism in general will influence the extent of reaction of the compound with DNA. As indicated by the work of Sega and Owens (5), DNA is not the only target for mutagenic chemical action, and reactions, for example with proteins, seem to be also important in the induction of certain genetic effects (e.g., dominant lethal events). For the induction of gene mutations, however, there is sufficient experimental evidence that the primary, initiating events induced by simple alkylating compounds such as EMS (ethyl methanesulfonate) are consequences of alkylation of specific DNA sites (6,21).

EMS was chosen as a model compound because it is a representative alkylating agent with an intermediate mechanism of chemical reactivity (7) and it is available as a radioactively labelled chemical (tritium labelling). Furthermore, extensive molecular dosimetry data exist that can be used for comparing the genetic effects induced in the mouse and in *Drosophila* (8,9). Finally, the activity of EMS in inducing a wide variety of genetic end

---

[1]Department of Radiation Genetics and Chemical Mutagenesis, The State University of Leiden, Leiden/The Netherlands
[2]National Institute of Public Health, Bilthoven/The Netherlands
[3]Laboratory of Molecular Genetics, The State University of Leiden, Leiden/ The Netherlands
[4]Department of Microbiology, University of Frankfurt/Main/FRG
[5]National Institute of Environmental Health Sciences, Research Triangle Park, North Carolina, USA
[6]The J.A. Cohen Interuniversity Institute for Radiopathology and Radiation Protection, Leiden/The Netherlands

points in different species has been amply documented from bacteriophages (10) to mammalian species (11).

In the present study, indicator organisms were used for which sensitive mutation systems have been elaborated and which are of actual or potential use in the different phases of testing strategies for environmental chemicals. The series includes bacteria such as *Escherichia coli* K-12 (12) and *Salmonella typhimurium* LT-2 (13), fungi such as *Saccharomyces cerevisiae* (14) and *Neurospora crassa* (15), as well as mammalian cells in culture, i.e., V-79 Chinese hamster cells (16) and L5178Y mouse lymphoma cells (17). The genetic end points vary but are measured as forward mutations rather than back mutations. Although back mutation assay systems are useful in the primary, qualitative detection of chemical mutagens due to their specific response to certain types of DNA alterations, this specific response is not desired in quantitative comparison of generalized genetic effects. Instead, forward mutation systems in which all known types of gene mutations (including deletions) will lead to viable, detectable mutant phenotypes appear more appropriate. Such systems include *galR⁻* and methyltryptophan-resistant mutations in *E. coli*, *ade*1, and *ade*2 mutations in yeast, and *ade--3* mutations in *Neurospora*. In mammalian cells, mutations to thioguanine resistance (HGPRT deficiency), ouabain resistance (changes in Na^+/K^+ ATPase activity), and 5-bromodeoxyuridine resistance (thymidine kinase deficiency) were measured, as well as the formation of sister chromatid exchanges (SCE; 22).

To obtain comparable results, the treatment conditions for measuring chemical reactivity of EMS with DNA and various genetic effects were similar. They involved treatment of stationary phase cells suspended in phosphate buffer (pH 7.2) for 120 min at 37°C in a final volume of 2.5 ml containing various concentrations of the mutagen. Concurrent parallel treatment with radiolabelled and unlabelled mutagen were used. After treatment the EMS was removed by washing and the genetic effects were measured from the unlabelled samples. The DNA was isolated from the samples which were radioactive and the number of ethylations per nucleotide was determined (18).

The results of mutation induction experiments performed under the standardized conditions mentioned above with the microbial indicators *E. coli*, *Salmonella*, yeast, and *Neurospora* (*Neurospora* experiments were performed under slightly different conditions, i.e., 300 min at 25°C) indicate that both prokaryotic and eukaryotic microbes have a similar pattern of biologic response, i.e., biphasic or exponential kinetics. In Fig. 1, for example, results with *E. coli* 343/113 are shown. It can be seen that under the present treatment regimen, exposure concentrations of EMS of up to 45 mM do not measurably inactivate the colony-forming ability of the cells. Mutation induction in the back mutation system (*arg⁺*) is less pronounced than in the two systems principally measuring forward mutations (in the *galR* gene and in several genes of the tryptophan biosynthesis pathway, MTR; see 12); all systems, in spite of quantitative differences probably due to the number of mutable loci affected by EMS action, exhibit

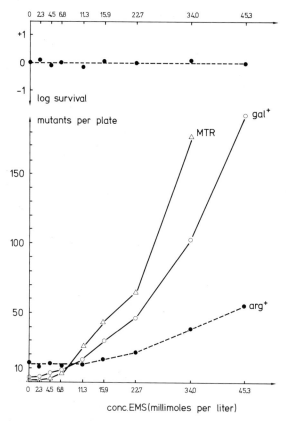

Fig. 1. Induction of mutations at three different loci in *E. coli* K-12 343/113 upon treatment with EMS under standardized conditions (stationary cell phase, 120 min, 37°C, in buffer pH 7.2). No decrease in survival occurs under these conditions. The experimental points are mean values of three plates in parallel of one representative experiment. Back mutations (*arg*⁺) and forward mutations (leading to MTR and *gal*⁺) were measured simultaneously by plating aliquots of the treated cell population on different selective media. Inoculum of bacterial cells per plate was ca. 10⁶

nonlinear induction kinetics. When his^+ back mutations in *Salmonella* LT-2/*his*G46 are measured under the same EMS treatment conditions as in *E. coli*, induction kinetics similar to the arg^+ system in *E. coli* are observed (data not shown). In Fig. 2, results of representative experiments with *Saccharomyces* are shown: Again, in the three genetic end points studied, i.e., forward mutations to ade_1^- and ade_2^- and back mutations to his^+ and lys^+, nonlinear or biphasic induction kinetics are observed; survival is ca. 100% at concentrations below 50 mM and decreases to 10% at 150 mM EMS. In *Neurospora crassa*, where conidia were treated at concentrations of up to 200 mM EMS a similar, exponential increase of forward mutations in the *ad*-3 locus (exponent is roughly 2.5) can be seen (Fig. 3).

In contrast to the microbial indicators, both the hamster cells and the mouse cells exhibit linear, i.e., dose proportional, mutation induction kinetics. This is clearly demonstrated in Fig. 4, for example, in which the induction of thioguanine-resistant mutations (arising as a consequence of forward mutations leading to loss of function of the HGPRT gene) is directly proportional to the applied concentration of EMS (up to 10 mM) as is the induction of SCEs. A further difference with the microbial indicators is the rather high frequency of gene mutations induced even at low-exposure concentrations of EMS:

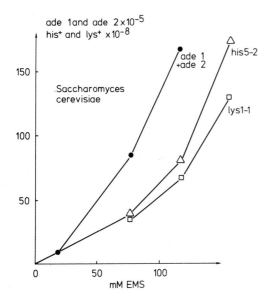

ade 1and ade 2×10^{-5}
his$^+$ and lys$^+$ ×10^{-8}

Saccharomyces cerevisiae

ade 1 +ade 2

his5-2

lys1-1

mM EMS

Fig. 2. Induction of mutations at four different loci in *S. cerevisiae* strain MB 1114-58 (RAD, REV) upon treatment with EMS under standardized conditions (see text). Survival was ca. 100% at 50 mM and ca. 60% at 100 mM of EMS. The experimental points for the induction of back mutations (*lys*1-1 and *his*5-2) are mean values of five plates in parallel of one representative experiment. Forward mutations (*ade*1 and *ade*2) were determined by plating aliquots of the treated yeast population on growth medium and observing red or sectored colonies upon incubation. Inoculum was ca. 10^8 per plate in back mutation experiments

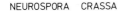

NEUROSPORA CRASSA

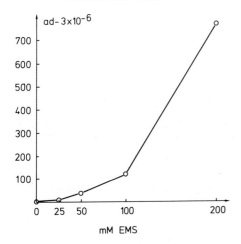

ad- 3×10^{-6}

mM EMS

Fig. 3. Induction of forward mutations in the *ad*-3 locus of *Neurospora crassa* heterokaryon 12 upon treatment with EMS. Treatment conditions of this preliminary experiment were different from the standardized treatment (see text) and included incubation of conidia for 300 min at 25°C and pH 7.0. Survival was 92% at 25 mM exposure, 84% at 50 mM, 71% at 100 mM, and 50% at 200 mM; *ad*-3 mutants were recorded as purple conidial colonies arising within the nonmutated, white colonies upon cultivation of the treated population in the dark at 30°C for 7 days

In the hamster cells, for example, approximately 100 induced thioguanine-resistant mutant clones are observed per 10^5 surviving cells after 100 mM EMS treatment (Fig. 4), whereas in all microbial indicators (Figs. 1-3) the recovered frequencies are much less. At the same exposure concentration differences in sensitivity are also reflected in survival, mammalian cells being more readily inactivated by EMS (65% survival at 10 mM EMS vs 100% survival with microbial cells).

These differences between mammalian and microbial indicators are not due to differences in penetration into the cells, since the measured levels of alkylation in DNA of *E. coli* and hamster

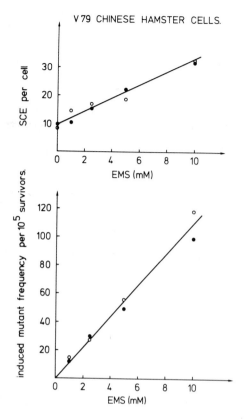

Fig. 4. Induction of HGRPT⁻ mutations and of SCEs in V-79 Chinese hamster cells upon treatment with EMS under standardized conditions (see text). Results of two independent experiments are shown (o and ●). HGPRT⁻ mutants were measured as 6-thioguanine-resistant clones upon cultivation of the treated cell population in medium devoid of the selective agent to allow for phenotypic expression. Survival of clone-forming ability was 65% at 10 mM of EMS. Induction of SCEs was determined after incubation of the treated cells for 2 cycles, with 5 µM 5-BrdUrd in the dark. The air-dried preparations of these cells were stained with Hoechst 33258 followed by Giemsa; 25 cells were scored for each experimental point

cells reported earlier (18) are similar under identical treatment with EMS at exposure concentrations of up to 50 mM. These chemical dosimetry experiments have been repeated and confirmed (to be published) and it has also been shown that *Saccharomyces* and *Neurospora* exhibit similar, i.e., linear, increase of alkylation in DNA with increasing exposure concentration of EMS. The question remains open, therefore, as to which physiologic differences are responsible for the qualitative and quantitative differences in biologic response observed between mammalian and microbial indicator cells.

Experiments conceived to explain the differences mentioned above were performed first with the *E. coli* indicator because experimental conditions such as growing cell stage can be easily varied and because the influence of different genetic backgrounds can be relatively easily studied. The results so far obtained clearly indicate that even slight variations of treatment procedure, experimental conditions, and genetic background can lead to large changes (increase) in recovered mutant frequencies. Two typical examples are shown in Fig. 5. If under otherwise identical, standardized EMS treatment, growing *E. coli* cells are used and compared with stationary phase cells, then a substantial increase in mutant colony frequency (Fig. 5a) can be observed. This difference between cell phase stages might be due to the fact that replicating (or derepressed) DNA is more accessible to EMS

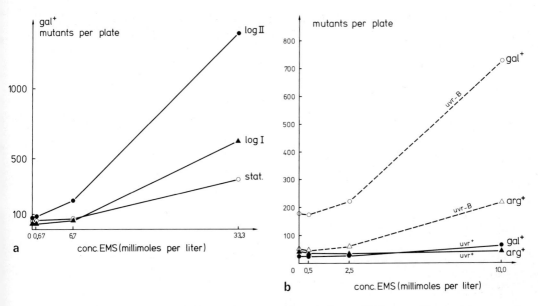

Fig. 5a and b. Influence of varying experimental conditions and genetic background on mutant yields in *E. coli* 343/113 upon treatment with EMS. (a) Induction of *gal*⁺ mutations in *E. coli* cells of different growth phase; *stat.*, stationary cells; *log I*, logarithmically growing cells (generation phase ca. 35 min) suspended in buffer during treatment (120 min at 37°C); *log II*, logarithmically growing cells suspended in fully supplemented growth medium during treatment with EMS (for 120 min at 37°C). (b) Induction of *gal*⁺ and of *arg*⁺ mutations in *E. coli* cells differing in their capacity to repair damage caused by alkylation of DNA: ●——● and ▲——▲, wild type bacteria; o-----o and Δ-----Δ, *uvr*-B derivative). The experimental points are mean values of three plates in parallel of one representative experiment. Inoculum per plate was ca. 10⁶ bacterial cells

alkylation reaction; alternatively, premutational damage can be fixed and expressed more rapidly in growing cells.

Another striking example of increased sensitivity to EMS muta-genicity is given when an excision-repair deficient mutation is introduced in the *E. coli* strain. In Fig. 5b, results of com-parative mutation experiments under identical EMS treatment con-ditions are shown for strain *E. coli* 343/113 (wild-type) and *E. coli* 343/113/*uvr*-B (excision-repair deficient); they clearly demonstrate a large increase in mutation frequency (especially in *gal*⁺ mutations) in the *uvr*-B background; this indicates and confirms that in wild-type *E. coli* strains a substantial part of EMS-induced premutational lesions is efficiently removed by ex-cision-repair systems (19). In further experiments not reported here, the influence of DNA adenine methylation potential on sen-sitivity to EMS (20) was confirmed by showing an increased mu-tability of strain *E. coli* 343/113 toward EMS in the presence of a *dam*-4 mutation. Using *Salmonella*, essentially the same results were obtained as with *E. coli*. For example, the induction of *his*⁺ back mutations (from *his*G46 auxotrophy) is greatly enhanced in a *uvr*-B derivative (Fig. 6) as compared with the wild-type strain; use of a permeable, deep rough derivative carrying an *rfa* mutation) does not measurably increase sensitivity to EMS in addition to the *uvr*-B effect, indicating that *rfa* and wild-type cells are of equal penetrability for small, lipid and water soluble molecules such as EMS. It appears thus that the increased sensitivity of hamster cells to the mutagenic and inactivating effects of EMS compared with microbial cells is probably due to differences in quality or magnitude of mutational repair pathways or to physiologic differences (growing stage of the cell).

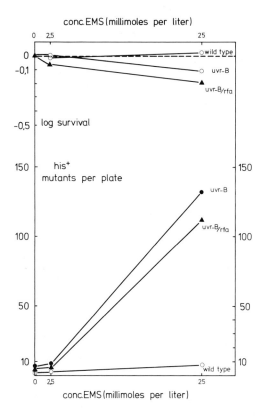

Fig. 6. Influence of DNA-repair capacity on mutant yield in *S. typhimurium his*G46 upon treatment with EMS under standardized conditions (incubation of stationary cells for 120 min at 37°C in buffer pH 7.2); (o————o), wild-type repair capacity; ●————●, *uvr*-B derivative; ▲————▲; *uvr*-B derivative with an additional mutation in lipolysaccharide core synthetizing gene *rfa*). Inoculum per plate was ca. 10⁶ bacterial cells

Concerning the mammalian/microbial differences in biologic dose-response kinetics (linear vs biphasic or exponential), experiments were performed with *E. coli* in the portion of the curve (up to 10 mM EMS) which is indistinguishable from linearity in the usual experiments (see Fig. 1). Results obtained with more than 100 plates in parallel to select for *gal*⁺ mutations indicate that, at low doses of up to 10 mM, the relative frequency of mutations observed may be proportional to dose with no clear indication of a threshold in *E. coli*, which resembles the results obtained with the mammalian cells.

Furthermore, experiments using the mouse cells indicate that the
response to mutagens varies greatly among different genetic
systems within the same population of treated cells. As shown
in Fig. 7, the induction by EMS of ouabain-resistant mutants,
thioguanine-resistant mutants, and BUdR-resistant mutants in
mouse lymphoma cells follows linear kinetics but the magnitude
of the effect varies strongly with the genetic end point used
and the frequencies are much lower than that observed in the
hamster cells, even when mutations in basically the same gene
(which codes for HGPRT) are scored as thioguanine-resistant
clones. This, again, indicates that the metabolic state of the
cell may influence the quantitative response to mutagens. It
also demonstrates that the differences between the microbial
indicators and the hamster cells are not greater than between
the mouse and the hamster cells under identical treatment conditions. In fact the mutation frequencies induced by EMS in
the microbial cells (Fis. 1-3) fall within the range of observed frequencies in the mammalian cells (Figs. 4 and 7).

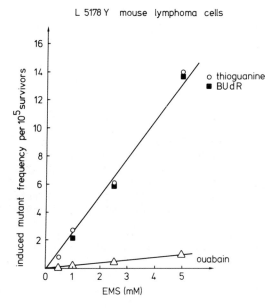

L 5178 Y   mouse lymphoma cells

Fig. 7. Induction of forward mutations at three different loci
in L5178Y mouse lymphoma cells
upon treatment with EMS under
standardized conditions (see text).
Mutations to 6-thioguanine resistance, BUdR resistance, and ouabain
resistance were determined as
drug-resistant clones after incubation of the treated cells in
media devoid of selective agent
to allow for phenotypic expression.
Each point represents mean values
of mutant clone number on selective
plates of one representative experiment. Survival was 65% at 5 mM
of EMS

In conclusion, these and previous results (see 8,9) show (a) that
molecular dosimetry is feasible in a wide range of organisms
varying from bacteria to animals; (b) that under identical treatment conditions using EMS, the dose in the DNA is similar in
organisms which widely differ in chromosome structure, DNA content, and metabolism and physiology; (c) that induction of genetic effects by EMS increases approximately linearly at low dose
in a variety of different organisms with no clear indication of
a threshold; and (d) that the variation between species is probably not greater than the variation within an organism with respect to mutation frequency per unit dose.

These findings, though preliminary, clearly indicate a way of quantitatively comparing genetic effects induced in a variety of test organisms. They permit the calculation of detection indices (as the ratio of relative frequency of observed mutations to the dose) which may allow extrapolation of results obtained with lower organisms to animals and ultimately to man.

Acknowledgments. The authors would like to express their deep gratitude to Professor Dr. F.H. Sobels for his support and continuous encouragement during this study. Part of the work reported here was supported by the Königin Wilhelmina Fonds, project LUKC SG-774.1, International Atomic Energy Agency contract 052-64-1 BIAN, and the European Community Environmental Research Programme contract O30-74-1-, ENVN.

References

1. Kilbey BJ, Legator M, Nichols V, Ramel C (eds) (1977) Handbook of mutagenicity test procedures. Elsevier, Amsterdam
2. Mohn GR (1978) An overview of animal and microbial test systems for carcinogenesis and mutagenesis. Human Genet 45:169-176
3. Sobels FH (1977) Some problems associated with the testing for environmental mutagens and a perspective for studies in "comparative mutagenesis". Mutat Res 46:245-260
4. Generoso WM, Russel WL (1969) Strain and sex variations in the sensitivity of mice to dominant lethal induction with ethylmethanesulfonate. Mutat Res 8:589-598
5. Sega GA, Owens JG (1978) Ethylation of DNA and protamine by ethyl methanesulfonate in the germ cells of male mice and the relevance of these molecular targets to the induction of dominant lethals. Mutat Res 52:87-106
6. Loveless A (1969) Possible relevance of O^6-alkylation of deoxyguanosine to the mutagenicity and carcinogenicity of nitrosamines and nitrosamines. Nature 223:206-207
7. Ostermann-Golkar S, Ehrenberg L, Wachtmeister CA (1970) Reaction kinetics and biological action in barley of monofunctional methanesulfonate esters. Radiat Bot 10:303-327
8. Sega GA, Cumming RB, Walton MF (1974) Dosimetry studies on the ethylation of mouse sperm DNA after in vivo exposures to ^{3}H ethyl methanesulfonate. Mutat Res 24:317-333
9. Aaron CS, Lee WR (1978) Molecular dosimetry of the mutagen ethyl methanesulfonate in *Drosophila melanogaster* spermatozoa. Linear relation of DNA alkylation per sperm cell (DOSE) to sex-linked recessive lethals. Mutat Res 49:27-44
10. Krieg DR (1963) Ethyl methanesulfonate-induced reversions of bacteriophage T4rII mutants. Genetics 48:561-580
11. Ehling UH, Russell WL (1969) Induction of specific locus mutations by alkyl methanesulfonates in male mice. Genetics 61:14-15
12. Mohn GR, Ellenberger J (1977) The use of *Escherichia coli* K-12/343/113 (λ) as a multipurpose indicator strain in various mutagenicity testing procedures. In: Kilbey BJ, Ramel C, Legator M (eds) Handbook of mutagenicity test procedures. Elsevier, Amsterdam, pp 95-108
13. Ames BN, McCann J, Yamasaki E (1975) Methods for detecting carcinogens and mutagens with the *Salmonella*/mammalian microsome mutagenicity test. Mutat Res 31:347-364

14. Mortimer RK, Manney TR (1971) Mutation induction in yeast. In: Hollaender A (ed) Chemical mutagens. Principles and methods for their detection, Vol 1, Plenum Press, New York, pp 289-310
15. De Serres FJ, Malling HV (1971) Measurement of recessive lethal damage over the entire genome and at two specific loci in the *ad*-3 region of a two-component heterokaryon of *Neurospora crassa*. In: Hollaender A (ed) Chemical mutagens. Principles and methods for their detection. Plenum Press, New York pp 311-342
16. Van Zeeland AA (1978) Post-treatment with caffeine and the induction of gene mutations by ultraviolet irradiation and ethyl methanesulfonate in V-79 Chinese hamster cells in culture. Mutat Res 50:145-151
17. Knaap AGAC (1978) The simultaneous determination of induced mutant frequencies at two loci in mouse lymphoma cells (L5178Y). Mutat Res 53:211-220
18. Aaron CS, Van Zeeland AA, Mohn GR, Natarajan AT (1978) Molecular dosimetry of the chemical mutagen ethyl methanesulfonate in *Escherichia coli* and in V-79 Chinese hamster cells. Mutat Res 50:419-426
19. Ishii Y, Kondo S (1975) Comparative analysis of deletion and base change mutabilities of *Escherichia coli* B strains differing in DNA repair capacity (wild type, *uvr*-A, *pol*-A, *rec*-A) by various mutagens. Mutat Res 27:27-44
20. Glickman B, Van den Elsen P, Radman M (1978) Induced mutagenesis in *dam⁻* mutants of *Escherichia coli*: a role for 6-methyladenine residues in mutation avoidance. Mol Gen Genet 163:307-312
21. Loveless A (1958) Increased rate of plaque-type and host-range mutations following treatment of bacteriophage in vitro with ethyl methanesulfonate. Nature 181:1212-1213
22. Natarajan AT, Tates AD, Van Buul PPW, Meijers M, De Vogel N (1976) Cytogenetic effects of mutagens/carcinogens after activation in a microsomal system in vitro. I. Induction of chromosome aberrations and sister chromatid exchanges by diethylnitrosamine (DEN) and dimethylnitrosamine (DMN) in CHO cells in the presence of rat-liver microsomes. Mutat Res 37:83-90

Comparative Results of Short-Term in Vitro and in Vivo Mutagenicity Tests Obtained with Selected Environmental Chemicals

D. Wild, K. Eckhardt, E. Gocke, and M. T. King[1]

Numerous short-term tests for detecting mutagens have been and are being developed, and with increasing knowledge of mutagenic chemicals a close correlation between mutagenic and carcinogenic properties —which has long been suspected —has become obvious. Therefore, short-term mutagenicity tests are now considered potentially useful for detecting carcinogens. The general validity of this correlation can, however, not be derived from our present understanding of mutagenesis and carcinogenesis, but it can be demonstrated for single test systems, mutagens, and carcinogens.

Extensive studies with the *Salmonella*/mammalian microsome test have clearly shown the mutagenic activity of most known carcinogens (and nonmutagenicity of noncarcinogens), but in most other test systems the mutagenicity of carcinogens has been validated less thoroughly.

The correlation of mutagenic and carcinogenic activities can alternatively be studied by use of short-term tests for screening of chemicals not studied before for mutagenic or carcinogenic potential. Thereby mutagens are discovered, and the carcinogenicity of these must be confirmed or rejected. This procedure requires long-term animal carcinogenicity tests and is therefore more time-consuming, but it has the advantage of revealing genotoxic properties of hitherto unsuspected chemicals and of visualizing potential risks to human health.

Here we report selected data obtained in the course of mutagenicity screening of environmental chemicals. The examples are chosen to demonstrate the efficiency of different test procedures and their combination. The following three short-term tests were routinely applied to all chemicals: the *Salmonella*/microsome test (Ames test), and two in vivo tests: the Basc test on *Drosophila* and the micronucleus test on the mouse.

We perform the Ames test as a plate incorporation test (1) using five mutation indicator strains of *Salmonella typhimurium*: TA 1535, TA 1537, TA 1538, and the plasmid strains TA 100 and TA 98. The strains are regularly checked for sensitivity to UV and crystal violet and for sensitivity or resistance to ampicillin. Experiments are run without and with metabolic activation. Metabolic activation is achieved by S-9 mix prepared from liver of

[1]Zentrallaboratorium für Mutagenitätsprüfung der Deutschen Forschungsgemeinschaft, Breisacher Straße 33, 7800 Freiburg/FRG

Aroclor-1254-pretreated rats (Sprague-Dawley SIV-50). The minimal medium contained per liter 15 g agar, 0.82 g trisodium citrate $\cdot 2H_2O$, 4.6 g $K_2HPO_4 \cdot 3H_2O$, 1.5 g KH_2PO_4, 1.0 g $(NH_4)_2SO_4$, 0.1 g $MgSO_4 \cdot 7H_2O$, and 15.0 g glucose.

In *Drosophila* we test for X-linked recessive lethal mutations in germ cells of male flies using the Basc test (2,3). Male flies of the Berlin wild strain are fed the test substance and crossed with virgin Basc females. The daughters carry the paternal treated X chromosomes. Crosses of the F_1 animals produce normally *four* visually distinguishable classes of animals in the F_2 generation; in case of a lethal mutation on the treated X chromosome of a male germ cell, red-eyed F_2 males are not viable and the F_2 cultures contain only *three* classes of animals. With this technique, a broad spectrum of gene mutations and mutagens can be detected (4).

The micronucleus test on mice is a cytogenetic test on bone marrow cells in vivo (5); its basis is shown in Fig. 1: acentric chromosome fragments occurring in erythroblast cells and lost chromosomes which do not become integrated into one of the daughter nuclei form "micronuclei." During nuclear expulsion, the micronucleus remains in the cell, and the outcome is an abnormal micronucleated erythrocyte. Micronuclei can very easily be recognized in erythrocytes; their spontaneous incidence in young (polychromatic) erythrocytes is about $2^o/oo$; chromosome-breaking chemicals can increase this incidence up to 50-fold.

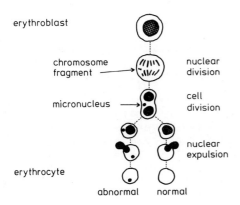

Fig. 1. Micronucleus test for the detection of chemically induced chromosome breaks and chromosome loss in erythroblasts of mouse bone marrow

Figure 2 presents the chemicals which will be discussed first: toluenesulfonamides, the ortho-toluenesulfonamide (OTS), and the isomeric para-toluenesulfonamide (PTS). They are impurities in saccharin which is produced according to the Remsen-Fahlberg synthesis. OTS is the major impurity; saccharin has been found to contain up to 5000 ppm of OTS (6).

Figure 3 gives results from using the Ames test. Both OTS and PTS induce revertants in strain TA 98 as shown here, but not in the parent strain TA 1538 or in the other tester strains. Neither

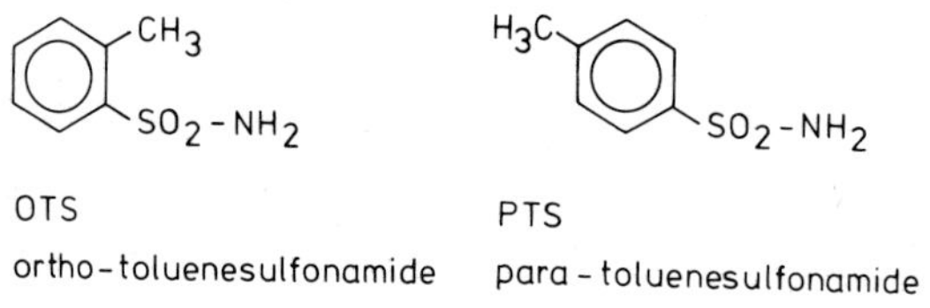

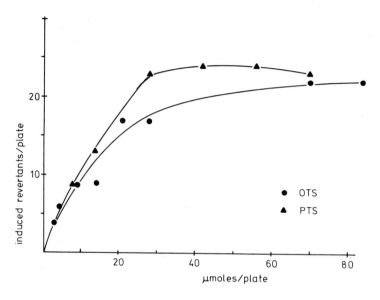

OTS
ortho-toluenesulfonamide

PTS
para-toluenesulfonamide

Fig. 2

Fig. 3. Mutagenic effect of OTS and PTS on *S. typhimurium* TA 98 in experiments with metabolic activation by S-9 mix prepared from Aroclor-pretreated rats. Each point is the mean value of three or four plates minus the spontaneous control value (12 revertants/plate)

chemical is mutagenic per se, but require metabolic activation mediated by the complete S-9 mix. A further parallel is expressed in the dose-effect curves: their shapes are very similar. Obviously, they are weakly, though significantly and reproducibly, mutagenic in this test, but this quantitative parameter should not be generalized, because these chemicals might not belong to one of the well-known chemical classes of mutagens and the conditions of the standard Ames test may be suboptimal for the detection of these mutagens.

The *Drosophila* data confirm the mutagenic potential of OTS and PTS. Table 1 presents the frequency of X-linked recessive lethal mutations in different broods or germ cell stages of the treated males. Either sulfonamide, at a concentration of 2.5 mM, increases highly significantly ($P \leq 1\%$) the frequency of recessive lethal mutations in brood I corresponding to mature sperm. In immature germ cells there is a sterilizing effect. Thus, the mutagenic effects of these two chemicals exhibit a high degree of similarity in *Drosophila*, as in *Salmonella*.

Table 1. Sex-linked recessive lethal mutations in *Drosophila*

Compound	Concentration (mM)	Recessive lethal mutations per X chromosomes		
		Brood 1	Brood 2	Brood 3
OTS	2.5	26/4310 0.60%[*]	7/2800 0.25%	10/1386 0.72%
PTS	2.5	25/3717 0.67%[*]	0/402 —	1/88 1.14%
Controls	0	19/7130 0.27%	8/5525 0.14%	19/4871 0.39%

*$P \leq 1\%$

Using the micronucleus test and oral and intraperitoneal administration of OTS and PTS, we could not find chromosome-breaking activity.

The *Salmonella* and *Drosophila* data are further supported by recent results with the mammalian spot test (7): if OTS is administered orally to pregnant mice, it induces specific locus mutations in embryonal prepigment cells, and these can be seen as coat color spots on the mice at the age of 3 weeks (8).

The demonstrated similarities between OTS and PTS may indicate that the metabolism and mutagenic mechanism of OTS and PTS are also very similar. In rats, OTS is metabolized by oxidation of the methyl group and converted to the corresponding sulfamoyl-benzyl alcohol and sulfamoylbenzoic acid (9). This acid is inactive in Ames tests (10). Possibly, an intermediate oxidation product is the ultimate mutagen.

The question of whether OTS and PTS are also carcinogenic cannot be answered at present. To our knowledge, only OTS has been studied. Whereas Canadian investigators did not find tumors in OTS-treated rats (11), Schmähl found several rats with bladder papillomas, which are considered as precancerous stages of bladder carcinomas, and one bladder carcinoma and concluded that "OTS may possibly have a weak carcinogenic effect" (12).

In summary, these data indicate that OTS and PTS are mutagenic in different organisms and that OTS may also be a weak carcinogen. Further studies on the metabolism of these compounds and on the mutagenicity of metabolites should help to estimate the potential relevance of OTS for the disputed genotoxic effect of saccharin.

A second group of chemicals to be discussed contains simple derivatives of benzene with hydroxy- and amino-substituents: phenol, the *p*-dihydroxybenzene hydroquinone, *p*-aminophenol, and *p*-phenylenediamine.

Phenol is one of the top 50 chemicals on the basis of its worldwide production volume. Hydroquinone is a metabolite of benzene and phenol in mammals. It is used, for instance, as photographic developer, as a hair dye component, and for skin bleaching. *p*-Aminophenol is a metabolite of aniline and of

p-nitrophenol and has similar uses as hydroquinone. p-Phenylenediamine is used for fur dyeing, while its use in hair dyes
has been discontinued in the Federal Republic of Germany because
of its allergenic properties.

Figure 4 shows the weak mutagenic activity of phenol in *Salmonella*
strain TA 98 in presence of S-9 mix. No effect was observed in
experiments without S-9 mix. These data parallel recent findings
of Bolt et al. that in vitro in presence of microsomes phenol
or rather a phenol metabolite binds irreversibly to liver microsomal protein (13). In *Drosophila* (10) and in mouse bone marrow
(Table 2) we found no mutagenic response to phenol. The mechanism
of this mutagenic effect in *Salmonella* is not understood, but a
highly unstable and reactive epoxide may be an intermediate.
The phenol metabolite hydroquinone is, however, not involved,
because hydroquinone is not mutagenic in strain TA 98 (see below). Likewise, phenol impurities are probably not responsible:
the phenol sample had a minimum content of 99.5% with 0.15%
cresols as main impurity. According to simultaneous studies on
the isomeric cresols, these could not have caused the observed
phenol effect (10).

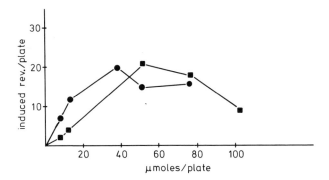

Fig. 4. Mutagenic effect of phenol on *S. typhimurium* TA 98 found in two
independent experiments with metabolic activation by S-9 mix prepared from
Aroclor-pretreated rats. Each point is the mean value of four plates minus
the spontaneous control value (●, 18 revertants/plate; ■, 14 revertants/plate)

Figure 5 demonstrates the mutagenic effects of hydroquinone,
p-aminophenol, and p-phenylenediamine in *Salmonella typhimurium*
strain TA 1535. It is emphasized that these results were found
in experiments without S-9 mix. With S-9 mix, hydroquinone and
p-aminophenol, even at high concentrations, were inactive.
Therefore, if experiments had been performed only with activation, we would have overlooked these effects and would have
classified p-aminophenol as nonmutagenic as McCann et al. did
(14) [p-phenylenediamine differs from the two other chemicals in
that it is active also with S-9 mix (15).]

These three compounds which are chemically closely related by
their hydroxy- or amino-substituents in 1,4- or para-position

Table 2. Micronucleus tests on mouse bone marrow

Chemical (solvent)	Number of mice	Dose (mg/kg)	Micronucleated PE (^{o}/oo)
Phenol	4	2 × 188	2.8
(Hanks sol.)	4	2 × 94	4.0
	4	2 × 47	1.2
	4	O	2.7
Hydroquinone	6	2 × 110	11.7*
(Hanks sol.)	6	2 × 55	4.1
	6	O	2.6
p-Aminophenol	4	2 × 436	14.5*
(3% gum arabic)	4	2 × 327	14.3*
	4	2 × 218	14.0*
	4	2 × 109	10.0*
	4	O	2.9
p-Phenylene-diamine	4	2 × 32.4	1.7
(0.9% NaCl)	4	2 × 21.6	2.6
	4	2 × 10.8	1.6
	4	O	1.2

*$P < 1\%$; PE, polychromatic erythrocytes

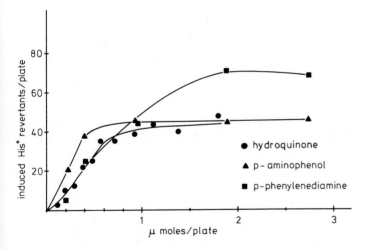

Fig. 5. Mutagenic effect of hydroquinone, p-aminophenol, and p-phenylene-diamine on S. typhimurium TA 1535. Each point is the mean value of four plates minus the spontaneous control value (23 revertants/plate)

of the benzene ring have also very similar characteristic mutagenic effects: (a) they are direct mutagens, (b) they mutate strain TA 1535 and thus induce base-pair substitutions, and (c) their dose-effect curves are very similar.

Therefore, it appears likely that these effects have a common basis. Some potential mechanisms can be excluded in view of the *direct* mutagenic activity, viz., epoxidation, C-hydroxylation, and N-hydroxylation. The most likely is a semiquinone/quinone mechanism. All three chemicals can be oxidized to radical semiquinones and further to quinone, or quinone derivatives.

Semiquinones as well as quinones can react with macromolecules and could be the "ultimate mutagens". Their formation requires oxygen, and can be catalyzed in an unspecific way by widespread metal-containing enzymes.

In *Drosophila*, hydroquinone was inactive, *p*-aminophenol is still under study in our laboratory, and *p*-phenylenediamine was reported as being weakly mutagenic by Blijleven (16).

The results of the cytogenetic tests are shown in Table 2: hydroquinone and *p*-aminophenol, applied intraperitoneally, increased the frequency of micronucleated polychromatic erythrocytes; they are, therefore, chromosome-breaking or spindle-inhibiting chemicals. In contrast to this, Hossack and Richardson, using high oral doses of *p*-aminophenol, did not detect micronucleus induction in rats (17).

The dose-effect relations of hydroquinone and *p*-aminophenol are again similar and might also suggest a basic similarity in the mode of action of these two chemicals. These results show clearly that mutagens which are inactivated by S-9 mix in the Ames test can nevertheless induce mutations in a mammal. *p*-Phenylenediamine differs again markedly from the two other compounds: it was more toxic and did not induce chromosomal abnormalities at the tolerated doses; a comparable result was found in rats (17).

It is remarkable that the mutagenicity of these long-known and broadly used chemicals has not been noticed previously, even though Mitra and Manna in 1971 published on mutagenic (cytogenetic) effects of *p*-aminophenol in mice (18).

Carcinogenicity data on these chemicals are very sparse. In bladder implantation studies, hydroquinone in cholesterol pellets increased the incidence of bladder carcinomas in mice (19), but feeding studies have not been performed. *p*-Aminophenol gave a negative result when fed to small groups of rats (20). Carcinogenicity studies on *p*-phenylenediamine are inconclusive (21). Therefore, carcinogenicity studies on these chemicals appear urgently needed. Furthermore, the mechanism(s) of the observed mutagenic effects and relations between chemical structure and mutagenic effect deserve detailed study.

In summary, all six mutagenic chemicals selected for this presentation were detected by use of the *Salmonella*/microsome test. The mutagenic activity of phenol could not be confirmed by use of the other tests, whereas up to now three of these mutagens have been confirmed by the *Drosophila* test and two by the micronucleus test. These examples and test results obtained with numerous other chemicals show the high efficiency of the *Salmonella*/microsome test for mutagen screening. Drosophila and micronucleus tests are valuable in claryfying the mutagenic potential in higher organisms of those substances found positive in bacterial systems. Mutagenicity tests can be combined with studies on the metabolism and mutagenic mechanism of newly detected mutagens; the collected information from those studies should be taken into account in the planning of carcinogenicity tests.

Addendum. In addition to the experiments reported, Salmonella tests on OTS and PTS have been performed on *Vogel-Bonner E*-medium under otherwise identical conditions. With the use of this medium, no mutagenic effect of OTS and PTS was detected. This medium dependence cannot be explained at present. We observed, however, that the colony size of TA 98 revertants is larger and the revertant frequency is higher on *Vogel-Bonner E*-medium.

To our knowledge this is the first example for the nonequivalence of different but related selective media in the Ames test. Currently we are trying to elucidate the basis of this phenomenon and are comparing mutagenic effects of other chemicals on either medium.

References

1. Ames BN, McCann J, Yamasaki E (1975) Methods for detecting carcinogens and mutagens with the Salmonella/mammalian-microsome mutagenicity test. Mutat Res 31:347-364
2. Abrahamson S, Lewis EB (1971) The detection of mutations in Drosophila melanogaster. In: Hollaender A (ed) Chemical mutagens, Vol 2. Plenum Press, New York, pp 461-487
3. Würgler FE, Sobels FH, Vogel E (1977) Drosophila as assay system for detecting genetic changes. In: Kilbey BJ et al. (eds) Handbook of mutagenicity test procedures. Elsevier, Amsterdam, pp 335-373
4. Vogel E, Sobels FH (1976) The function of Drosophila in genetic toxicology testing. In: Hollaender A (ed) Chemical mutagens, Vol 4. Plenum Press, New York, pp 93-142
5. Schmid W (1976) The micronucleus test for cytogenetic analysis. In: Hollaender A (ed) Chemical mutagens. Plenum Press, New York, pp 31-53
6. Stavrič B, Klassen R (1975) O-Toluenesulfonamide in saccharine preparations. J Assoc Off Anal Chem 58:427-432
7. Fahrig R (1978) The mammalian spot test: a sensitive in vivo method for the detection of genetic alterations in somatic cells of mice. In: Hollaender A, De Serres FJ (eds) Chemical mutagens, Vol 5. Plenum Press, New York, pp 151-176
8. Fahrig R, submitted
9. Renwick AG, Ball LM, Corina DL, Williams RT (1978) Fate of saccharin-impurities —Excretion and metabolism of toluene-2-sulfonamide in man and rat. Xenobiotica 8:461-474
10. King MT, Eckhardt K, Gocke E, Wild D (1978) unpublished
11. Arnold DL, Charbonneau SM, Moodie CA, Munro IC (1977) Long-term toxicity study with orthotoluenesulfonamide and saccharin (abstract). Toxicol Appl Pharmacol 41:164

12. Schmähl D (1978) Experiments on the carcinogenic effect of ortho-toluolsulfonamid (OTS). Z Krebsforsch 91:19-22
13. Bolt HM (1977) Structural modifications in contraceptive steroids altering their metabolism and toxicity. Arch Toxicol 39:13-19
14. McCann J, Choi E, Yamasaki E, Ames BN (1975) Detection of carcinogens as mutagens in the Salmonella/microsome test: assay of 300 chemicals. Proc Natl Acad Sci USA 72:5135-5139
15. Venitt S, Searle CE (1976) Mutagenicity and possible carcinogenicity of hair colourants and constituents. INSERM Symposia Series, Vol 52, pp 263-272
16. Blijleven WGH (1977) Mutagenicity of four hair dyes in Drosophila melanogaster. Mutat Res 48:181-186
17. Hossack DJN, Richardson JC (1977) Examination of the potential mutagenicity of hair dye constituents using the micronucleus test. Experientia 33:377-378
18. Mitra AB, Manna GK (1971) Effect of some phenolic compounds on chromosomes of bone marrow cells of mice. Indian J Med Res 59:1442-1447
19. IARC-Monographs on the evaluation of the carcinogenic risk of chemicals to man, Vol 15. IARC, Lyon (1977), pp 155-175
20. IARC-Monographs on the evaluation of the carcinogenic risk of chemicals to man, Vol 4. IARC, Lyon (1974), pp 27-39
21. IARC-Monographs on the evaluation of the carcinogenic risk of chemicals to man, Vol 16. IARC, Lyon (1978), pp 125-142

Correlations Between Primary Effects of Xenobiotics on Liver Cells in Vitro and Their Mutagenicity and Carcinogenicity in Vivo

R. Rickart, K. E. Appel, M. Schwarz, G. Stöckle, and W. Kunz[1]

Numerous studies have established a high degree of correlation between the carcinogenicity of chemical compounds and their mutagenic potential. This fact not only supports the somatic mutation theory, but has also been successfully used to identify and eliminate carcinogenic compounds from the human environment (1).

A general disadvantage of these in vitro systems used to detect genetic damage is that both microbial and eucaryotic indicator cells lack metabolizing enzymes possessed by the mammalian target cells which are necessary to convert procarcinogens to their ultimate active forms.

In consequence, subcellular-bioactivating fractions have to be added. As the active metabolites are generated outside the indicator cells, high yields of metabolites are usually needed to reach the critical target molecules.

Liver microsomes are generally induced by pretreatment with such agents as phenobarbital, 3-methylcholanthrene (3-MC), and polychlorinated biphenyls, and are used in conjunction with high concentrations of the compounds under test (2,3).

However, this procedure is not without problems, especially with regard to quantitative aspects. An example is shown in Fig. 1, which demonstrates the alkylating activity of dimethylnitrosamine (DMN) incubated in vitro with microsomes from animals pretreated with inducers mentioned above. Alkylation rates were measured by determining the specific radioactivities of microsomal proteins after exhaustive solvent extraction. DMN was administered over a wide concentration range, as shown in the double-logarithmic plot. A dose-dependent relationship for the activation of nitrosamines was found following pretreatment with phenobarbital, halothane, or 3-MC. Alkylation was less intensive in the low dose range in the cases of phenobarbital and halothane, whereas an enhanced alkylation rate was found at high doses. Administration of 3-MC led to diminished alkylation rates. However, the inhibition became less marked with increasing dosages, but did not exceed control values.

It is suggested that the main reason for this unusual behavior might be that various cytochrome P-450 species with different kinetic parameters catalyze the bioactivation of DMN. Additional causes cannot, however, be excluded (4-6).

---

[1] Deutsches Krebsforschungszentrum, Institut für Biochemie, Im Neuenheimer Feld 280, 6900 Heidelberg/FRG

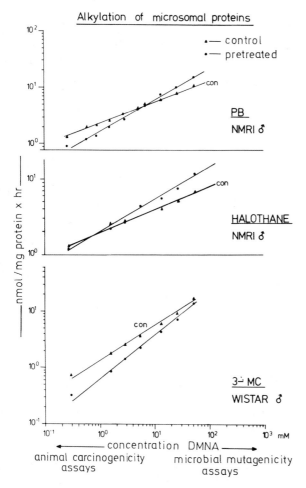

Fig. 1. Dependence of protein alkylation on ^{14}C-DMN concentrations in incubation samples of liver microsomes from NMRI mice pretreated with phenobarbital (*PB*) or *halothane* or from Wistar rats pretreated with 3-methylcholanthrene (*3-MC*). The microsomal incubation mixtures contained 4 mg protein/ml. The values are expressed as nmol [14]CH$_3$ groups covalently attached to microsomal proteins

The changes in intensity of alkylation under these conditions depend on the concentration of this promutagen, as well as on the inducer, the sex, and the species of the animals used. When an attempt is made to correlate the bioactivation of DMN in vitro with its carcinogenicity in vivo, the data obtained in vitro at high substrate concentrations are questionable. Since it is unlikely that hepatic DMN concentration approaches the high doses of the in vitro test, it is probable that the alkylation rate is in vivo more relevant to the results obtained at the lower DMN concentrations.

Furthermore, since it is well established that not only exogenous but also endogenous factors such as oxygen pressure and NADPH regeneration are responsible for the variable biologic effects of chemicals in vivo, the picture of the mutagenic effects of chemicals obtained by using in vitro techniques is necessarily incomplete. We therefore attempted to correlate alkylation rates found in vitro with those obtained in vivo by combining modifiers of the monooxygenase system with DMN.

Figure 2 shows the changes in the alkylation rates of bases in DNA in the presence of DMN as influenced by phenobarbital, 3-MC, SKF 525A, and halothane. Phenobarbital and 3-MC were found to diminish the alkylation rate, whereas SKF 525A and halothane produced an enhancement. These findings were expected on the basis of in vitro results obtained with DMN at low concentrations.

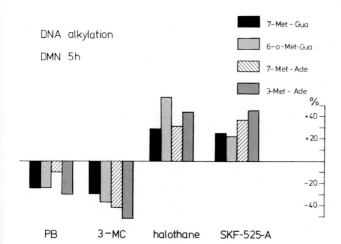

Fig. 2. Methylated bases eliminated from mouse liver DNA 5 h after i.p. injection of ^{14}C-DMN (10 mg/kg = 1 mCi/kg) and simultaneous application of various drugs. The changes are expressed as percentages of the controls. DNA was hydrolyzed under mild acidic conditions; base analyses were performed by ion-exchange chromatography on Aminex A 6 columns

Covalent binding of mutagens or carcinogens can lead to single-strand breaks in DNA (7). This sequential step has been measured at the cellular level by means of two in vivo techniques capable of detecting DNA damage (8,9).

Results obtained when carcinogen-treated DNA is passed through a filter under alkaline conditions are presented in Table 1. About 95% of untreated DNA (control) remains on the filter, whereas when the DNA is obtained from rat liver after treatment with various carcinogens in vivo, more nucleic acid passes through. However, this simple method is somewhat insensitive, as the inability of the carcinogen acetylaminofluorene to modify DNA shows. This technique has therefore not been used to study the quantitative extent of drug-carcinogen interaction.

Centrifugation of DNA through alkaline sucrose gradients offers a more sensitive method of investigating the extent of DNA breakage. Centrifugation profiles of rat liver DNA after treatment in vivo with increasing doses of DMN are shown in Fig. 3. Relative amounts of DNA are given on the ordinate, while the abscissa represents fractions of the gradient. The shift of the DNA peak to the top (left) indicates a lowering of the average molecular weight due to single-strand breakage.

The gradients were calibrated with SV 40 DNA in order that molecular weights might be determined. This centrifugation technique enabled us to study the influence of microsomal

Table 1. Effect of various foreign compounds administered in vivo on the alkaline elution characteristics of mouse liver DNA. Controls received vehicles only. DNA was measured colorimetrically by the diphenylamine method

Compound	Dose (mg/kg)	Duration of treatment (h)	% remaining on the filter $\pm$ SD	n
Control			96 ± 2.8	15
DMN	1	4	81 ± 3.5	5
DMN	5	4	62 ± 8.5	5
DMN	10	4	42 ± 6.5	5
DEN	100	1	56 ± 7.9	5
Nitrosomorpholine	100	4	61 ± 3.8	5
MMS	150	4	18 ± 2.3	5
AAF	20-100	4-24	98 ± 2.1	10
DAB	100	4	92 ± 2.5	5
CCL_4	2.5	4	95 ± 3.8	5

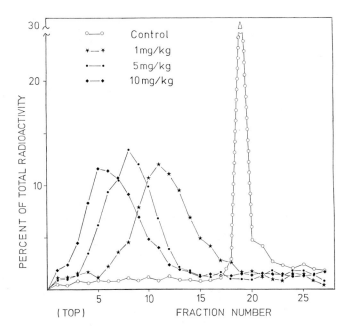

Fig. 3. Alkaline sucrose sedimentation profiles of hepatocellular DNA 4 h after treatment of rats with various doses of DMN. Cells were isolated and lysed on top of alkaline sucrose gradients through which the ^{3}H-thymidine-labelled DNA was centrifuged. Sedimentation was from *left to right*

inducers on the appearance and extent of carcinogen-induced single-strand breaks in DNA.

As shown in Fig. 4, pretreatment of the animals with phenobarbital results in a decreased number of DMN-induced strand breaks, here expressed as percentage of reduction of the weight-average

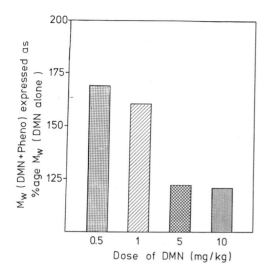

Fig. 4. Effect of phenobarbital pretreatment on the extent of DMN-induced DNA breakage. The data are expressed as percentages of the weight-average molecular weights (M_w) after DMN had been given in combination with phenobarbital in relation to M_w values obtained after DMN treatment alone. The rats were injected i.p. on 3 successive days with 80 mg/kg phenobarbital in order to induce cytochrome P-450. The M_w value of the control was 1.4×10^9 (n = 5)

molecular weights (M_w). This difference becomes progressively higher as the DMN dose is lowered. This inverse relationship is also in accordance with studies on alkylation rates of hepatic biopolymers (10).

Attention was then focused on in vivo conditions in tumor development, where it appears conceivable that cell proliferation kinetics are operative.

The irreversible enzyme-deficient foci of the liver provided a suitable tool for this study. Such foci are known to appear after the administration of nitrosamines and other carcinogens (Table 2). These enzyme-deficient areas (Fig. 5), commonly called "islands," some of which not only lack one or more enzymes but also show glycogen storage and/or positive gamma-glutamyltransferase (GGT) reaction, can be used as a cellular indicator of the mutagenic effect of the carcinogen in vivo. In our investigations we were measuring the ATPase-deficient foci as was originally done by Schauer and Kunze (11).

As we wanted to study the modifying effects of the drugs mentioned earlier, it was necessary at first to establish the relationship between amount and duration of carcinogen administration and the number and extent of these mutagenic lesions. Figure 6 shows the results of such an experiment, in which the animals received doses of diethylnitrosamine (DENA) from 2 to 10 mg/kg/day for periods of 2-6 weeks. The total size of the enzyme-deficient areas, as well as the number and the average size of the islands, increase linearly with time when recorded in a double-logarithmic plot. The slopes of the regression lines are different for each parameter, but are nearly parallel one with another. How small the variation proved to be becomes particularly evident in the narrow range of the 95% confidence interval for the mean regression line, which is hatched in. The inclination of the lines is independent of the doses given, the mode of application, and interference by other compounds.

Table 2. Comparisons of covalent binding to DNA, induction of single-strand breaks in DNA, appearance of enzyme deficiency in the liver, and carcinogenic capacity after in vivo administration of various well-established carcinogens and other miscellaneous compounds, including drugs and food additives

Compound	Covalent binding to DNA	DNA-strand breaks Filter elution	DNA-strand breaks Alk. gradient centrifugation	Enzyme-deficient cell areas	Carcino-genicity
DMN	+	+	+	+	+
DEN	+	+	+	+	+
Nitrosomorpholine	+	+	+	+	+
Nitrosopiperazine	+	O	+	+	+
Nitrosopyridine	+	O	+	+	+
Aminopyrine (1000 PPM)	O	O	O	-	-
Aminopyrine nitrite (>100 PPM)	O	O	O	+	+
Nitrite (>500 PPM)	O	O	O	+	+
DAB	+	-	O	+	+
Amaranth	O	O	O	-	?
Ponceau R6	O	O	O	-	-
Orange GGN	O	O	O	-	-
Chrysoine S	O	O	O	-	-
Sunset yellow	O	O	O	-	-
Fast yellow	O	O	O	-	-
AAF	+	-	+	+	+
Aflatoxin B_1	+	+	O	+	+
Ethionine	+	O	O	+	+
Vinylchloride	+	O	O	+	+
CCL_4	-	-	O	+	+
Phenobarbital	-	-	-	-	?
Halothane	-	-	-	-	?

+ = Positive, - = Negative, O = Not determined, ? = Questionable

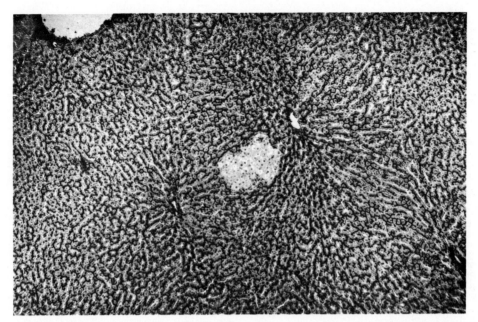

Fig. 5. Enzyme-histochemical demonstration of an ATPase-deficient area in rat liver

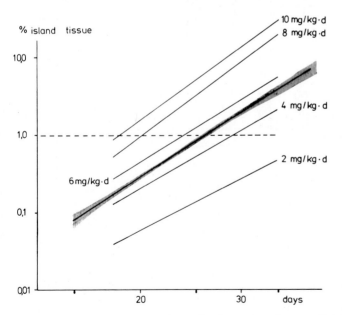

Fig. 6. Dependence of % island tissue on dose and time of DENA treatment. Female Sprague-Dawley rats were given the indicated dosages of DENA daily by stomach tube. After 2-6 weeks the animals were sacrified, and the relative extents of ATPase-deficient areas in the liver were determined morphometrically. The *hatched area* represents the 95% confidence interval of the mean regression line

The changes in total island tissue and island number were investigated using this method with regard to the influence of the same drugs that were used in the earlier experiments (Fig. 7). Phenobarbital and 3-MC decrease island formation, whereas halothane and SKF enhance it. In both instances we found a dose dependency of these changes which was the same as that found in our earlier experiments in vivo and in vitro. The lower the DENA dose given, the greater was the decreasing effect of phenobarbital and the greater was the increasing effect of halothane.

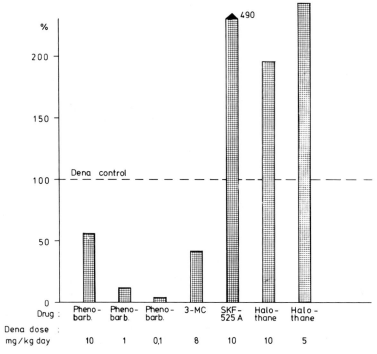

Fig. 7. Changes in total island tissue in the liver under the influence of various agents, as compared with DENA alone (*control*). The higher dosages of the carcinogen (5,7, and 10 mg/kg) were administered daily by stomach tube, whereas the lower doses were given continually in the drinking water. Phenobarbital-Na (0.1%) was included in the drinking water, whereas 3-MC (50 mg/kg i.p. twice weekly), SKF 525A (100 mg/kg i.p. 5 times weekly), and halothane (1%, 1h/day) were given in 1 h prior to carcinogen treatment over periods of 1-4 weeks

As our aim was to quantitate the effects of interfering substances a dose-time relationship had to be established for the carcinogen alone. This required an arbitrary response parameter as a reference. We chose the time that is needed to induce a 1% proportion of island tissue as a parameter of the preneoplastic effect of the carcinogen at various dose levels. For each daily dosage this "1% induction time" was derived from the data shown in Fig. 6. Then, in a second step of evaluation, these "1% induction times" (Fig. 8, abscissa) were plotted against the daily dosages (Fig. 8, ordinate). In a double-logarithmic plot there results a linear relationship between decreasing daily dose and increasing "1% induction time" (Fig. 8).

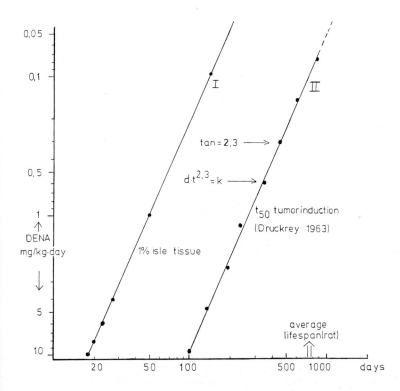

Fig. 8. Dose-time relationship of DENA-induced preneoplastic cell areas compared with that of liver tumors induced with the same carcinogen. We chose as arbitrary response parameter for the preneoplastic alterations that time required to induce a 1% proportion of island tissue in the liver (derived from the data in Fig. 6). Theses "1% induction times" are plotted against the daily dosages (I). The induction of liver tumors in 50% of the animals, found by Druckrey et al. (12), served as the parameter for tumor development (II). The "reinforcing action" of time is extremely similar in both instances

With this information the effective DENA dose can be calculated in experiments in which the carcinogen was combined with the interfering agents mentioned above. The time at which 1% island tissue was reached is marked on the abscissa in Fig. 8; then the corresponding value on the ordinate is taken as the effective DENA dose.

The second line in the graph (Fig. 8) shows the dose-time relationship for t_{50}, the induction time of liver tumors in 50% of the animals, a value which was determined by Druckrey et al. for DENA-induced liver tumors (12,13). The development of the total island size shows approximately the same "reinforcing action" of time as was found valid for tumor induction. So it is possible to draw quantitative conclusions from changes in preneoplastic lesions to tumor appearance independent of the causal or statistical basis of the similarity of the slopes.

The results of the experiments presented here can be summarized as follows:

The initial effects of various carcinogens in vitro and their mutagenic action in vivo have been studied under the influence of several modifying factors. The alteration in the mutagenic effect produced by the various modifying factors over the relevant concentration ranges of the carcinogen has always been in the same direction as that observed in corresponding long-term carcinogenicity studies. Two main conclusions can be drawn from these findings:

1. The concept that the initial effect of carcinogens is essentially a mutagenic one has been confirmed.
2. The experimental models presented here provide a means of studying in vivo the action of carcinogens as well as the influence of modifying endogenous and environmental factors. This can be done within relevant dose ranges and in much shorter times than those required in conventional carcinogenicity studies.

Acknowledgments. The authors gratefully acknowledge Dr. R. Jones for helpful discussions.

References

1. Bartsch H, Malaveille C, Montesano R (1976) The predictive value of tissue-mediated mutagenicity assays to assess the carcinogenic risk of chemicals. In: Montesano R, Bartsch H, Tomatis L (eds) Screening tests in chemical carcinogenesis. International Agency for Research on Cancer, Lyon
2. Makiura S, Aoe H, Sugihara S, Hirao K, Arai M, Ito N (1974) Inhibitory effect of polychlorinated biphenyls on liver tumorigenesis in rats treated with 3'-methyl-4-dimethylaminoazobenzene, N-2-fluorenylacetylamide and diethylnitrosamine. J Natl Cancer Inst 53:1253
3. Czygan P, Greim H, Garro JA, Utterer F, Schaffner E, Popper M, Rosenthal O (1973) Microsomal metabolism of dimethylnitrosamine and the cytochrome P-450 dependency of its activation to a mutagen. Cancer Res 33:2983
4. Arcos SC, Bryant GM, Venkatesan N, Argus MF (1975) Repression of dimethylnitrosamine-demethylase by typical inducers of microsomal mixed-function oxidases. Biochem Pharmacol 24:1544
5. Arcos SC, Davies DL, Brown GEL, Argus MF (1977) Repressible and inducible enzymic forms of dimethylnitrosamine-demethylase. Z Krebsforsch 89:181
6. Appel KE, Kunz HW (1978) Differences in binding of nitrosamines to cytochrome P-450. Possible relevance for their activation and inactivation. Naunyn Schmiedebergs Arch Pharmacol 302:R 20

7. Farber E (1973) Carcinogenesis — cellular evolution as a unifying thread: Presidential address. Cancer Res 33:2537
8. Petzold GL, Swenberg JA (1978) Detection of DNA damage induced in vivo following exposure of rats to carcinogens. Cancer Res 38:1589
9. Cox R, Damjanov I, Abanobi SE, Sarma DSR (1973) A method for measuring DNA damage and repair in the liver in vivo. Cancer Res 33:2114
10. Kunz W, Appel KE, Rickart R, Schwarz M, Stöckle G (1978) Enhancement and inhibition of carcinogenic effectiveness of nitrosamines. In: Remmer H, Bolt HM, Bannasch P, Popper H (eds) Primary liver tumours. MTP Press Ltd, Lancaster
11. Schauer H, Kunze E (1968) Enzymhistochemische and autoradiographische Untersuchungen während der Cancerisierung der Rattenleber unter Diäthylnitrosamin. Z Krebsforsch 70:252
12. Druckrey H, Schildbach A, Schmähl D, Preußmann R, Ivankovic S (1963) Quantitative Analyse der carcinogenen Wirkung von Diäthylnitrosamin. Z Arzneim Forsch 13:841
13. Druckrey H, Preußmann R, Ivankovic S, Schmähl D (1967) Organotrope carcinogene Wirkungen bei 65 verschiedenen N-Nitroso-Verbindungen an BD-Ratten. Z Krebsforsch 69:105
13a. Kunz W, Stöckle G, Appel K (1976) Quantitative analyses of enzyme-deficient cell areas to assess early precancerous alterations of hepatocarcinogenic substances. Naunyn Schmiedebergs Arch Pharmacol 293:R 65
13b. Schieferstein G, Pirschel S, Frank W, Friedrich-Freksa H (1974) Quantitative Untersuchungen über den irreversiblen Verlust zweier Enzymaktivitäten in der Rattenleber nach Verfütterung von Diäthylnitrosamin. Z Krebsforsch 82:191

The Microbial Host-Mediated Assay in Comparison with in Vitro Systems: Problems of Evaluation, Predictive Value and Practical Application

P. Arni[1]

Abstract

The purpose of investigations on mutagenicity using the host-mediated assay is, on the one hand, to demonstrate metabolites of those substances which are not mutagenic themselves. On the other hand, by applying this test system, relationship may be established between the mutagenic effect of a test substance in the animal and the dosage which is required to produce it.

The applicability of this test system is demonstrated by results which were obtained from different well-known mutagenic or carcinogenic substances. In addition, these results are compared with the data which were obtained with the Ames test, i.e., in vitro. The host-mediated assay proves to be a more suitable system for demonstrating conditions in vivo.

A comparison of the sensitivity of different indicator organisms in the host-mediated assay does not as yet allow definite conclusions with regard to the selection of the indicator organism of choice. For this reason it is advisable at present to use that indicator organism which has proved to be suitable for the respective substance or group of substances, in an in vitro assay.

At present, microorganisms are commonly employed in order to test chemical substances with regard to their mutagenic activity. For this purpose, bacteria and fungi are used with particular, genetically fixed properties. Induced mutants as well as those which developed spontaneously are visualized on selective media. Any mutagenic effect of the chemical substance tested is demonstrable by a comparison of the number of mutants in the treated and control cultures. These investigations are mostly carried out in vitro, and by addition of mammalian liver microsomes, metabolic activation of the test substance to mutagenic metabolites which possibly occurs in the mammalian organism is simulated. There is also the possibility to inject microorganisms into animals — preferably mice or rats — which have been treated with the test substance previously. When the cells after a certain length of time are recovered from the host organism, they can be examined as to whether the test substance or its metabolites have induced any mutations. In this approach, which is described as the "host-mediated assay", it is possible, on the one hand, to obtain mutagenic metabolites of an originally

---

[1]Ciba-Geigy AG, CH-4002 Basel/Switzerland

nonmutagenic substance which are formed either in the liver or in another organ of the host organism. On the other hand, a relationship can be established between the mutagenic action of a substance and a dose being effective within the animal, and this applies as well to direct mutagens as to metabolites.

The usefulness of a test system is generally judged by the amount of information obtainable therefrom, but even more by its sensitivity with regard to well-known mutagenic or carcinogenic substances. The reliability of the results which are obtained by a system of this kind depends essentially on the methods of investigation. Special significance should be attached to experiences which were made with a test system and equally to the interpretation of the results.

The host-mediated assay which we would like to discuss in this presentation is carried out in our laboratory with male NMRI mice (1). The test substance is given orally, subcutaneously, or intraperitoneally by administering one or three doses (Fig. 1). The strains of *Salmonella typhimurium* which were developed by Ames and co-workers are used as indicator organisms. 0.2 or 0.3 ml of a bacterial suspension containing approximately 10^{11} cells/ml is injected into the lateral tail vein immediately after administration of the last dose of the substance. The animals are killed 1 h after bacterial administration. The livers are removed and homogenized. Subsequently, the bacteria contained in the livers are recovered by centrifugation. For determination of the histidine prototrophic mutants, the undiluted bacterial suspensions are spread on minimal agar. This determination is carried out separately for each animal. Subsequently, two dilutions of the suspensions are spread on complete agar to obtain the total number of viable bacteria present in the livers. The results are given as either the number of mutants per plate or the number of mutants in respect to the number of bacteria which have survived, i.e., by mutant frequencies.

Investigations were performed with eight substances which are known to be mutagenic to *S. typhimurium*: diethylnitrosamine (DENA), isopropylmethanesulfonate (iPMS), cyclophosphamide, β-naphthylamine, 2-acetylaminofluorene, nitrofurantoin, FANFT, and 4-nitroquinoline-N-oxide.

After a single intraperitoneal (IP) administration of 2-acetylaminofluorene, no mutagenic effect was seen in this test system (Fig. 2). The same result was obtained with β-naphthylamine. After oral (PO) administration of a freshly prepared solution of the substance, there was no proof of mutagenic action either. When the experiment was carried out with a solution of β-naphthylamine that had been prepared the day before, an obvious dose-dependent effect occurred. Isopropylmethanesulfonate (iPMS) showed a clearly mutagenic action at the highest dose administered (1170 mg/kg). The mutagenic property of the substance was not seen after the administration of lower doses (390 and 130 mg/kg). Diethylnitrosamine (DENA) showed an obvious dose-dependent mutagenic effect when applied in this system (Fig. 3).

192

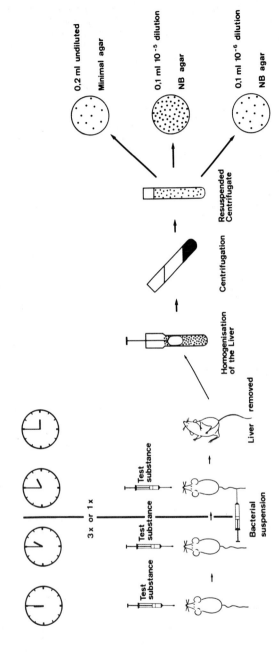

Fig. 1. Protocol for the host-mediated assay

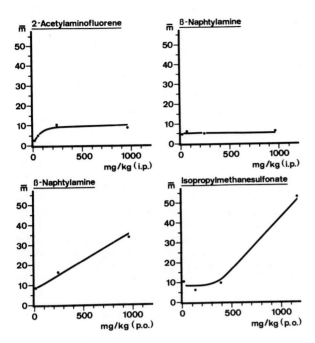

Fig. 2. Intrasanguine host-mediated assay with *S. typhimurium* TA 100; $\bar{m}$, mean number of mutant colonies per plate

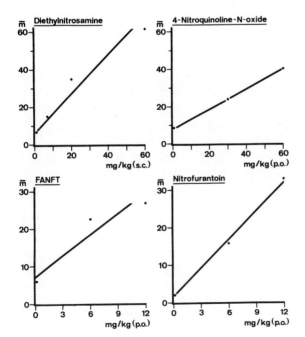

Fig. 3. Intrasanguine host-mediated assay with *S. typhimurium* TA 100; $\bar{m}$, mean number of mutant colonies per plate

Even when the lowest dose of 6.67 mg/kg was administered, a mutagenic effect was clearly recognizable. Cyclophosphamide, however, proved to have a relatively weak mutagenic action in this system. A mutagenic effect could be demonstrated when a dose of 390 mg/kg was administered. Clear relationships between dose and effect were seen with the direct mutagens FANFT and nitrofurantoin. Both substances showed clearly positive results after administration of a total dose of 6 mg/kg, the lowest dose tested in this experiment. Also, 4-nitroquinoline-N-oxide showed a mutagenic action after administration of doses of 30 and 60 mg/kg, respectively.

In Tables 1 and 2, the results which were obtained with the host-mediated assay, on the one hand, and the Ames test, on the other, are compared. The lowest doses are shown which were administered in the respective system and with which it was possible to demonstrate the mutagenic property of the corresponding substance. Some results of the Ames test which were obtained by employing S-9 liver fractions of noninduced mice are also shown.

Table 1. Intrasanguine host-mediated assay with *S. typhimurium* and Ames test, strain TA 100. Comparison of results obtained with promutagens

	Host-mediated assay mouse		Ames test Mouse liver microsomes Not induced		Rat liver microsomes Induced	
		mg/kg		mg/plate		mg/plate
Diethyl-nitrosamine	+ SC	6.7	+	5	+	~ 2.5
Isopropyl-methane-sulfonate	+ PO	<1170			+	~ 0.5
Cyclophospha-mide	+ PO	390	(+)	0.4	+	~ 0.2
β-Naphthyl-amine	− IP + PO	960 240	+	0.1	+	0.01
2-Acetyl-amino-fluorene	(−) IP	960			+	< 0.005 (TA 1538)

Table 1 shows the results obtained with indirect mutagens. When carrying out the experiments with the host-mediated assay, the findings resulting from the administration of DENA may be interpreted more easily than those obtained with the Ames test. Obviously, the short-lived metabolites can be better demonstrated in vivo than in vitro. This does not apply to the same extent to iPMS since in this case a certain concentration of the mutagenically effective metabolites is apparently needed for demonstrating mutagenic action with *S. typhimurium*. Another route of

Table 2. Intrasanguine host-mediated assay with *S. typhimurium* and Ames test, strain TA 100. Comparison of results obtained with ultimate mutagens

	Host-mediated assay, mouse		mg/kg	Ames test Without activation mg/Plate		With activation mg/Plate
FANFT	+	PO	< 6	+	$\sim 5 \times 10^{-6}$	+ $\quad 1.6 \times 10^{-3}$
Nitrofurantoin	+	PO	< 6	+	$\sim 6.25 \times 10^{-4}$	+ $\quad \sim 6.25 \times 10^{-4}$
4-Nitroquinoline-N-oxide	+	PO	~ 30	+	$\sim 6.25 \times 10^{-5}$	

administration would possibly show different results in the host-mediated assay.

As far as cyclophosphamide is concerned, we have already reported on the effectiveness of this substance and on variations with regard to the mutagenic effect which occurred with *S. typhimurium* within the intrasanguine host-mediated assay (1). In more recent investigations a weaker effect was observed than in earlier ones when this substance was administered PO in the same test system. An effect was obtained, repeatedly, however, with a single dose of 390 mg/kg. Within the host-mediated assay, cyclophosphamide is a relatively weak mutagen although this substance is satisfactorily absorbed and rapidly metabolized and excreted as well. 2-Acetylaminofluorene showed no clearly mutagenic action in the host-mediated assay, which may possibly be due to the insufficient absorption of the substance within the host animal.

β-Naphthylamine showed no mutagenic effect either after it had been administered IP. When the highest dose was administered, the substance was absorbed, however, since the animals showed symptoms of poisoning after they had been treated. With the PO administration of a substance solution which had been prepared the day before, a clearly mutagenic effect was proved. An explanation for these results can be given when they are compared with those that were obtained from long-term carcinogenicity tests carried out by Bonser et al. (3). In a freshly prepared solution the substance will produce only a weak carcinogenic effect after having been administered IP. A distinct effect could be observed, however, when the substance was administered PO or after IP administration of a solution which was allowed to age before injection. These findings may be explained by the fact that oxidation products of the substance are said to be responsible for the carcinogenic effect which will not develop with an IP administration of a freshly prepared substance solution. The same seems to apply to the mutagenic effectiveness of the substance.

Table 2 shows the results for three direct mutagens: the intrasanguine host-mediated assay using *S. typhimurium* as an indicator organism proves to be as suitable when applying FANFT and nitrofurantoin as it is when using DENA. Even a very small dose, far

below the LD50, is able to produce sufficient concentrations in
the animal to cause mutations, at least within the indicator
organism. When administering 4-nitroquinoline-N-oxide, a higher
dose is, however, necessary for proving the mutagenic property
with the host-mediated assay. For all three substances the Ames
test appears to be a very sensitive system.

At present, the sensitivity of various indicator organisms within
the host-mediated assay can only be compared to a limited degree. Too few substances have so far been examined under the
same conditions within this test system using different microorganisms. We have tested DENA with strain *S. typhimurium* TA 100
by administering doses similar to those employed by Mohn and
Ellenberger (4) with *Escherichia coli* 343/113. If one compares the
mutation frequency of *S. typhimurium* with those of the arginine
mutants reported by Mohn and Ellenberger, a similar relationship
appears to exist with regard to dose and effectiveness. Malling
and Frantz (5) demonstrated a weak mutagenic effect when they
administered IP 150 mg/kg DENA and used *Neurospora* as the indicator organism. It appears that under these circumstances bacteria
are much more sensitive than *Neurospora* or *Saccharomyces*. DENA,
however, is only mutagenic in the host-mediated assay when the
indicator organisms are administered by intravenous (IV) injection. Several investigators have examined cyclophosphamide in
the host-mediated assay by giving IP administrations of *S. typhimurium* strains or IV injections of *S. cerevisiae*. Relatively
high doses were administered since this substance has a relatively weak effect in the host-mediated assay. Braun and
Schöneich (6) were successful, however, in obtaining an effect
with strain *S. typhimurium* TA 1950 when they administered the substance subcutaneously (SC) at a dose of 200 mg/kg. 4-Nitroquin-
oline-N-oxide which was tested in the intrasanguine host-mediated
assay with *S. cerevisiae* by Fahrig (7) showed positive results.

Generally there is as no yet preferred indicator organism for
the host-mediated assay, although it would be desirable to
employ the most sensitive microorganism in respect to a substance or a group of substances within this system. Since, however, the host-mediated assay is relatively expensive compared
with investigations made in vitro, it is not possible to test
all substances with different indicator organisms. For common
usage that indicator organism should be employed which proved
to be suitable for the respective substance or group of substances when applied in the test in vitro.

At least for certain groups of substances the host-mediated
assay has proved to be a useful means of evaluating the mutagenic properties of chemical substances. We would like to
emphasize, however, that the results should be interpreted very
cautiously. Quite a number of factors may misrepresent the
evaluation or make it impracticable. The latter applies to
animals suffering from infectious diseases. This was observed
occasionally in our investigations. Furthermore, sometimes the
spontaneous mutation rate increases within a dosage group. This
was seen particularly when employing strains TA 98 and TA 1537.
It can be avoided, however, by using pooled bacterial suspensions

which have been prepared under exactly the same conditions for all groups of an experiment. If plates are incubated for more than 2 days, sometimes additional small colonies may grow on the minimal agar. These mutants have very probably developed later on the plate and should not be counted. The results may also be misinterpreted by the fact that there is no exact correlation between the number of surviving cells in the animal and the number of spontaneously developing revertants. A significant increase of the mutation frequency may be caused by a slight growth-inhibiting action of a substance or by an inaccurately prepared dilution for the determination of the total number of cells, there being no increase in the actual number of revertants. It is possible, however, to avoid false-positive results if one observes that in order to show a positive result not only must the mutation frequencies be increased but also the frequency of the revertants per plate in comparison with the control groups.

As to the information obtainable from the host-mediated assay and its practicable application we can say that, for substances which are not metabolized in the liver but in other organs, this method is the only possibility to see the effects of mutagenic metabolites for these substances with regard to microorganisms. These substances are, however, relatively rare. It would therefore not be justified to routinely test in the host-mediated assay each substance which showed negative results in the Ames test. The assay would only have an advantage if metabolic activation is expected outside of the liver, e.g., the alteration of a substance or the interaction of different substances in the alimentary tract.

An investigation using the host-mediated assay can provide valuable additional information on those substances which proved to be mutagenic in the Ames test by direct action as well as on those which need metabolic activation in order to demonstrate a mutagenic effect. As already explained, for some substances, a dose may be determined which shows an acute mutagenic effect in the animal.

Valuable information may also be obtained by the host-mediated assay after uncertain findings resulting from investigations made in vitro. Particularly, positive results may be confirmed with the host-mediated assay.

It is often said that the host-mediated assay is less sensitive in comparison to in vitro investigations. This consideration is, however, not justified, since the host-mediated assay does not only examine the mutagenic effect of a substance or of its metabolites on microorganisms. Other factors, such as absorption and detoxification, also play a decisive role. The results should, however, be very carefully evaluated and for the interpretation it would be desirable to know the kinetic properties of the test substance within the host organism.

In summary, we would like to state that the host-mediated assay may be recommended under the following conditions:

1. If metabolic activation of the test substance external to the liver is to be considered.
2. When a relationship is to be established between the effective dose in the whole animal and the positive results obtained in investigations made in vitro.
3. If questionable results from investigations made in vitro need to be confirmed.

For these reasons this test system should not be limited to basic research. It would be desirable to enlarge the data-base using well-known mutagenic or carcinogenic substances within the host-mediated assay. Negative findings are as important as positive ones and the results should be published.

Generally, the search for particular sensitive test methods should not be the only objective, but attempts should be made to evaluate more thoroughly the obtainable information of existing systems.

References

1. Arni P, Mantel Th, Deparade E, Müller D (1977) Intrasanguine host-mediated assay with Salmonella typhimurium. Mutat Res 45:291-307
2. Ames BN, McCann J, Yamasaki E (1975) Methods for detecting carcinogens and mutagens with the Salmonella/mammalian-microsome mutagenicity test. Mutat Res 31:347-364
3. Bonser GM, Clayson DB, Jull JW, Pyrah LN (1956) The carcinogenic activity of 2-naphthylamine. Br J Cancer 10:533
4. Mohn GR, Ellenberger J (1977) The use of Escherichia coli K 12/343/113 (λ) as a multipurpose indicator strain in various mutagenicity testing procedures. In: Kilbey BJ, Legator M, Nichols W, Ramet C (eds) Handbook of mutagenicity test procedures. Elsevier/North-Holland Biomedical Press, Amsterdam, pp 95-118
5. Malling HV, Frantz CN (1973) In vitro versus in vivo metabolic activation of mutagens. Environ Health Perspect 6:71-82
6. Braun R, Schöneich J (1975) The influence of ethanol and carbon tetrachloride on the mutagenic effectivity of cyclophosphamide in the host-mediated assay with Salmonella typhimurium. Mutat Res 31:191-194
7. Fahrig R (1975) Development of host-mediated mutagenicity tests —yeast systems. II. Recovery of yeast cells out of testes, liver, lung and peritoneum of rats. Mutat Res 31:381-394

Mutagenic and Carcinogenic Effects of Antimetabolites

E. V. GOLOVINSKY[1]

We are witnessing the total investigation of the carcinogenic
effect of organic compounds. The substances studied are of different molecular structures, varying both chemically (here we
could mention various azo, nitro, and nitroso compounds, metal
complexes with organic ligands, acids and their numerous derivatives, etc.) and biologically active substances (such as
pesticides, herbicides, industrial poisons, pharmaceutical and
perfumery products, and chemotherapeutic preparations).

I would like to discuss here some considerations concerning those
organic compounds which by their mechanism of action are referred to as the antimetabolites.

It is known that from the viewpoint of both theory and practice
that biologically active substances are usually classified by
the kind of effect they produce. Thus, drugs are divided into
substances influencing the regulation of physiologic functions,
substances influencing the function of organs, substances influencing tissue metabolism, chemotherapeutic preparations, etc.
On the other hand the substances used in agriculture as growth
and development regulators of plants are divided for instance
into auxins, cytokinins, retardants, defoliants, etc. In agriculture, pesticides, fungicides, insecticides, and many other
compounds are widely used.

The biologically active substances known at present and those
having biologic potential can be grouped not only according to
the effect they induce, but also by other criteria. One of
these criteria, the applications of which has become possible
due to the achievements of modern biochemistry, is the molecular
mechanism of action of the biologically active substances. The
most investigated at this time and the best delineated group
of these substances consists of the structural analogues-anta-
gonists of metabolites, viz. antimetabolites.

An antimetabolite's effect depends on its similarity in chemical
structure to normal intermediary metabolites, which leads to
biologic competition (antagonism) between the metabolite and its
structural analogue. A quantitative measurable manifestation of
this antagonism is the inhibition of one or more enzyme reactions as a result of which the growth of a cell or of an organism
is delayed. In this sense, antimetabolites are metabolic inhibitors.

---

[1] Institute of Molecular Biology, Bulgarian Academy of Sciences, 1113 Sofia/
Bulgaria

Usually, antimetabolites compete with a substrate of an enzyme reaction. This means that no covalent bonds are formed between any part of the enzyme molecule and the substrate analogue. Contrary to these "classic antimetabolites" there exist also those, both of natural and synthetic origin, which react with the enzyme. An example of metabolic analogues of this type are "the active-site-directed irreversible metabolic inhibitors" developed by Baker (10).

Antimetabolites are applied in different fields, but mainly as chemotherapeutic agents for the treatment of infectious diseases, (e.g., sulphonamides and nicotinic acid analogues), of viral infections (e.g., 5-bromo- and 5-iododeoxyuridine, p-fluorophenylalanine), and of malignant formations (e.g., 6-mercaptopurine, 5-fluorouracil, methotrexate, and cytarabine). Antimetabolites have been applied also as immunosuppressive drugs (e.g., Imuran), in agriculture (e.g., maleic acid hydrazide), etc. A number of antibiotics (e.g., penicillin, puromycin, and toyocamycin) are typical antimetabolites by their molecular mechanism of action (2).

Antimetabolites have an especially strong position in the cancer chemotherapy. They have been applied successfully together with groups of chemotherapeutic preparations such as the alkylating agents and the antibiotics. All antitumor agents affect one or the other of the metabolic links of information macromolecules (Fig. 1). This biochemical effect is the basis of the antitumor action of the agents investigated, but it is responsible for two other — unwelcome — effects: mutagenic and carcinogenic activity.

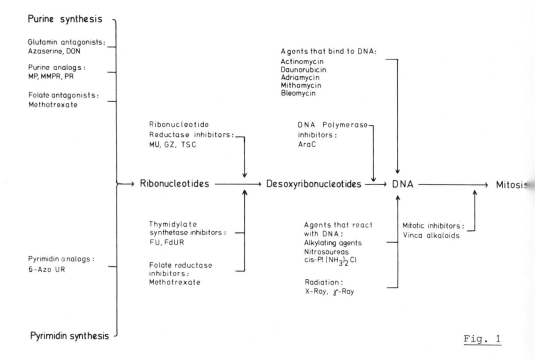

Fig. 1

Many authors find a parallelism between the carcinogenic and the mutagenic action of chemical compounds. If the carcinogenic and mutagenic actions are represented graphically by circles (3), then the overlapping of these circles increases every year. Only one antimetabolite, 5-bromodeoxyuridine, always remains outside the overlapping region. This substance has shown mutagenic activity, but appears not to be carcinogenic (3).

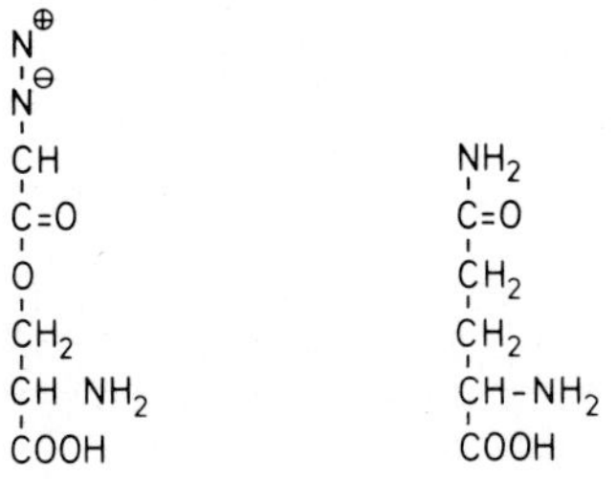

L-AZASERINE   L-GLUTAMINE

Fig. 2a

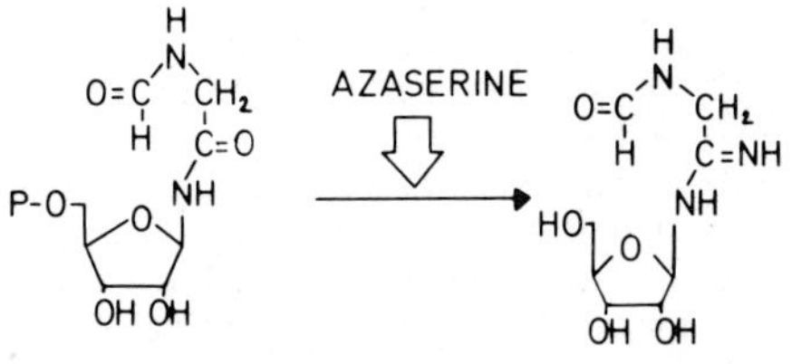

Fig. 2b

The same authors, basing their conclusions on the experimental material obtained with 240 compounds studied both for their carcinogenic and mutagenic actions, have found that in most cases mutagens are also carcinogens; the case of mutagens without a carcinogenic effect is most rare.

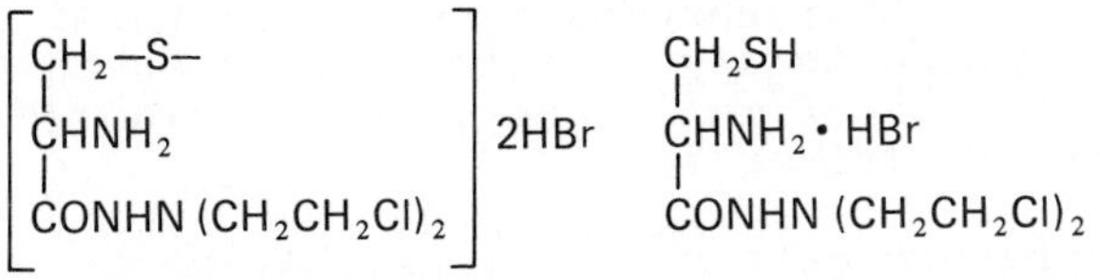

Fig. 3. A new substance effective against transplantable tumors in vivo: L-cystine-bis-(N,N-β-chloroethyl)-hydrazide (see 12)

The antimetabolites best characterized for their mutagenic action are predominantly the nucleoside analogues of pyrimidine and purine bases. It has been known for a long time that their mutagenic action is due to the possibility of the analogue being incorporated into DNA. Under appropriate conditions this incorporation could lead to point mutation (2).

Besides 5-bromodeoxyuridine, which already has been mentioned, mutagenic action has been shown for 5-bromouracil itself, and also for 5-iodouracil, 5-trifluoromethyluracil, 5-aminouracil and their 2'-deoxynucleosides, cytosine arabinoside, and a number of purine analogues, etc.

Recently some authors have demonstrated that many of the effective antitumor preparations have carcinogenic activity (4). Many of these substances have been proved to exert a carcinogenic effect in animals, and for some of them arguments have been presented on their possible carcinogenic action in man. It should be noted that the antitumor substances having a carcinogenic action are chiefly alkylating agents. Evidence for this can be found in the Programme of the International Agency for Cancer Research (5). It has been shown that, for instance, cyclophosphamide and melphalan have a carcinogenic effect, as do other alkylating agents, such as nitrogen mustard, aziridine and its derivatives, and other substances with an alkylating action. Marquardt (4) has observed that the antimetabolites used in the chemotherapy of cancer, i.e., methotrexate and purine and pyrimidine analogues, are able to induce malignant transformations in vitro, but the carcinogenic action of these substances has not yet been determined in vivo. In fact, these authors point out that only relatively few carcinogenicity tests of cytostatics have been performed (4). A similar conclusion about the absence of a carcinogenic effect of 6-mercaptopurine and methotrexate is reported by Benedict et al. (6), in spite of the literature evidence of lymphomas and lymphosarcomas in experiments with mice after 6-mercaptopurine administration.

In animals, Schmähl and Osswald (16) have compared the effect of alkylating agents nitrogen mustard (HN$_2$), its oxide Mitomen, cyclophosphamide (Cytoxan), mannomustin, thiotepa, triaziquone, procarbazine, and mitomycin C with that of the antimetabolites 5-fluorouracil, 6-mercaptopurine, methotrexate, vinblastine, and colchicine on the induction of tumors in rats and mice. The alkylating agents varied in their carcinogenic potency from the low activity of busulphan to high potency, as might have been expected for earlier experiments with procarbazine, whereas none of the antimetabolites were tumorigenic, Schmähl's colleagues failed to find any correlation between the carcinogenicity of these compounds and their immunosuppressive action. This work confirms the general impression that the reactive electrophilic biologic alkylating agents, which occupy a central position in modern concepts of the initiation of malignancy, are carcinogenic, whereas antimetabolites are not (after 7).

One way or another the literature data convince us that antimetabolites, at least those applied in cancer chemotherapy, contrary to the other preparations used for the same purposes, do not have a carcinogenic action or their carcinogenic action is weakly expressed.

It is necessary, however, to dwell longer on two antimetabolites, which have been shown to be carcinogenic and in this sense are an exception to the other representatives of this group, ethionine and azaserine.

Ethionine is the ethyl analogue of methionine. Its diverse biologic effects are attributed mainly to the fact that ethionine can substitute for methionine in enzyme reactions which use the latter amino acid. The ethionine is activated to S-adenosylethionine. This activated form of the antimetabolite does not transfer methyl, but ethyl, groups to the corresponding acceptors, which results in abnormal modified metabolites. Owing to this mechanism ethionine can "ethylate," or otherwise alkylate proteins, nucleic acids, choline, creatine, and many other substrates. The carcinogenic action of ethionine may be due to this ethylating property, and not to the formal structural analogy with the metabolite (1).

Therefore, in this case we do not have an effect due to competition with a substrate or to incorporation into a biopolymer as with "classic" antimetabolites, but to alkylation. The alkylating action of a series of substances including cytostatics is known to be the cause of their carcinogenic action (8).

L-Azaserine, on the other hand, which is an analogue of L-glutamine (Fig. 2a) also is not a "classic" antimetabolite. On the contrary, unlike competitive inhibitors, azaserine binds covalently to the enzyme inhibited, phosphoribosylformylglycineamine synthetase (Fig. 2b). The interaction of azaserine with the active site of the enzyme is an alkylation of the catalytic protein through the reactive diazo group (9).

Table 1. L-Cystine-bis-(N,N-β-chloroethyl)-hydrazide

Tumor	Dose (mg/kg)	Application in successive days	% Suppression
1. Myeloma P-8	6	8	100
2. Sarcoma 180	12	8	100
(Crocker)	8	10	50
3. Carcinosarcoma Walker	10	8	100
4. Lymphosarcoma Pliss	5	9	60
	10	10	100
5. Sarcoma Yoshida[a]	5	10	100
6. Sarcoma Jensen	5	10	75
7. Ehrlich ascites tumor	5	10	No suppression

[a]The animals under observation for a 120-day period: 5 survived without traces of tumor tissue; 1 died on the 35th day (recurrence?). All control animals died between the 18th and 26th day

Thus, in the case of azaserine we do not have an ordinary antimetabolite, but rather a typical "active-site-directed irreversible inhibitor" in the sense propounded by Baker (10). Though I am not in the possession of data about the carcinogenic effect of "nonclassic antimetabolites" of the type of Baker's inhibitors, it may be assumed that these substances could exhibit a definite carcinogenic action similar to azaserine. The same carcinogenic effect might be expected with antimetabolites having a molecule with alkylating residues.

An example is the cytostatic agent developed by our research team: L-cystine-Bis-N,N-(2-chloroethyl)-dihydrazide ("cydrine"). This substance is a modified antimetabolite (like cystine hydrazide) but with two alkylating (2-chloroethyl) groups (Fig. 3). This agent has shown a high antitumor activity with transplantation tumors in vivo (11,12) (Table 1). It also had alkylating reactivity under the conditions of the reaction with NBP reagent (13) and suppressed DNA biosynthesis to a considerable degree (14). Taking into consideration all these data, we investigated the mutagenic action of the substance (15).

For the investigation of the mutagenic action of "cydrine" we used an auxotrophic strain of *Escherichia coli* 3462 of genotype his^-, lac^+, mal^+, rha^+, str^s, fla^+, wF^+. In a mutagenicity test we expected the appearance of changes in the genome of the auxotrophic strain under the effect of cydrine and its reversion to prototrophy. We established that in fact the strain investigated did revert to prototrophy under the action of the substance studied. The reversion rate expressed as the ratio of the number of reverted cells to the number of cells inoculated initially (in percentage) was determined in several ways: by inoculation in a minimal nutritional medium; by inoculation in a histidine-enriched medium and after cell growth the colonies were replica plated according to Lederberg on Petri dishes containing minimal agar; and by inoculation in tubes with liquid histidine-enriched medium in which case after the growth of the culture the contents of each tube was inoculated in a Petri dish with a histidine-enriched agar, wherefrom the colonies cultivated were printed in dishes containing minimal agar. The results showed that in the first case the reversion rate was 0.3×10^{-6}%; in the second, 0.2×10^{-6}%; and in the third, 0.7×10^{-6}%.

Cydrine has most probably also a carcinogenic action considering its marked alkylating activity due to the presence of two reactive alkylating groups. Investigations in this respect are presently being carried out.

Summing up the examples presented it might be predicted with a considerable degree of certainty that in the synthesis of a new antimetabolite, in particular a pyrimidine or purine analogue, if it is found that the analogue is incorporated into DNA (or at least there are theoretical considerations for such an incorporation), then the analogue might be expected to be mutagenic also. At the same time it could be asserted with almost complete certainty that this analogue should not show a carcinogenic action. An exception in this respect might be the case when the analogue has also an alkylating action, or otherwise is able to react irreversibly with biopolymers.

It seems to me that the experimental evidence, already quite impressive today, suggests that similar predictions could not be made for any other group of mutagens.

References

1. Golovinsky E (1975) Biochemistry of antimetabolites. Nauka i Izkustvo, Sofia (Bulg, Summary in Engl)
2. Langen P (1975) Antimetabolites of nucleic acid metabolism. Gordon and Breach, New York, London, Paris
3. Sugimura T, Sato S, Nagao M, Yahagi T, Matsushima T, Seino Y, Takeushi M, Kawachi K (1976) In: Magee PN et al. (eds) Fundamentals in Cancer Research. University Park Press, Baltimore
4. Marquardt H (1930) Induction of malignant transformation and mutagenesis in cell cultures by cancer chemotherapeutic agents. Cancer 40:1930
5. Tomatis L, Agthe C, Bartsch H, Huff J, Montesano R, Saracci R, Walker W, Willbourn J (1978) Evaluation of the carcinogenicity of chemicals: a review of the Monography Program of the International Agency for Research on Cancer (1971-1977). Cancer Res 38:877
6. Benedict W, Baker M, Hauroun L, Choi E, Ames B (1977) Induction of morphological transformation in mouse C3H/10T1/2 clone 8 cells and chromosomal damage in hamster a(T1)C1-3 cells by cancer chemotherapeutic agents. Cancer Res 37:2209
7. Clayson DB, Shubik P (1976) The carcinogenic action of drugs. Cancer Detect Prevent. 1:43
8. IARC Monographs on the evaluation of cancerogenic risk of chemicals to man. IARC Lyon 1975
9. Gale E, Reinolds P, Cundliffe E, Richmond M, Waring M (1972) The molecular basis of antibiotic action. Wiley and Sons, New York
10. Baker B (1967) Design of active-site directed irreversible enzyme inhibitors. Wiley and Sons, New York
11. Aleksiev B, Stoev S, Spassov, Maneva L, Emanuilov E, Golovinsky E (1972) Amino acid derivatives. Bulg Pat 21479, US Pat 3897494, 1975
12. Golovinsky E, Aleksiev B, Spassov A, Stoev S, Emanuilov E, Angelov I, Maneva L, Stoychev Ts (1977) A new substance effect against transplantable tumors in vivo L-cysteine-bis-(N,N-betachloroethyl)-hydrazide. Neoplasma 24:401
13. Lozeva S, Golovinsky E (1975) C R Acad Bulg Sci 28:947
14. Rousev G, Emanuilov E, Angelov I, Golovinsky E (1974) Rapid procedure for the determination of DNA synthesis inhibition by cytostatic in Ehrlich ascites tumor cells. C R Acad Bulg Sci 27:1815
15. Markov K, Shivarova N, Maneva L, Golovinsky E (1975) C R Acad Bulg Sci 28:1549
16. Schmähl D, Osswald H (1970) Experimentelle Untersuchungen über carcinogene Wirkungen von Krebs-Chemotherapeutica und Immunosuppressiva. Arzneim Forsch 20:1461-1467

Section III

Use of Mammalian Cells for Short-Term Testing of Carcinogens

Mutagen-Metabolizing Enzymes in Mammalian Cell Cultures: Possibilities and Limitations for Mutagenicity Screening

F. J. Wiebel[1], L. R. Schwarz[1], and T. Goto[2]

Introduction

A large variety of mammalian cells in culture are available which could serve as sensitive indicators for the mutagenic action of chemicals. A critical factor for their applicability as screening systems for mutagenicity is their capacity to metabolize premutagens to their reactive forms. Indeed, in cultured mammalian cells as well as in other in vitro test systems the metabolic activation of chemicals is the facet which most frequently gives rise to misinterpretation of their mutagenic potential. Many cultured cell lines of interest for mutagenicity studies were found to activate premutagens or carcinogens very poorly if at all (1-4). To overcome this defect, test cells were fortified with extraneous activation systems which consist either of "feeder" cells that actively metabolize xenobiotics (3,4) or of cell fractions such as postmitochondrial supernatant and microsomes from rodent liver (5-8). Although both approaches proved to be satisfactory for the detection of many premutagens, they are limited by some inherent deficiencies, primarily by the possible failure of reactive intermediates formed outside the cell to reach the target either because they are too short-lived or are trapped by intracellular inactivation reactions. Optimally, in screening for potential mutagens, the test cells used as indicators for genetic damage should be fully competent in the activation of the test compounds. The use of intact cells in culture which mimic the in vivo conditions more closely may also be helpful in obtaining some information on the potency of a mutagenic compound.

The following discussion concerns the possibilities and limitations of using mammalian cells in culture for mutagenicity testing, i.e., possibilities and limitations arising from the specificity and level of their mutagen-metabolizing enzymes.

The activation of the majority of premutagens and precarcinogens occurs via the oxidative metabolism by microsomal monooxygenases (2,9,10). These enzymes are therefore of crucial importance for setting up any mutagenicity test systems and will be in the foreground of this presentation. Enzymes which convert the primary oxidation products to usually more polar metabolites such as

[1]Abteilung für Toxikologie, Gesellschaft für Strahlen- und Umweltforschung, Ingolstädter Landstr. 1, D-8042 Neuherberg/München/FRG

[2]Salem GmbH, Forschungslaboratorium, D-8000 München/FRG
Present address: National Defense Medical College, Dept. Biochem. Tokorosawa, Japan

conjugases or hydratase require attention as well in view of both their deactivating functions and their occasional involvement in the activation of chemicals (11-13). They will be the subject of the latter part of this presentation.

Monooxygenase Activity in Mammalian Cells in Culture

In the majority of studies in cultured cells, monooxygenase activity is determined by the oxygenation of benzo(a)pyrene (BP) to fluorescent phenolic products, which is variously called BP hydroxylase, aryl hydrocarbon hydroxylase, or BP monooxygenase. (In the present report the terms aryl hydrocarbon hydroxylase and BP monooxygenase are used interchangeably.) This reaction was preferentially used not only because it offered the most sensitive assay for monooxygenase activity but also because it is carried out by at least two different forms of the enzyme (14,15). In the following, the oxygenation of BP will serve as an example for quantitative and qualitative aspects of monooxygenase activity in cultured cells to point out some of their principal features in regard to mutagen metabolism. However, it is important to realize that this activity is unlikely to be representative of all monooxygenase forms (see below) that are possibly contained in cultured cells.

Table 1 shows the spectrum of cells which contain BP monooxygenase. The activity occurs in cell lines from rodents and man, from fetal, newborn, and adult organisms, from hepatic and extrahepatic tissues, and in cells transformed by chemicals or by viruses. Highest enzyme activities are generally found in newly isolated embryonic cells from rodents. In established cell lines the monooxygenase activity is usually 1-2 orders of magnitude lower, with some exceptions, notably the hepatoma cells, H-4-II-E. Whenever monooxygenase activity is detectable in tissue culture cells it is also inducible by polycyclic hydrocarbon type inducers. Furthermore, Table 1 shows that cells used in mutagenicity and transformation assays contain widely varying levels of monooxygenase activities. Thus, primary embryonic hamster cells (16) exhibit relatively high enzyme activity which at the induced level is comparable to the activity in the liver of untreated rodents (Table 1). BHK21 and 3T3 cells (17-19) show intermediate monooxygenase levels, and in V79 cells (20) no BP monooxygenase activity is detectable (Table 1). A number of observations have shown that monooxygenase activity in cultured cells may increase beyond the maximal level induced by polycyclic hydrocarbons upon exposure to dexamethasone (21) or cyclic AMP as well as to inhibitors of cyclic nucleotide phosphodiesterase (22,23,24). Alteration of the cyclic AMP level was found to enhance significantly cellular susceptibility to carcinogenic polycyclic hydrocarbons (22).

Table 1. Benzo(a)pyrene monooxygenase activity in cultured cells

Cultures	BP monooxygenase activity (pmol/mg protein/30 min)	
	Control	Induced[a]
Short-term cultures		
1. Secondaries, fetal, golden hamster[b]	80	600
2. Secondaries, fetal, BALB/C mouse[c]	95	420
3. Epithelial, skin, newborn BALB/C mouse[c]	26	181
4. Fibroblast, skin, newborn BALB/C mouse[c]	11	114
5. Lymphocytes, human[d]	<1	2
6. Lymphocytes, mitogen-treated, human[d]	2	12
7. Monocytes, human[d]	<1	7
Cell lines		
8. H-4-II-E, hepatoma, rat[c]	230	3000
9. JEG-3, choriocarcinoma, human[e]	4	150
10. OBP, fetal, golden hamster[c]	2	110
11. BRL 3C4, epithelial, liver, rat[e]	5	80
12. 3T3-4C2, fibroblast, Swiss mouse[e]	10	75
13. 3T3-A31, fibroblast, BALB/C mouse[e]	3	20
14. JLSV-5, spleen-thymus, mouse[e]	5	50
15. BHK21 (C13) newborn, Syrian hamster[f]	3	48
16. A-549, epithelial, lung, human[c]	2	24
17. DON-C, Chinese hamster[c]	4	20
18. RBM 2454, mouse x human hybrid[e]	<1	11
19. XP-2, skin, fibroblast, human[c]	<1	14
20. FIII, fibroblast, rat[c]	<1	12
21. BHK-TK⁻, fetal, golden hamster[e]	<1	3
22. VA-2, newborn, Syrian hamster[e]	<1	2
23. RAG, carcinoma, kidney, BALB/C mouse[e]	<1	<1
24. V-79, lung, Chinese hamster[c]	<1	<1
25. L-A9, fibroblast, C3H/An mouse[e]	<1	<1

[a] Cultures were exposed to benz(a)anthracene (1 µg/ml growth medium) for 18 h. BP monooxygenase activity was determined as described by Wiebel et al. (24)
[b] Cultures were prepared as described by Nebert and Gelboin (32)
[c] Cell lines (cf. numbers of first column) were kindly provided: [19] by Dr. R.S. Day III; [13] by Dr. T. Kakunaga; [3,4,17,24] by Dr. S.H. Yuspa; all NCI, Bethesda; [8] by Dr. B. Thompson; [16] by Dr. S. Brown, NIH, Bethesda; [20] by Dr. G. DiMayorca, University of Illinois
[d] [5,6] data from Whitlock et al. (63); and [7] from Bast et al. (64)
[e] The source of these cultures is described: [9,10,12,21,22,25] in Wiebel et al. (33); [14] in Wiebel et al. (34); [11] in Whitlock et al. (65); [23] in Brown et al. (61)
[f] [15] from American Type Tissue Culture Collection

BP Monooxygenase in Human Primary Amnion Cells

Ideally, mutagen metabolism and genetic effects are assessed in competent *human* cells. However, in regard to mutagen activation the prospects of using human cells in established cultures appear not to be very bright. Monooxygenase activity in human cells in culture which are mostly of fibroblastoid nature was found to be very low or undetectable (1,26, and Table 1). The epitheloid choriocarcinoma cells JEG (Table 1) which exhibit appreciable enzyme levels (15) are difficult to grow and are unsuitable for large-scale or routine investigations.

Thus, the use of primary epithelial cells, if they are readily obtainable, might be of considerable interest and has been explored by various groups (27-29). Recently we have described the culturing of human amnion cells from placenta at term (30). These cells form confluent monolayers of epithelial appearance and contain only a very few fibroblastlike cells during the first week in culture. Figure 1 shows the time course of induction of aryl hydrocarbon monooxygenase in amnion cultures on the 2nd and 5th days after plating. Enzyme activity increases rapidly in the presence of the inducer, benz(a)anthracene, from very low levels to activities which are in the range of those in rodent fibroblasts in culture or in primary fetal human liver cells (31). The time course of induction was similar to that in other established or short-term cultures (21,32-34).

Although these data are promising, some obstacles to the use of these cells in genetic toxicology will have to be overcome. One apparent drawback is the limited life span of these epithelial cells in culture, which does not exceed a few weeks. The short life span is accompanied by a decrease in monooxygenase activity with time in culture as shown in Fig. 2. The enzyme inducibility remains fairly stable during the first 5 days in culture to decrease to about 1/3 on the 8th day. If cultures are subdivided and subcultured, the enzyme levels are reduced further. Under these conditions the primary amnion cells may readily be

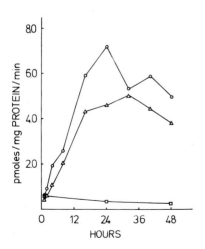

Fig. 1. Kinetics of aryl hydrocarbon hydroxylase induction in human amnion cells in primary culture [Goto and Wiebel (30)]. Cells were exposed to 13 µM BA on the 2nd (o) and 5th (Δ) days in culture. Control plates received DMSO (□) on the 2nd day. Cells were harvested at times indicated and assayed for in vitro enzyme activity. Other conditions as described by Goto and Wiebel (30)

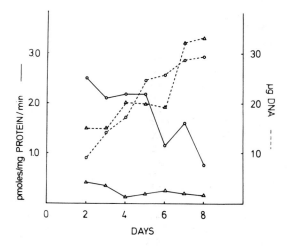

Fig. 2. Inducibility of aryl hydrocarbon hydroxylase activity and DNA content of cell cultures at various times after plating (30). BA was added to 1-8-day-old cultures for 24 h. Controls received DMSO. DNA determination and enzyme assays were performed on the same cell homogenates. (Δ) DMSO-treated cells; (o) BA-treated cells; ——— aryl hydrocarbon hydroxylase activity; ----- DNA content. Other conditions as described by Goto and Wiebel (30)

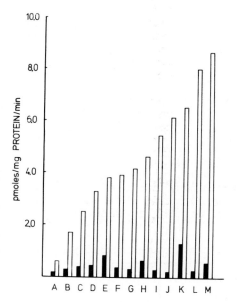

Fig. 3. Induction of aryl hydrocarbon hydroxylase activity in cultured amnion cells from 13 individuals (30). Cell inocula ranged from 4×10^5 to 1.2×10^6 cells/ml. Cultures were incubated for 24 h except from donors B and J (48 h and 72 h, respectively) and exposed to 13 μM BA (□) or DMSO (■) for 24 h. Values represent the mean of duplicate determinations from 2 to 4 cultures. Other conditions as described by Goto and Wiebel (30)

used to assess genetic damage by chemicals during their first few days in culture but not at later times. A more serious complication is presented by the variability of the enzyme activity in cultures derived from different donors. As shown in Fig. 3, "constitutive" and induced enzyme levels vary by a factor of 10. In amnion cells from one placenta (donor A) the activity is exceptionally low. Presently, we do not know the reasons for the variability in enzyme levels, whether it is of experimental, genetic, or environmental origin. Obviously, the variability precludes the application of human amnion cells in standard tests unless large batches of cells from many individuals have been pooled and stored. So far, this has not been achieved with these cells. Although these cultures are not suit-

able for screening of mutagens, they appear to be very useful
to study the intracellular activation and the interaction of
mutagens with cellular components of human cells and specifically epithelial cells which are major targets of chemical carcinogens.

Specificity of Monooxygenases in Cell Cultures

The observations presented in the foregoing have been concerned
merely with quantitative aspects of monooxygenase activity in
cultured cells. It is well established that monooxygenases comprise a whole family of enzymes which differ in their catalytic,
spectral, electrophoretic, and immunologic properties (35-37).
Two points are of particular relevance in this context: (a) the
monooxygenases have a broad but overlapping substrate specificity,
and (b) the different enzyme forms may oxygenate substrates preferentially in specific positions of the molecule. For the purpose of the following discussion roughly two groups of monooxygenases will be distinguished (Table 2) which are characterized,
for example, by their induction by phenobarbital or by a polycyclic hydrocarbon such as 3-methylcholanthrene (MC) and by their
spectral properties from which the two groups derive their names:
cytochrome P-450-dependent and cytochrome P-448-dependent monooxygenases, respectively.

The low content of monooxygenases in cultured cells and the small
amount of material available renders a purification and proper
identification of various enzyme forms virtually impossible. To
date, the characterization of the monooxygenases in cultured
cells depends largely on indirect evidence. Presently, all observations suggest that cells in continuous culture contain predominantly, if not exclusively, the cytochrome P-448-dependent
monooxygenase form(s). One indication for the presence of this

Table 2. Some properties of two major forms of microsomal monooxygenases[a]

	Cytochrome(s) "P-450"	Cytochrome(s) "P-448"
Inducer	Phenobarbital	3-Methylcholanthrene
Time course of induction	Several days	$\sim$ 24 h
Inducibility	2-3-fold	3-100-fold
Main tissue localization	Liver	Liver and extrahepatic tissues
In vitro modification	Stimulation by 7,8-BF	Inhibition by 7,8-BF
Typical Substrates	Nitrosamines, cyclophosphamide	Polycyclic aromatic hydrocarbons

[a]Each of the monooxygenase forms may comprise more than one enzyme entity.
The properties of the two forms listed should not be taken as exclusive
since for all of them some overlap has been observed

form is the selective inducibility by polycyclic hydrocarbon
type inducers and the lack of response to phenobarbital-type
inducers in established cells in culture. A second line of
evidence comes from the susceptibility to modifiers of the enzyme, such as the synthetic flavonoid, 7,8-benzoflavone (15,38).
This compound strongly inhibits polycyclic hydrocarbon induced
aryl hydrocarbon hydroxylase (cytochrome P-448 forms) but stimulates or does not affect cytochrome P-450-dependent hydroxylase of liver. As shown in Fig. 4, benzoflavone inhibits the
enzyme of both untreated and benz(a)anthracene-treated H-4-II-E
hepatoma cells to a similar degreee, suggesting a predominance
of cytochrome P-448 type monooxygenases independently of the
state of induction. Similar results have been obtained in all
cells in long-term culture studied so far (38,39). It is of
interest that the MC-inducible monooxygenase form apparently
predominates also in most extrahepatic tissues of rodents (15,
for review see Wiebel, 38).

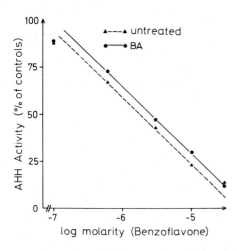

Fig. 4. In vitro effect of 7,8-benzo-
flavone on aryl hydrocarbon hydroxylase activity of untreated and inducer-
treated H-4-II-E cells. Cultures were
exposed to 13 µM BA for 18 h. 7,8-
Benzoflavone (50 µM, final) was added
in 40 µl methanol together with the substrate, BP (100 µM, final). In vitro
aryl hydrocarbon hydroxylase activity
was determined as described earlier
(24). 100% of control corresponds to
monooxygenase activity in the absence
of 7,8-benzoflavone

A third indication for the presence of specific forms of monooxygenase in cultured cells is derived from the metabolite
pattern of BP. Table 3 summarizes the oxidative attack in
various regions of the BP molecule by preparations of cultured
cells and liver microsomes. It is apparent that the oxygenation
of BP by the enzymes from these two sources differs greatly:
The monooxygenases of hamster and mouse embryo cells attack
more strongly the benzo ring of BP, i.e., positions 7-10, whereas
the enzymes of hepatic microsomes of rat, mouse, and hamster predominantly oxygenate the pyrene side of the molecule. It remains
to be established how representative the metabolic profile of
BP in these secondary embryo cells is for other cell lines in
culture. Striking in these and in other cells in culture (27,
40,41) is the apparent lack of formation of 4,5-dihydrodiol
which is a major product in hepatic microsomes particularly
after treatment with phenobarbital (42,43), and the substantial
formation of the 7,8- and 9,10-diols which are preferably produced in hepatic microsomes after MC treatment (42-44).

Table 3. Position-specific benzo(a)pyrene metabolism in cultured cells and liver microsomes (41)

Cells in culture	(% of total metabolites)[a]	
Hamster embryo	55	18
Mouse embryo	58	21
Liver microsomes		
Hamster	12	84
Mouse	34	62
Rat[b]	30	54

[a] Numbers represent the sum of phenols and dihydrodiols as percent of total metabolites in the two major regions of the BP molecule indicated. BP metabolites were separated by HPLC (41)
[b] Data from Selkirk et al. (41)

The data clearly show that the metabolism of BP in cultured cells and in microsomes from liver may significantly differ, suggesting the presence or predominance of different forms of monooxygenases in the two systems. This obviously has major implications for the activation of chemicals to their mutagenic or carcinogenic forms in view of the position-specific oxidation of chemicals by different monooxygenase forms to products of widely differing biologic activity. A case may be made for BP. A growing number of observations indicate that 7,8-diol-9, 10-epoxides are the most mutagenic and possibly the ultimate carcinogenic forms of BP (45,46), i.e., those BP metabolites which are preferentially formed in the cultured cells. Thus, these cells in culture offer an excellent activation system for BP and most likely for other polycyclic hydrocarbons such as MC and 7,12-dimethylbenz(a)anthracene which undergo similar activation steps as BP (47,48). However, although the presence of the MC-inducible cytochrome P-448 form may insure the activation of polycyclic hydrocarbons and of other substrates, the apparent lack of phenobarbital-inducible cytochrome P-450 form(s) is bound to mask the mutagenicity of those chemicals which are substrate for the latter monooxygenases as, for example, the nitrosamines. The incompetence of established cell lines, at least of those investigated so far and employed in the detection of mutagens, to metabolize all classes of premutagens renders these cells unsuitable as self-reliant, general test systems of mutagenicity. Presently, the lack of some monooxygenase forms, notably the phenobarbital-inducible cytochrome P-450-dependent form in established cell cultures, appears to be the single major drawback to their usefulness as mutagenicity testers.[1]

[1] See note added in proof (page 225).

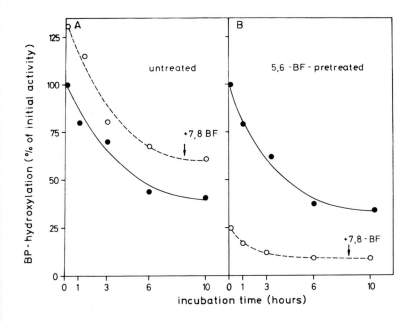

Fig. 5A,B. Aryl hydrocarbon hydroxylase activity of cultured hepatocytes
(51). Hepatocytes were isolated following the method of Baur et al. (62)
from (A) untreated rats or (B) rats treated with 5,6-benzoflavone. In vitro,
7,8-benzoflavone was added together with the substrate in 50 µl of acetone
to give a final 50 µM. Values represent the percent of initial enzyme activities which were determined immediately after isolation of the hepatocytes. Initial activities in cell preparations (A) and (B) were 15 and 70
pmol/min/mg protein, respectively. Other conditions as described by Schwarz
et al. (51)

BP Monooxygenase Activity in Short-term Cultures of Hepatocytes

The problem outlined above may possibly by overcome by using
newly isolated hepatocytes which immediately after isolation
express the liver-specific monooxygenase functions (49-51).
Hepatocytes have been explored as test system for chemical
carcinogens and found to be suitable to detect the DNA-damaging
action of a variety of known carcinogens (52,53). But, aside
from the fact that primary hepatocytes are only capable of giving
indirect evidence for mutagenicity of chemicals, two objections
to their use may be raised based on the properties of their drug
metabolizing enzymes. One drawback may be that liver cells possess not only high monooxygenase activities but are also rich in
inactivating enzymes potentially leading to false-negative
results (cf. below). More importantly, monooxygenase activities
are prone to change rapidly soon after isolation of the hepatocytes. This is illustrated in Fig. 5 for hepatocytes isolated
from untreated rats and from rats treated with the MC-type
inducer, 5,6-benzoflavone. The presence of different forms of
BP monooxygenases in these two hepatocyte preparations is in-

dicated by the in vitro effect of 7,8-benzoflavone, i.e., the
stimulation of the BP monooxygenase from untreated animals and
the strong inhibition of the induced enzyme. "Constitutive"
as well as induced monooxygenase activities decrease rapidly
during the first hours of culture to reach 50% of their initial
activity after about 10 h. Similar results have been obtained
for the epoxidation of aldrin (51). Observations of others
have shown that monooxygenase activities are largely lost from
hepatocytes after 24 h of culturing (50). Thus, using conventional culture techniques the lability of the monooxygenases
sets fairly narrow limits to the applicability of newly isolated
hepatocytes in activation studies. Recently, the culturing of
primary hepatocytes has been described which maintain monooxygenase activities and inducibilities for several days (54) and
hence partially lift the temporal restrictions pointed out
above.

UDP-Glucuronyltransferase Activity in Cell Cultures

In cells in culture, the steady-state level of reactive intermediates of chemicals is strongly influenced by the presence
of inactivating enzymes which in isolated cell fractions are
largely inoperative due to the lack of cofactors. One of the
major groups of inactivating enzymes are the UDP glucuronyltransferases.

Table 4 shows a comparison of UDP-glucuronyltransferase and
monooxygenase activities in various cell lines. It is apparent
that the activities of the two enzymes differ greatly, the
glucuronyltransferase being 2-3 orders of magnitude more active than the BP monooxygenase in all the cell lines examined
except for the hepatoma line, H-4-II-E, even though the monooxygenase activities were previously induced by treatment with
a polycyclic hydrocarbon inducer (cf. Table 1). A second fact
demonstrated by these observations is that no correlation exists
between the expression of the two enzymes. For example, the
renal adenoma cell line, RAG, which has the highest glucuronyltransferase activity of the lines tested, does not possess detectable monooxygenase activity. On the other side, the exceptionally high BP monooxygenase activity in H-4-II-E cells is
not matched by an equally high level of glucuronyltransferase
activity. The human lymphoblastoid cell NC37 BaEV and the
hamster cell line V79 are both devoid of either glucuronyltransferase or monooxygenase activities. As shown in Table 5,
the state of induction may drastically alter the ratio of the
activating and inactivating enzymes. Exposure of BHK21(C13)
cells to benz(a)anthracene causes a 20-fold increase in monooxygenase activity which increases again by a factor of about
10 when aminophylline, an inhibitor of cyclic nucleotide phosphodiesterase, is included in the medium. In contrast, glucuronyltransferase activity remains unaltered in the presence of the
polycyclic hydrocarbon inducer and doubles after additional
aminophylline treatment. This results in an almost 100-fold reduction in the ratio of inactivating to activating pathways.

Table 4. UDP glucuronyltransferase and monooxygenase activities
in various cell lines[a]

| Cell line[b] | (pmol/min/mg protein) | |
	3-OH-BP glucuronyl-transferase	BP monooxygenase[c]
RAG, rat	679	ND[d]
H-4-II-E, rat	776	80.00
A549, human	199	0.30
L-A9, rat	182	ND
3T3/BALB, mouse	133	0.66
BHK-TK⁻, hamster	96	0.27
NC37 BaEV, human	<0.5	ND
V79, hamster	<0.5	ND

[a] UDP glucuronyltransferase activity and BP monooxygenase activities were determined according to Singh and Wiebel (66) and Wiebel et al. (24), respectively
[b] The source of the cell lines is given in legend to Table 1
[c] BP monooxygenase activities in cells treated with benz(a)-anthracene (13 µM) for 24 h
[d] ND, not detectable

Table 5. UDP glucuronyltransferase and monooxygenase activities in BHK(21) (C13) cells: Effect of benz(a)anthracene and aminophylline treatment[a]

| Treatment | (pmol/min/mg protein) | | |
	3-OH-BP glucuronyl-transferase	BP monooxygenase	Glucuronyl-transferase/monooxygenase
DMSO	703	0.08	8800
Benz(a)anthracene	760	1.65	460
Benz(a)antracene + aminophylline	1630	14.05	120

[a] Cells were treated with benz(a)anthracene (13 µM) added in DMSO (final 0.1%) and aminophylline (0.7 mM) for 18 h. UDP glucuronyltransferase and BP monooxygenase activities were determined according to Singh and Wiebel (66) and Wiebel et al. (24), respectively

It should be noted that the glucuronidation of 3-OH-BP may be
representative only of the form(s) of transferases which are
typified by the substrate 1-naphthol (55,56). Preliminary evidence (Schwarz LR, personal communication, 1978) indicates
that the activity of the transferase form typified by the substrate morphine (55,56) is either very low or lacking in all
the cell lines listed in Table 4.

Epoxide Hydratase Activity in Cell Cultures

Another important drug-metabolizing enzyme with predominantly inactivating functions is the microsomal hydratase (57). Table 6 shows the hydratase activity toward the substrate BP-4, 5-oxide in three cell lines together with the activity of the BP monooxygenases. All three cell lines, the rat adenoma cells, the hybrid cell line containing human bone marrow, and the baby rat liver cells, exhibit considerable hydratase activity. The findings are in two respects similar to those seen with the glucuronyltransferases: (a) the maximum activity of the hydratase is by some orders of magnitude greater than that of the monooxygenase, and (b) the expression of hydratase is independent of the presence of monooxygenase activity. A number of observations indicate that cell lines which contain BP monooxygenase activity also form dihydrodiols from BP (27,40,41, 58-60) presenting indirect evidence for the widespread presence of the hydratase in cultured cell lines.

Table 6. Comparison of hydratase and monooxygenase activity in various cell lines[a,b]

Cell line[c]	(pmol/min/mg protein)	
	BP-4,5-oxide hydratase	BP monooxygenase
BRL 3C4	410	0.30
RBM 24S4	80	0.04
RAG	180	0.002

[a] Leutz, Gelboin, and Wiebel, unpublished
[b] In vitro activities of BP-4,5-oxide hydratase and of BP monooxygenase were determined according to Leutz and Gelboin (67) and Wiebel et al. (24), respectively
[c] The source of the cells is given in legend to Table 1

Conclusions and Outlook

Although the enzymes described above represent only part of the complex web of drug-metabolizing enzymes, a general picture emerges from the data. We are confronted with a variety of cell lines or short-term cultures which exhibit highly diverse ratios of activating and inactivating enzymes leading to greatly differing steady-state levels of reactive metabolites. In view of these differences, it seems nearly impossible to extrapolate the findings on the action of chemicals from one cell type to another, even more, to make an extrapolation to the in vivo situation unless more is known about these enzymes in cultures and the in vivo counterpart.

As pointed out above, presently a most serious shortcoming of mammalian cells in established cultures as test systems for mutagenicity is their lack of some major forms of monooxygenases, i.e., the phenobarbital-inducible cytochrome P-450-dependent forms. Another potential source for the misjudgment of mutagenic chemicals may be an abundance of inactivating enzymes. This applies not only to metabolically self-reliant test cells but also to cellular test systems which include subcellular fractions or feeder cells. However, we feel that with the advancement of tissue culture techniques both shortcomings are likely to be overcome once closer attention is paid to the problems. The large variety in the complement of drug-metabolizing enzymes in different cell types and the possibility to evoke and to eliminate the expression of these enzymes by alteration of the genotype, e.g., by cell hybridization (25,61), hold great promise to select or construct cell lines with distinct pharmacologic and toxicologic properties.

Metabolism by monooxygenases as well as by conjugases or hydratase may cause the conversion of some chemicals to their mutagenic forms and the deactivation of others to harmless products. This dual function of drug-metabolizing enzymes in the activation and inactivation of mutagens a priori precludes the development of a single universally applicable culture system for mutagenicity testing. It will be necessary to develop a battery of cell lines which are well defined in their make-up in drug-metabolizing enzymes and are competent in handling the widest spectrum possible of mutagenic chemicals. Such a set or sets of cell lines should also prove to be very useful to dissect the metabolic pathways of chemicals in intact cells and to study the mechanism of their activation. Finally, cells in culture which reflect more closely the in vivo conditions than, for example, in vitro systems using subcellular fractions may provide the means to approach the problem of organ specificity in chemical carcinogenesis and help to estimate the risk of exposure to environmental chemicals.

Abbreviations: BA, benz(a)anthracene; BP, benzo(a)pyrene; DMSO, dimethylsulfoxide; MC, 3-methylcholanthrene.

Acknowledgments. We thank Dr. H. Greim for the critical reading of the manuscript. The expert help of Ms. Judy Byers in preparing the manuscript is gratefully acknowledged.

References

1. Diamond L (1971) Metabolism of polycyclic hydrocarbons in mammalian cell cultures. Int J Cancer 8:451-462
2. Gelboin HV, Wiebel FJ (1971) Studies on the mechanism of aryl hydrocarbon hydroxylase induction and its role in cytotoxicity and tumorigenicity. Ann NY Acad Sci 179:529-547
3. Marquardt H, Heidelberger C (1972) Influence of "feeder" cells and induction and inhibition of microsomal mixed-function oxidases on hydrocarbon-induced malignant transformation of cells derived from C3H mouse prostate. Cancer Res 32:721-725
4. Huberman E, Sachs L (1974) Cell-mediated mutagenesis of mammalian cells with chemical carcinogens. Int J Cancer 13:326-333

5. Umeda M, Saito M (1975) Mutagenicity of dimethylnitrosamine to mammalian cells as determined by the use of mouse liver microsomes. Mutat Res 30: 249-254

6. Bimboes D, Greim H (1976) Human lymphocytes as target cells in a metabolizing test system in vitro for detecting potential mutagens. Mutat Res 35:155-160

7. Krahn DF, Heidelberger C (1977) Liver homogenate-mediated mutagenesis in Chinese hamster V79 cells by polycyclic hydrocarbons and aflatoxins. Mutat Res 46:27-44

8. Kuroki T, Drevon C, Montesano R (1977) Microsome-mediated mutagenesis in V79 Chinese hamster cells by various nitrosamines. Cancer Res 37: 1044-1050

9. Miller J (1970) Carcinogenesis by chemicals: an overview. G.H.A. Clowes memorial lecture. Cancer Res 30:559-576

10. Heidelberger C (1975) Chemical oncogenesis in culture. Adv Cancer Res 18:317-366

11. Bentley P, Oesch F, Glatt H (1977) Dual role of epoxide hydratase in both activation and inactivation of benzo(a)pyrene. Arch Toxicol (Berl) 39:65-75

12. Mulder GJ, Hinson JA, Gillette JR (1977) Generation of reactive metabolites of N-hydroxy-phenacetin by glucuronidation and sulfation. Biochem Pharmacol 26:189-196

13. Rannug U, Sundvall A, Ramel C (1978) The mutagenic effect of 1,2-dichloroethane on Salmonella typhimurium I. Activation through conjugation with glutathione in vivo. Chem Biol Interact 20:1-16

14. Alvares AP, Schilling GR, Kuntzman R (1968) Differences in the kinetics of benzpyrene hydroxylation by hepatic drug-metabolizing enzymes from phenobarbital and 3-methylcholanthrene-treated rats. Biochem Biophys Res Commun 30:588-593

15. Wiebel FJ, Leutz JC, Diamond L, Gelboin HV (1971) Aryl hydrocarbon (benzo(a)pyrene) hydroxylase in microsomes from rat tissues: differential inhibition and stimulation by benzoflavones and organic solvents. Arch Biochem Biophys 144:78-86

16. DiPaolo JA, Donovan PJ (1967) Properties of Syrian hamster cells transformed in the presence of carcinogenic hydrocarbons. Exp Cell Res 48: 361-377

17. Newbold RF, Wigley CB, Thompson MH, Brookes P (1977) Cell-mediated mutagenesis in cultured Chinese hamster cells by carcinogenic polycyclic hydrocarbons: nature and extent of the associated hydrocarbon-DNA reaction. Mutat Res 43:101-116

18. Styles JA (1977) A method for detecting carcinogenic organic chemicals using mammalian cells in culture. Br J Cancer 36:558-563

19. Kakunaga T (1973) A quantitative system for assay of malignant transformation by chemical carcinogens using a clone derived from BALB/3T3. Int J Cancer 12:463-473

20. Chu EHY (1971) Induction and analysis of gene mutations in mammalian cells in culture. In: Hollaender A (ed) Chemical mutagenesis, principles and methods of their detection, Vol 2. Plenum Press, New York, pp 411-444

21. Whitlock JP, Jr, Miller H, Gelboin HV (1974) Induction of aryl hydrocarbon (benzo(a)pyrene) hydroxylase and tyrosine aminotransferase in hepatoma cells in culture. J Cell Biol 63:136-145

22. Huberman E, Yamasaki H, Sachs L (1974) Genetic control of the regulation of cell susceptibility to carcinogenic polycyclic hydrocarbons by cyclic AMP. Int J Cancer 14:789-798

23. Yamasaki H, Huberman E, Sachs L (1975) Regulation of aryl hydrocarbon (benzo(a)pyrene) hydroxylase activity in mammalian cells. Induction of

hydroxylase activity by dibuturylcyclic AMP and aminophylline. J Biol Chem 250:7766-7770

24. Wiebel FJ, Brown S, Waters HL, Selkirk JK (1977) Activation of xenobiotics by monooxygenases: cultures of mammalian cells as analytical tool. Arch Toxicol (Berl) 39:133-148

25. Wiebel FJ, Brown S, Minna JD, Gelboin HV (1977) Assignment of a human gene for aryl hydrocarbon hydroxylase expression to chromosome 2. In: Ullrich V, Estabrook RW (eds) Microsomes and drug oxidations. Pergamon Press, Oxford, pp 426-434

26. San RHC, Stich HF (1975) DNA repair synthesis of cultured human cells as a rapid bioassay for chemical carcinogens. Int J Cancer 16:284-291

27. Fox CH, Selkirk JK, Price FM, Croy RG, Sanford KK, Cottler-Fox M (1975) Metabolism of benzo(a)pyrene by human epithelial cells in vitro. Cancer Res 35:3551-3557

28. Freeman AE, Lake RS, Igel HJ, Gernand L, Pezzutti MR, Malone JM, Mark C, Benedict WF (1977) Heteroploid conversion of human skin cells by methylcholanthrene. Proc Natl Acad Sci USA 74:2451-2455

29. Lake RS, Kropko ML, Pezzutti MR, Shoemaker RH, Igel HJ (1978) Chemical induction of unscheduled DNA synthesis in human skin epithelial cell cultures. Cancer Res 38:2091-2098

30. Goto T, Wiebel FJ (to be published) Aryl hydrocarbon (benzo(a)pyrene) monooxygenase activity in human primary amnion cell cultures. Europ J Cancer

31. Pelkonen O, Korhonen P, Jouppila P, Kärki N (1975) Induction of aryl hydrocarbon hydroxylase in human fetal liver cell and fibroblast cultures by polycyclic hydrocarbons. Life Sci 16:1403-1410

32. Nebert DW, Gelboin HV (1968) Substrate-inducible microsomal aryl hydroxylase in mammalian cell culture. I. Assay and properties of induced enzyme. J Biol Chem 243:6242-6249

33. Wiebel FJ, Gelboin HV, Coon HG (1972) Regulation of aryl hydrocarbon hydroxylase in intraspecific hybrids of human, mouse, and hamster cells. Proc Natl Acad Sci USA 69:3580-3584

34. Wiebel FJ, Matthews EJ, Gelboin HV (1972) Ribonucleic acid synthesis-dependent induction of aryl hydrocarbon hydroxylase in the absence of ribosomal ribonucleic acid synthesis and transfer. J Biol Chem 247:4711-4747

35. Haugen DA, Hoeven TA van der, Coon MC (1975) Purified liver microsomal cytochrome P-450. Separation and characterization of multiple forms. J Biol Chem 250: 3567-3570

36. Wiebel FJ, Selkirk JK, Gelboin HV, Haugen DA, Hoeven TA van der, Coon MJ (1975) Position-specific oxygenation of benzo(a)pyrene by different forms of purified cytochrome P-450 from rabbit liver. Proc Natl Acad Sci USA 72:3917-3920

37. Lu AYH (1976) Liver microsomal drug-metabolizing enzyme system: functional components and their properties. Fed Proc 35:2460-2463

38. Wiebel FJ (1980) Activation and inactivation of carcinogens by microsomal monooxygenases: modification by benzoflavones and polycyclic aromatic hydrocarbons. In: Slaga TJ (ed) Carcinogenesis, Vol 5. Modifiers of chemical carcinogenesis. Raven Press, New York, pp 57-84

39. Owens IS, Nebert DW (1975) Aryl hydrocarbon hydroxylase induction in mammalian liver-derived cell cultures. Stimulation of "cytochrome P_1-450-associated" enzyme activity by many inducing drugs. Mol Pharmacol 11:94-104

40. Sims P (1970) The metabolism of some aromatic hydrocarbons by mouse embryo cell cultures. Biochem Pharmacol 19:285-297

41. Selkirk JK, Croy RG, Wiebel FJ, Gelboin HV (1976) Differences in benzo(a)pyrene metabolism between rodent liver microsomes and embryonic cells. Cancer Res 36:4476-4479

42. Holder G, Yagi H, Dansette P, Jerina DM, Levin W, Lu AYH, Conney AH (1974) Effects of inducers and epoxide hydrase on the metabolism of benzo(a)pyrene by liver microsomes and a reconstituted system: analysis by high pressure liquid chromatography. Proc Natl Acad Sci USA 71: 4356-4360

43. Pezzuto JM, Yang CS, Yang SK, McCourt DW, Gelboin HV (1978) Metabolism of benzo(a)pyrene and (-)-trans-7,8-dihydroxy-7,8-dihydrobenzo(a)pyrene by rat liver nuclei and microsomes. Cancer Res 38:1241-1245

44. Yang SK, Selkirk JK, Plotkin EV, Gelboin HV (1975) Kinetic analysis of the metabolism of benzo(a)pyrene to phenols, dihydrodiols, and quinones by high-pressure chromatography compared to analysis of aryl hydrocarbon hydroxylase assay, and the effect of enzyme induction. Cancer Res 35: 3642-3650

45. Huberman E, Sachs L, Yang SK, Gelboin HV (1976) Identification of mutagenic metabolites of benzo(a)pyrene in mammalian cells. Proc Natl Acad Sci USA 73:607-611

46. Levin W, Wood AW, Yagi H, Dansette PM, Jerina DM, Conney AH (1976) Carcinogenicity of benzo(a)pyrene 4,5-, 7,8-, and 9,10-oxides on mouse skin. Proc Natl Acad Sci USA 73:243-247

47. King HWS, Osborne MR, Brookes P (1978) The identification of 3-methylcholanthrene-9,10-dihydrodiol as an intermediate in the binding of 3-methylcholanthrene to DNA in cells in culture. Chem Biol Interact 20:367-371

48. Dipple A, Nebzydoski JA (1978) Evidence for the involvement of a diolepoxide in the binding of 7,12-dimethylbenz(a)anthracene to DNA in cells in culture. Chem Biol Interact 20:17-26

49. Vadi H, Moldéus P, Capdevila J, Orrenius S (1975) The metabolism of benzo(a)pyrene in isolated rat liver cells. Cancer Res 35:2083-2091

50. Guzelian PS, Bissell DM, Meyer UA (1977) Drug metabolism in adult rat hepatocytes in primary monolayer culture. Gastroenterology 72:1232-1239

51. Schwarz LR, Götz R, Wolff T, Wiebel FJ (1979) Monooxygenase and glucuronyltransferase activities in short term cultures of isolated rat hepatocytes. FEBS Lett 98:203-206

52. Williams GM (1976) Carcinogen-induced DNA repair in primary rat liver cell cultures: a possible screen for chemical carcinogens. Cancer Lett 1:231-236

53. Michalopoulous G, Sattler GL, O'Conner D, Pitot HC (1977) Unscheduled DNA synthesis induced in hepatocellular suspensions and primary cultures of hepatocytes by procarcinogens. Proc Am Assoc Cancer Res 18:246

54. Michalopoulous G, Sattler GL, O'Connor L, Pitot HC (1978) Unscheduled DNA synthesis induced by procarcinogens in suspensions and primary cultures of hepatocytes on collagen membranes. Cancer Res 38:1866-1871

55. Bock KW, Clausbruch UC von, Josting D, Ottenwälder H (1977) Separation and partial purification of two differentially inducible UDP-glucuronyltransferases from rat liver. Biochem Pharmacol 26:1097-1100

56. Wishart GJ (1978) Demonstration of functional heterogeneity of hepatic uridine diphosphate glucuronosyltransferase activities after administration of 3-methylcholanthrene and phenobarbital to rats. Biochem J 174:671-672

57. Oesch F (1973) Mammalian epoxide hydrases: inducible enzymes catalyzing the inactivation of carcinogenic and cytotoxic metabolites derived from aromatic and olefinic compounds. Xenobiotica 3:305-340

58. King HWS, Osborne MR, Beland FA, Harvey RG, Brookes P (1976) (+)-7α, 8β-Dihydroxy-9β,10β-epoxy-7,8,9,10-tetrahydrobenzo(a)pyrene is an intermediate in the metabolism and binding to DNA of benzo(a)pyrene. Proc Natl Acad Sci USA 73:2679-2681
59. Baird WM, Diamond L (1977) The nature of benzo(a)pyrene-DNA adducts formed in hamster embryo cells depends on the length of time of exposure to benzo(a)pyrene. Biochem Biophys Res Commun 77:162-167
60. Shinohara K, Cerutti PA (1977) Formation of benzo(a)pyrene-DNA adducts in peripheral human lung tissue. Cancer Lett 3:303-309
61. Brown S, Wiebel FJ, Gelboin HV, Minna JD (1976) Assignment of a locus required for flavoprotein-linked monooxygenase expression to human chromosome 2. Proc Natl Acad Sci USA 73:4628-4632
62. Baur H, Kasperek S, Pfaff E (1975) Criteria of viability of isolated liver cells. Hoppe Seylers Z Physiol Chem 356:827-838
63. Whitlock JP, Jr, Cooper HL, Gelboin HV (1972) Aryl hydrocarbon (benzo-(a)pyrene) hydroxylase is stimulated in human lymphocytes by mitogens and benz(a)anthracene. Science 177:618-619
64. Bast RC, Jr, Whitlock JP, Jr, Miller H, Rapp HJ, Gelboin HV (1974) Aryl hydrocarbon (benzo(a)pyrene) hydroxylase in human peripheral blood monocytes. Nature 250:664-665
65. Whitlock JP, Jr, Gelboin HV, Coon HG (1976) Variation in aryl hydrocarbon (benzo(a)pyrene) hydroxylase activity in heteroploid and predominantly diploid rat liver cells in culture. J Cell Biol 70:217-225
66. Singh J, Wiebel FJ (1979) A highly sensitive and rapid fluorometric assay for UDP-glucuronyltransferase activity using 3-hydroxybenzo(a)-pyrene as substrate. Anal Biochem 97:394-401
67. Leutz JC, Gelboin HV (1975) Benzo(a)pyrene-4,5-oxide hydratase: Assay, properties, and induction. Arch Biochem Biophys 168:722-725

Note Added in Proof: A report on the metabolism of bile acids that appeared during the preparation of the manuscript suggests that some hepatoma cell lines derived from H-4-II-E may express cytochrome P-450-dependent monooxygenases (Lambiotte and Sjövall, (1979) Biochem. Biophys. Res. Commun. 68:1089-1095). This is supported by further observations on the activation of aflatoxin B_1 (Lambiotte and Thierry (1979) Biochem. Biophys. Res. Commun. 89:933-942) and on the substrate, inhibitor and inducer specificities of aryl hydrocarbon hydroxylase and aldrin epoxidase in these cell lines (Wiebel and Wolff, unpublished).

Studies on the Detection of Carcinogens Using a Mammalian Cell Transformation Assay with Liver Homogenate Activation

J. A. STYLES[1]

Summary

The transformation of mammalian cells in vitro has been used to study the mechanism of carcinogenesis. There are many cell transformation assays, each having a different end-point such as changes in morphology, plating efficiency, serum requirement, nuclear size, enzyme activity, growth in semi-solid agar, cytoskeletal structure and antigenicity. These changes appear to be acquired by primary cells at different times following exposure to a carcinogen and may not all be mutational in origin. Growth in semi-solid agar is usually the last characteristic to appear in transformed cells and appears to be a mutational event. The only unequivical end-point in relation to tumorigenesis is transplantation of transformed cells into a suitable host followed by the evolution on an invasive tumour. While there is a close relationship between growth in semi-solid agar and tumour formation following transplantation this correlation is not of overriding importance in the use of in vitro transformation as a short-term predictive assay for chemical carcinogens. A test method using BHK C1 13 cells in semi-solid agar and including liver homogenates for metabolic activation has been used to screen organic chemicals and found to be very accurate in discriminating between carcinogens and non-carcinogens and has detected several classes of carcinogen which were not identified by the *Salmonella* reverse mutation assay. Our experience with the cell transformation assay so far indicates that it cannot be used for predicting the potency of a carcinogen.

Introduction

A number of cell culture systems have been developed over the past ten years in which normal or non-malignant cells have been changed ("transformed") with respect to various test markers, including malignancy in the whole animal following injection of the cells after exposure in vitro to chemical carcinogens. The prime purpose of these methods was analysis of the mechanisms involved in chemical carcinogenesis, but because of their obvious connection with cancer, they also showed great promise as rapid tests to detect potential carcinogens.

---

[1] Imperial Chemical Industries, Limited, Central Toxicology Laboratory, Alderley Park, MacClesfield, Cheshire/UK

The early investigations into the phenomenon of cell transformation were concerned with observing changes in morphology of the test cells and alterations in the growth patterns of the colonies formed following exposure to carcinogens. Two morphological transformation systems have been studied extensively, the first, using Syrian hamster embryonic cells, has been reviewed by Di Paolo (1,2) and the second, using mouse cells (C3H/10T½) has been reviewed by Heidelberger (3-5). Many carcinogens have been correctly identified using this type of assay as a screen [R.J. Pienta (41)].

Other investigations into cell transformation observed different test end-points and some of these are listed in Table 1. Most of the data on the various indicators of transformation are based on embryonic fibroblast cells, although more recent work on these end-points has concentrated on epithelial cells, since it has been estimated that 85% of human cancers are epithelial in origin (6,7). The relevance of any in vitro transformation end-point to cancer can be tested by taking the cells, implanting them into suitable animal hosts and observing the appearance of tumours. Growth in semi-solid agar appears, at the moment, to be the most reliable criterion for transformation of both fibroblast and epithelial cultures and has the best correlation with tumorigenicity (0.98), whereas the other test end-points have correlation coefficients of less than 0.75 (8,9). Growth in agar is a simple objective criterion of transformation but does not detect early changes in cells following exposure to a chemical carcinogen (10,11). The different markers of neoplastic transformation listed in Table 1 are acquired by primary or early passage cells after various population doublings following exposure to a carcinogen, but the last characteristic to appear is the ability to grow in semi-solid agar (9). It is assumed from these studies that the lesion caused by the carcinogen in primary or early passage cells is mutagenic and is followed by a series of epigenetic steps leading to malignant transformation. These epigenetic steps may be changes in control mechanisms which suppress the expression of mutations. If established cell lines such as BHK21 Cl 13 or CHO-K1 cells are exposed to a carcinogen, then transformation occurs rapidly, indicating that these cells have already undergone epigenetic changes and express mutations very rapidly (Fig. 1). This is borne out by the observation that BHK cells have a relatively high spontaneous transformation frequency and can produce tumours in hamsters if large numbers of cells are inoculated, whereas primary cells show little or no spontaneous transformation and are not tumorigenic.

Of the available short-term predictive tests for carcinogens which have been validated [12-21; R.J. Pienta (41)], cell transformation assays have an obvious and demonstrable connection with cancer, which may be useful when relating the in vitro positive test result of a compound to the induction of a tumour. However, desirable it may be to have a short-term test which is related to cancer, for the purposes of a screen the main concern should be initially an ability to discriminate between carcinogens and non-carcinogens.

Table 1. Properties of transformed cells in culture [Weinstein et al. (10)]

Cell properties	Fibroblasts	Epithelial cells	Correlation with tumorigenicity
Tumorigenicity	+	+	
Growth in agar or methocel	+	+	0.98
Morphological changes	+	−	< 0.75
Increased saturation density and piling-up	+	+	< 0.75
Decreased serum requirement	+	$\bar{?}$	< 0.75
Altered cell-surface glycoproteins and glycolipids	+	?	?
Lectin agglutination	+	+	?
Increased membrane transport	+	?	?
Decreased cAMP	+	?	?
Increased protease production	+	?	< 0.75
Decreased microfilament sheaths	+	?	?

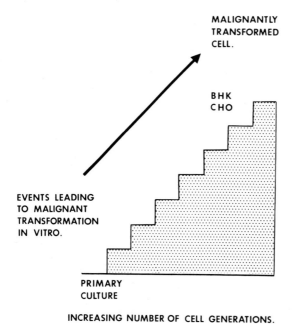

MALIGNANTLY TRANSFORMED CELL.

BHK CHO

EVENTS LEADING TO MALIGNANT TRANSFORMATION IN VITRO.

PRIMARY CULTURE

INCREASING NUMBER OF CELL GENERATIONS.

Fig. 1. Schematic diagram of malignant transformation in vitro. The events leading to transformation, some of which are listed in Table 1, are known to occur after a single exposure to a carcinogen. The last event is thought to be growth in semi-solid agar

A clear distinction must be drawn, for the present, between in vitro cell transformation studies which are directed towards understanding the mechanisms of carcinogenesis and those which are used to detect chemical carcinogens, particularly when established cell lines are used. These cells are metabolically abnormal and may be used in conjunction with liver homogenates (S-9 mix) or with feeder layers to augment metabolism, in which case the magnitude of the test response will be determined largely by the balance between activating and detoxifying enzymes

in the S-9 mix (22). It must also be borne in mind that any
cell culture model is a simplified version of the intact animal,
and while models may be useful as a means of solving specific
problems in toxicology, the results derived from in vitro
studies must not be extrapolated beyond the limits of the system. The cell culture transformation models described above are
closed systems and are lacking in most of the barriers that a
chemical must pass through in an animal before reaching the
target macromolecules critical to cancer induction (route of
entry, absorption, "real" metabolism, detoxification and excretion) and the barriers that a population of exposed cells
must negotiate before a malignant tumour appears (selective
pressure, cellular repair, immunosurveillance, humoural controls).

BHK Cell Transformation Assay

The BHK transformation system, using growth in semi-solid agar
as an end-point, will serve as an example of how cell transformation assays can be used to screen chemicals for carcinogenic
potential and to gather experimental evidence for structure-
activity studies (23,24). The BHK-agar transformation assay (25-
27) has been modified to include auxiliary metabolic activation
(21) and has been subjected to a validation study using 120
chemicals (19,20) where it was found to be capable of discriminating between carcinogens and non-carcinogens with about 90%
accuracy. Similar accuracy has been reported by Pienta (unpublished work) using Syrian hamster embryo cells and observing
morphological transformation. Figures indicating predictive accuracy in short-term tests must be treated with caution since
they can be drastically altered by the choice of chemicals used
(28). It has been proposed (20,29) that maximum reliance can be
placed on the prediction from a short-term test only if carcinogenic and non-carcinogenic structural analogues of the test
chemical are assayed at the same time and give the correct response. Obviously, if the control analogues behave incorrectly
in the assay, little reliance can be placed on the result generated by the test compound.

The reliability of the cell transformation test using BHK cells
can be seen from Figs. 2-4. The results of testing benzidine on
10 separate occasions are shown in these figures. It can be seen
from the survival curve in Fig. 2 that the accuracy declines at
low survival but that it is possible to determine the LC_{50} within
a tenfold dose range. All test results are compared at the LC_{50}
so that differences in toxicity between compounds are eliminated.
Figure 3 shows the number of transformed colonies found in semi-
solid agar following incubation of BHK cells with benzidine.
The transformation frequency derived from the previous two sets
of data is shown in Fig. 4, where it can be seen that transformation and survival are interdependent since the errors at all
doses are greatly reduced. Similar results have also been obtained with 2-acetylaminofluorene and benzo(a)pyrene (23).

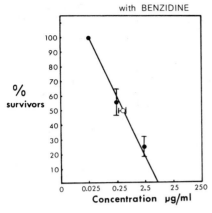

Fig. 2. Survival curve of BHK cells exposed to benzidine. Mean of 10 experiments ± SD

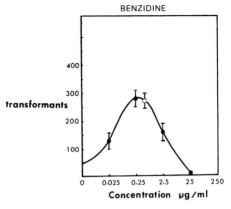

Fig. 3. Number of colonies BHK cells growing in semi-solid agar after treatment with benzidine. Mean of 10 experiments ± SD

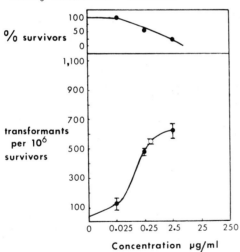

Fig. 4. Transformation frequency of BHK cells after treatment with benzidine. Mean of 10 experiments ± SD

Since BHK cells transform spontaneously, a population of BHK cells maintained continuously in culture will accumulate transformants, so re-cloning and selection must be carried out regularly (30,31). Re-cloning does not appear to affect the sensitivity of the cells as can be seen in Fig. 5 where the results of testing 4-aminobiphenyl in a clone of cells having a spontaneous transformation frequency of 50 per 10^6 cells, i.e., a

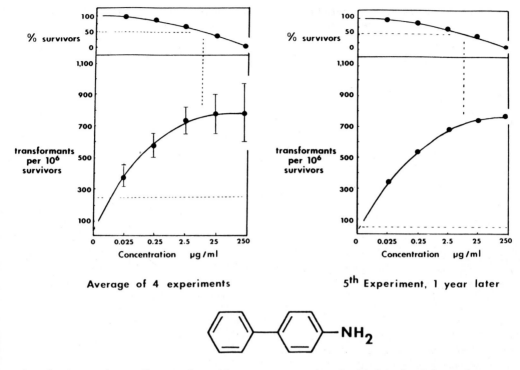

Fig. 5. Comparison of transformation assays on 4-aminobiphenyl with a clone
of BHK cells which had a spontaneous transformation frequency of 50 per
10^6 cells and with a clone having a spontaneous frequency of 10 per 10^6 cells

threshold frequency of 250 per 10^6 survivors at the LC_{50} (21),
are compared with the results of a test carried out about a
year later on 4-aminobiphenyl, using a clone of cells with a
spontaneous transformation frequency of 10 per 10^6 cells, i.e.,
a threshold frequency of 50 per 10^6 survivors at the LC_{50}. These
results are a further demonstration of the reproducibility of
the test.

Comparison with Bacterial Assay

There are many classes of chemical carcinogens which are correctly distinguished by both the cell transformation assay and the
Salmonella test, [83% of compounds tested by Purchase et al. (20)],
examples being tobacco smoke condensate (Fig. 6) *para* nitrosodimethylaniline (Fig. 7), vinyl chloride (Fig. 8), unstabilised
trichlorethylene (Fig. 9), ethylene dichloride (Fig. 10), and
chloroform (Fig. 11). However, when compared with the *Salmonella*
assay it can be seen that for certain classes of chemicals the
cell transformation assay can discriminate between carcinogens
and non-carcinogens which are not detected by the bacterial assay.
For example, the cell transformation assay distinguished between
the non-carcinogen aniline and the closely related carcinogen
o-toluidine. The response of this test for an untested aniline

232

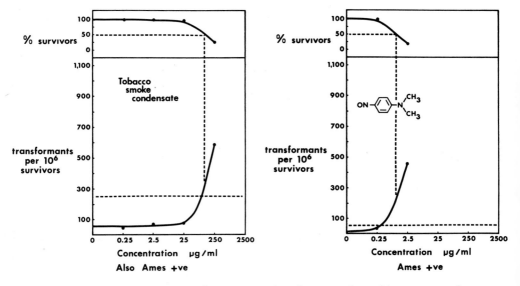

Fig. 6. Transformation assay of tobacco smoke condensate. A positive
result was also found in the Ames
assay

Fig. 7. Transformation assay of
*para*nitrosodimethylaniline showing
positive result. The Ames assay was
also positive

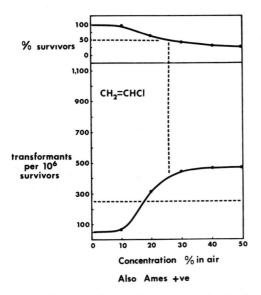

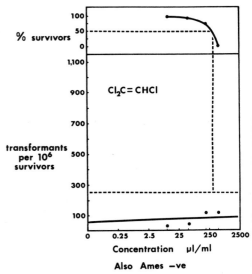

Fig. 8. Transformation assay of vinyl
chloride gas. Both the transformation
and Ames assays gave positive results

Fig. 9. Negative result given by
unstabilised trichloroethylene in
transformation assay. Unstabilised
TCE also gave a negative result in
Ames assay

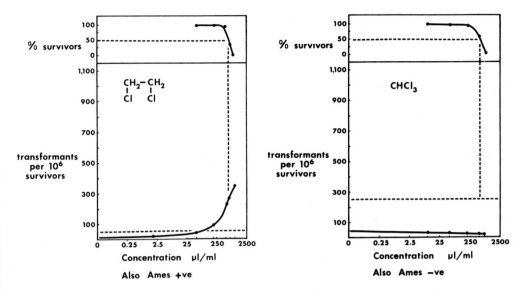

Fig. 10. Positive transformation result with ethylene dichloride which
was also positive in the Ames assay

Fig. 11. Negative result in transformation assay of chloroform which
was also negative in the Ames assay

is therefore credible, in contrast to the *Salmonella* assay which
registers both aniline and *o*-toluidine as negative or positive
depending on the test condition, i.e., whether or not norharman
is included (32-34). In both situations the result from the
Salmonella assay for a previously untested aniline is of inde-
terminate significance (Figs. 12 and 13). A further example of
a carcinogen which the cell transformation assay is capable of
detecting correctly, but which gave negative results in the
Salmonella assay, was 2-aminotriazole. Based on this test response
it is possible to predict that a structurally related, but untested, analogue of 2-aminotriazole, guanazole, will be non-
carcinogenic (Figs. 14 and 15).

There are compounds such as saccharin and cyclamate which have
produced tumours in animals but which are negative in both the
Salmonella and cell transformation assays (35) (Figs. 16 and 17).
It has been argued that these compounds are epigenetic carcinogens or promoters or co-carcinogens and would not be expected
to register in short-term test such as those which are probably
sensitive to genotypic carcinogens (35). Saccharin has been
shown by Mondal et al. (36) in a transformation assay to be
capable of promoting the action of 20-methylcholanthrene. This
observation indicates that some mammalian cell transformation
assays involve both genetic and epigenetic changes.

Further categories give reproducible positive results in the
cell transformation assay whilst giving erratic but mainly negative results in the *Salmonella* test, examples being hexamethylphosphoramide (Fig. 18) (37,38), butter yellow (Fig. 19) (39,40),
dimethylnitrosamine and hydrazine. However, it must be noted

234

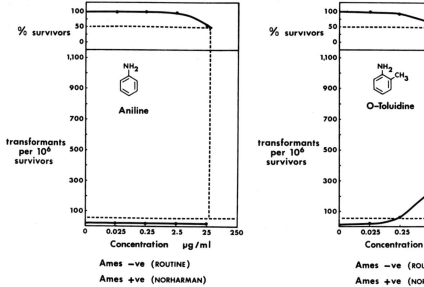

Fig. 12. Negative result in transformation assay of aniline. Aniline was
negative in Ames assay but positive
if tested in the presence of norharman

Fig. 13. Positive test result in
transformation assay by *o*-toluidine.
This compound, like aniline, gave a
negative result in the Ames assay but
was positive in the presence of norharman

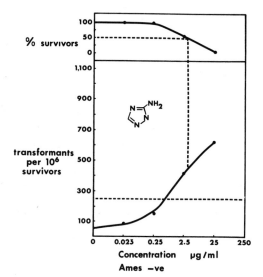

Fig. 14. Positive transformation
assay result given by 2-aminotriazole
which is Ames negative

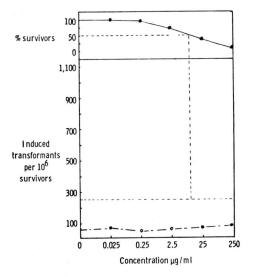

Fig. 15. Negative transformation assay result given by guanazole, a non-carcinogenic analogue of 2-aminotriazole. Guanazole was also negative in the Ames assay

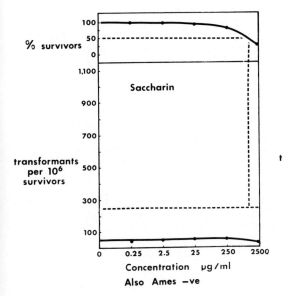

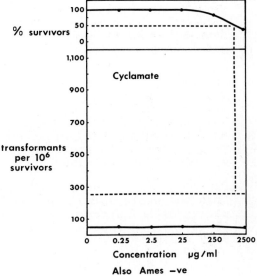

Fig. 16. Negative test results given in cell transformation assay and Ames test with saccharin

Fig. 17. Negative test result given in cell transformation assay and Ames test with cyclamate

that the cell transformation assay failed to detect some other classes of carcinogen, such as the flame-retardant tris (2,3-dibromopropyl) phosphate and trimethyl phosphate, which are correctly identified by the *Salmonella* assay.

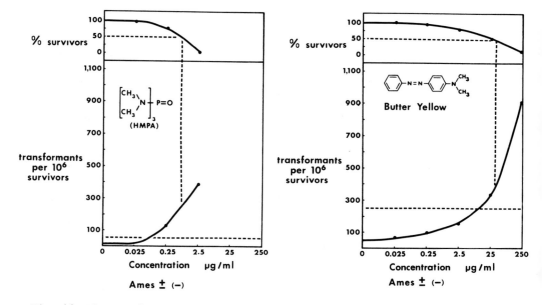

Fig. 18. The carcinogen hexamethyl-phosphoramide (HMPA) is consistently positive in the cell transformation assay but is erratic and mainly negative in the Ames test

Fig. 19. The carcinogen butter yellow gives a consistently positive result in the cell transformation assay but is erratic and mainly negative in the Ames test

In summary, the BHK cell transformation test, as an example of mammalian cell transformation assays, is reproducible and gives good discrimination between carcinogens and non-carcinogens of many classes. The assay should be used, where possible, with appropriate chemical class controls (as should any short-term test) in order to increase the credibility of the test result for a compound of undefined activity.

Finally, since the cell transformation test is a simpler system than the whole animal and does not employ the full metabolic capacity of an intact mammal, the magnitude of the test response is of unknown relevance and should not be assumed, in the present state of knowledge, to define the potency of a carcinogen.

References

1. Di Paolo JA (1974) Quantitative aspects of in vitro chemical carcinogenesis. Biochem Dis 4:433
2. Di Paolo JA (1974) Quantitative aspects of in vitro chemical carcinogenesis. In: Ts'o Po, Di Paolo JA (eds) Chemical carcinogenesis (Part B). Dekker, New York, pp 443-455
3. Heidelberger C (1973) Chemical oncogenesis in culture. Adv Cancer Res 18:317-366
4. Heidelberger C (1973) Current trends in chemical carcinogenesis. Fed Proc 32:2154-2161
5. Heidelberger C (1975) Chemical carcinogenesis. Annu Rev Biochem 44:79-121

6. Cairns J (1975) The cancer problem. Sci Am 233:64-72
7. Higginson J, Muir CS (1973) Epidemiology. In: Holland JF, Frei E III (eds) Cancer medicine, Lea and Febiger, Philadelphia, p 241
8. Ts'o POP (1977) Some aspects of the basic mechanisms of chemical carcinogenesis. J Toxicol Environ Health 2:1305-1315
9. Ts'o POP (1978) The relationship between neoplastic transformation and the cellular genetic apparatus. Abstract No 209 In Vitro 14:385
10. Weinstein IB, Wigler M, Stadler U (1976) Analysis of the mechanism of chemical carcinogenesis of epithelial cell cultures. In: Montesano R, Bartsch, H, Tomatis L (eds) Screening tests in chemical carcinogenesis. IARC Scientific Publication 12:355-387
11. Weinstein B, Yamaguchi N, Gebert R, Kaighn ME (1975) Use of epithelial cell cultures for studies on the mechanism of transformation by chemical carcinogens. In Vitro 11:130-141
12. Brookes P, Serres F de (1976) Report on the workshop on the mutagenicity of chemical carcinogens. Mutat Res 38:155-160
13. Stoltz DR, Poirier LA, Irving CC, Stich HF, Weisburger JH, Grice HC (1974) Evaluation of short term tests for carcinogenicity. Toxicol Appl Pharmacol 29:157-180
14. Montesano R, Bartsch H, Tomatis L (1976) Screening tests in chemical carcinogenesis. IARC/WHO Sci Publ 12
15. Ames BN, Durston WE, Yamasaki E, Lee FD (1973) Carcinogens are mutagens: a simple test system combining liver homogenates for activation and bacteria for detection. Proc Natl Acad Sci USA 70:2281-2285
16. Ames BN, McCann J, Yamasaki E (1975) Methods for detecting carcinogens and mutagens with the Salmonella/mammalian-microsome mutagenicity test. Mutat Res 31:347-364
17. McCann J, Choi E, Yamasaki E, Ames BN (1975) Detection of carcinogens as mutagens in the Salmonella/microsome test, part 1. Assay of 300 chemicals. Proc Natl Acad Sci USA 72:5135-5139
18. McCann J, Ames BN (1976) Detection of carcinogens as mutagens in the Salmonella/microsome test: assay of 300 chemicals: part II. Discussion. Proc Natl Acad Sci USA 73:950-954
19. Purchase IFH, Longstaff E, Ashby J, Styles JA, Anderson D, Lefevre PA, Westwood FE (1976) Evaluation of six short term tests for detecting organic chemical carcinogens and recommendation for their use. Nature 264:624-627
20. Purchase IFH, Longstaff E, Ashby J, Styles JA, Anderson D, Lefevre PA, Westwood FR (1978) Evaluation of six short term tests for detecting organic chemical carcinogens and recommendations for their use. Br J Cancer 37:873-959
21. Styles JA (1977) A method for detecting carcinogenic organic chemicals using mammalian cell in culture. Br J Cancer 36:558-563
22. Ashby J, Styles JA (1978) Does carcinogenic potency correlate with mutagenic potency in the Ames assay? Nature 271:452-455
23. Styles JA (1978) Cell transformation assays. In: Paget GE (ed) Mutagenesis in sub-mammalian systems, status and significance. Lancaster, MTP Press Limited, pp 147-163
24. Styles JA (1979) Tissue culture methods for evaluating biocompatibility of polymers. In: Williams DF (ed) CRC reviews in biocompatibility, Vol 1. Fundamental aspects of biocompatibility. Florida, CRC Press Inc
25. MacPherson I, Montagnier L (1964) Agar suspension culture for the selective assay of cells transformed by polyoma virus. Virology 23:291-294
26. Di Mayorca G, Greenblatt M, Trauthen T, Soller A, Giordano R (1973) Malignant transformation of BHK 21 clone 13 cells in vitro by nitrosamines — a conditional state. Proc Natl Acad Sci USA 70:46-49

27. Mishra NK, Di Mayorca G (1974) In vitro malignant transformation of cells by chemical carcinogens. Biochim Biophys Acta 355:205-219

28. Ashby J (1978) Implications of Carcinogenicity. In: Paget GE (ed) Mutagenesis in sub-mammalian systems, status and significant. Lancaster, MTP Press Limited, pp 165-189

29. Ashby J, Purchase IFH (1977) The selection of appropriate chemical controls for use with short term tests for potential carcinogenicity. Ann Occup Hyg 20:297-301

30. Bouck N, Di Mayorca G (1976) Somatic mutation as the basis for malignant transformation of BHK cells by chemical carcinogens. Nature 264:722-727

31. Ishii Y, Elliott JA, Mishra NK, Lieberman MW (1977) Quantitative studies of transformation by chemical carcinogens and ultraviolet radiation using a subclone of BHK 21 clone 13 Syrian hamster cells. Cancer Res 37:2023-2029

32. Sugimura T, Kawachi T, Matsushima T, Nagao M, Sato S, Yahagi T (1977) A critical review of submammalian systems for mutagen detection. In: Scott D, Bridges BA, Sobels GH (eds) Progress in genetic toxicology. Elsevier/North Holland Biomedical Press, Amsterdam, pp 126-154

33. Nagao M, Yahagi T, Honda M, Seino Y, Matsushima T, Sugimura T (1977) Demonstration of mutagenicity of aniline and o-toluidine by norharman. Proc Jpn Acad 53:34-37

34. Nagao M, Yahagi T, Kawachi T, Sugimura T, Kosuge T, Tsuji K, Wakabayashi K, Mizusaki S, Matsumototo T (1977) Comutagenic action of norharman and harman. Proc Jpn Acad 53:95-98

35. Ashby J, Styles JA, Anderson D, Paton D (1978) Saccharin: an epigenetic carcinogen/mutagen? Fd Cosmet Toxicol 16:95

36. Mondal S, Brankow DW, Heidelberg C (1978) Enhancement of oncogenesis in C3H/10T½ mouse embryo cell cultures by saccharin. Science 201:1141-1142

37. Ashby J, Styles JA, Anderson D (1977) Selection of an in vitro carcinogenicity test for derivatives of the carcinogen hexamethylphosphoramide. Br J Cancer 36:564-571

38. Ashby J, Styles JA, Paton D (1978) Potentially carcinogenic analogues of the carcinogen hexamethylphosphoramide: evaluation in vitro. Br J Cancer 38:418-427

39. Ashby J, Styles JA, Paton D (1978) In vitro evaluation of some derivatives of the carcinogen butter yellow: implications for environmental screening. Br J Cancer 38:34-50

40. Ashby J, Styles JA (1978) Comutagenicity, competitive enzyme substrates, and in vitro carcinogenicity assays. Mutat Res 54:105-112

41. Pienta RJ (1979) A hamster embryo cell model system for identifying carcinogens. In: Griffin AC, Shaw CR (eds) Carcinogens: identification and mechanisms action. Raven Press, New York, pp 121-141

Effects of Different Polycyclic Aromatic Hydrocarbons on Cultured Fetal Hamster Lung Cells and Tracheal Explants

H. B. Richter-Reichhelm, M. Emura, and U. Mohr[1]

Abstract

A number of polycyclic aromatic hydrocarbons have been suspected of playing a role in human pulmonary carcinogenesis. In order to test the biologic effects of pure single compounds we have developed a new test system which combines a cell transformation and an organ culture assay.

Short-term cultured lung cells, isolated from fetuses which were dissected aseptically from pregnant female Syrian golden hamsters at the 15th day of gestation, were plated at a density of $3-6 \times 10^3$ into 60 mm Petri dishes. Test substances dissolved in not more than 0.5% DMSO were added to the cells 1 day after plating; 24 h later, the cultures were washed three times with Hanks' solution and re-fed with normal medium. After 10-14 days, the cultures were fixed with methanol and Giemsa stained.

The evaluation showed a dose-related toxicity of all tested compounds (i.e., benzo(a)pyrene, benz(a)anthracene, benzo(e)pyrene, and chrysene). Transformation could be obviously detected with benzo(a)pyrene, while the other test compounds induced only weak or no transformation.

Tracheal pieces from the same fetuses were dissected and transferred to organ culture. Morphological alterations caused by the same test compounds were examined on serial sections of the explants after a cultivation time of 4-8 weeks. The exposure to chemicals started 1 day after the beginning of cultivation and lasted 1 week.

As this system has been initiated very recently, the results are only preliminary and have to be improved upon. Our primary concern has been directed at the consistency of correlations between the results of lung cell and tracheal explant cultures. Therefore, the feasibilities for standardizing the in vitro conditions as well as the advantages of adopting the system for other tissues (human) will be discussed.

[1]Abteilung für experimentelle Pathologie, Medizinische Hochschule Hannover, Karl-Wiechert-Allee 9, D-3000 Hannover 61/FRG

Introduction

For a number of years, efforts have been made to determine just
how hazardous the variety of chemical compounds in the environment are for man. As well as studies in experimental animals,
in vitro tests were developed which were expected to demonstrate
the biologic effect of such chemicals, mainly in terms of mutagenicity and carcinogenicity (1-4). However, the results of
only some of these tests corresponded to the in vitro data,
while others produced false-positive and false-negative results
in relation to the individual chemical structure of the test
compound. Obviously data from prescreening is necessary and relatively short-term tests should be performed. These could be
used by public health bodies as a basis for regulatory activities.
At present, there are no specific in vitro methods. Although the
Ames' system is currently the most popular, its relation to the
human situation seems very remote. There is thus an enormous
gap between microorganism tests and human carcinogenesis, and
this must be crossed before a valid judgment can made. In this
respect, all transformation tests and organ culture assays could
form the bridge connecting the two situations.

This encouraged us to set up another test system, which was constructed, to some extent, as an imitation of conditions in the
respiratory tract of an individual exposed to polycyclic aromatic hydrocarbons. Human lung cancer is reported to be related
to environmental pollutants (5) and data are available which demonstrate that human lung tissue can metabolize polycyclic aromatic hydrocarbons into active metabolites (6). Thus the in vitro
system, which consisted of a fetal hamster lung cell transformation and a trachea organ culture assay, was preliminarily
tested with some common polynuclear hydrocarbons, but without
using an auxiliary activator (i.e., feeder cells or microsomal
liver cell fractions).

Methods

Lung Cell Preparation and Primary Culture. Lungs from Syrian golden
hamster fetuses were removed on the 15th day of gestation.
Isolated cells were obtained after cutting the pooled lung
lobes into small fragments and repeated trypsinization according to the technique described by Emura et al. (7). The cells
were resuspended in RPMI 1640 (Flow Lab., Bonn, FRG) supplemented with 100 IU/ml penicillin, 100 µg/ml streptomycin, and 20%
fetal bovine serum (FBS) (Flow Lab., Bonn, FRG) and seeded in
75 cm^2 plastic flasks (Falcon, Oxnard, California, USA) with
15 ml of medium at a density of 1-2 × 10^6/flask. They were then
cultivated at 37°C in a humidified incubator with 10% CO_2 in
air. On becoming 90% confluent, the cells were either subcul-
tivated by using a mixture of 0.225% trypsin and 0.02% EDTA, or
else stored frozen, with 5%-10% dimethylsulfoxide (DMSO) in the
medium, in liquid nitrogen.

Colony Forming and Transformation Assay. The cells were harvested
from the 2nd to 6th subcultures. They were plated at densities
of 4-8 × 10^3/20 cm^2 Falcon dish in 3 ml of medium. To achieve a

constant plating efficiency, insulin (Hoechst, Frankfurt, FRG) was added in concentrations of up to 0.8 IU/ml medium. Treatment of cells was started 24 h after cell plating, and test substances were dissolved in not more than 0.1% DMSO (Merck, Darmstadt, FRG) in concentrations of 0.05, 0.1, 0.25, 0.5, 0.75 and 1.0 μg/ml in medium were added under reduced light. The exposure to chemicals lasted 24 h. Five dishes were prepared for each concentration of the test substances and DMSO, and for an untreated control. After 10-14 days, the assay was stopped by fixing with methanol and staining with May-Grünwald Giemsa. Colonies consisting of more than 16 cells were considered positive for survival growth. They were counted with a stereo microscope and a New Brunswick electronic colony counter. Colonies were considered transformed when they consisted of densely growing fibroblastic cells possessing basophilic small cytoplasm, were spindle-shaped, grew randomly, one on top of another at the periphery, and were not found in untreated and DMSO cultures.

Soft Agar Test. Cell colonies morphologically consisting of epithelial or fibroblastic cells, treated or untreated, were transferred mechanically to dishes containing 0.33% agar in RPMI 1640 with 10% tryptosephosphate and 10% FBS. Antibiotics were added as previously described. The colony-forming ability was observed under a phase-contrast and dark-field microscope after a cultivation period of up to 42 days in semisolid medium.

Reimplantation. A total of 5×10^6 untreated or treated cells suspended in 0.1 ml RPMI 1640 were injected subcutaneously into newborn hamsters from the same breeding colony. The animals were palpated weekly for detectable neoplasms. After 3 months, they were killed and a histologic examination of grown tumors and site of cell injection was carried out.

Organ Culture of Trachea Explants. Fetal tracheae were dissected aseptically from the same fetuses, as described for the lung cell culture. After being divided into cranial and caudal halves, the explants were placed on cellulose nitrate filters (3-8 μm pore size) (Sartorius Membranfilter, Göttingen, FRG), which were fixed with heated glass beads onto the bottom of multiwells (3.5 cm Ø) of plastic organ culture dishes (Costar, Cambridge, Massachusetts, USA) (Fig. 1) (8). CMRL 1066 (Flow Lab., Bonn, FRG) supplemented with 0.2 μg/ml steptomycin and 5% FBS was used as the growth medium. The organ explants were cultured at 37°C in a humidified Bellco gas chamber with 5% CO_2 in air on a rocking platform (5 changes/min) (Bellco, Vineland, New Jersey, USA). Test substances dissolved in not more than 0.5% DMSO were added to the medium over a period of 7 days, 1 day after the start of cultivation, in concentrations of 0.75, 1.0, and 1.5 μg/ml. After 28 days, the assay was stopped by fixing the explants with Bouin's solution. Paraplast-embedded tracheae were totally cut as serial sections, then stained with hematoxylin-eosin and examined microscopically.

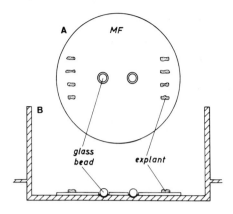

Fig. 1A and B. Schematic illustration of a Costar cluster dish well, equipped with a membrane filter (*MF*), on which explants are laid. (A) view of the membrane filter from above; (B) cross section of the well with an MF and glass beads

Results and Discussion

After adding insulin in concentrations of 0.025–0.2 IU/ml to the medium, a relatively constant plating efficiency was achieved (approx. 4%). The reasons for the stabilizing effects of insulin in relation to plating efficiency are still under investigation. As shown in Table 1, the colony-forming ability of fetal lung cells was reduced by increasing the insulin concentrations when the benzo(a)pyrene [B(a)P] treatment remained stable. Thus the toxic effect of B(a)P seemed to be enhanced by insulin. The total colony survival decreased with increasing concentrations of B(a)P (Fig. 2), i.e., 3% survival at 1.0 µg B(a)P/ml medium. Morphologically, only the fibroblastic cell colonies revealed detectable transformations. The frequency of those colonies was about 1% at dose levels of 0.05 and 0.25 µg/ml B(a)P. In Fig. 3, the normal monolayered growth pattern of an untreated colony of fetal hamster lung cells is depicted. Figure 4, on the other hand, shows the periphery of a transformed fibroblastic colony with "criss-crossing" and "piling-up", as well as a completely disoriented growth pattern. When benz(a)anthracene, benzo(e)pyrene, and chrysene were tested in the colony-forming assay, a dose-related, toxic effect of each substance was detectable (Table 2). In higher concentrations, chrysene and benzo(e)pyrene appeared to be more toxic than benz(a)anthracene. Since the latter polycyclic aromatic hydrocarbons induced either a very weak transformation or else none at all, the question arose as to what extent, and by which technical modifications of the system, transformations which were other than fibroblastic could be detected.

Thus epithelial-looking colonies, which were mechanically isolated were transferred to culture vessels where they were cultivated in soft agar (Table 3). Four out of six epithelial cell clones which were previously treated with 0.5 or 0.75 µg B(a)P showed proliferation and three formed colonies of 0.2 mm diameter. To determine whether the B(a)P-treated cells induced malignant tumors after they had formed colonies in soft agar, 5×10^6 untreated and chemically transformed cells were reimplanted into newborn hamsters from the same breeding colony. Four out of five treated developed tumors after having been injected with clone

Table 1. Insulin-enhanced toxicity of BP in an established line of fetal hamster lung cells[a]

Insulin (IU/ml)	No. of colonies per dish		
	None	DMSO (0.025%)	DMSO (0.025%) + BP (0.25 µg/ml)
0	206.8 + 9.2[b]	151.5 + 4.3	93.6 + 13.2
0.05	226.6 + 1.9	126.0 + 18.1	77.0 + 22.3
0.1	228.6 + 12.7	164.8 + 11.7	76.6 + 5.6
0.2	219.4 + 4.1	114.0 + 14.1	22.8 + 9.1

[a] Mixed cell population at 13 passages. Cells were seeded at 3×10^3/dish
[b] Mean + standard error

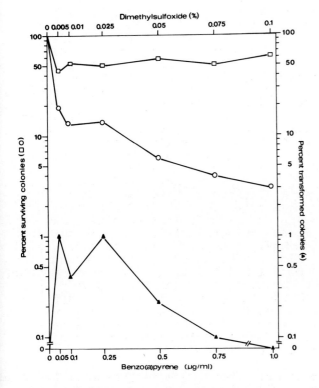

Fig. 2. Toxic and transforming effects of benzo(a)pyrene. Toxicity is calculated as of mean value of surviving colonies in 5 untreated control dishes. Transformation is calculated as percent of counts of fibroblastic transformed colonies in relation to the mean of total colonies in the controls

5-2/22b cells, while no tumors were observed in the controls. The histologic pattern of the tumors was that of a fibro- or endotheliosarcoma, with areas of epithelial features. A further attempt to select epithelial cells from mixed lung cell populations was recently initiated, and studies are now under way to determine whether these cells may be used as targets in the transformation assay. Due to the different metabolizing activities

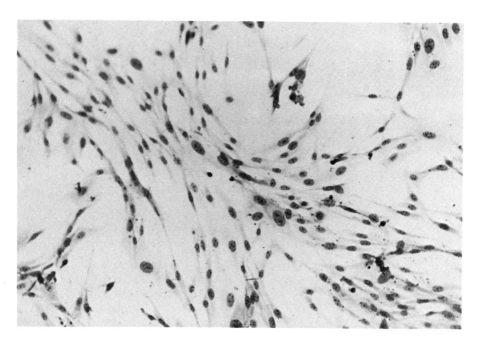

Fig. 3. Fetal hamster lung cell culture; periphery of a normal colony with oriented monolayered growth ability. x 140

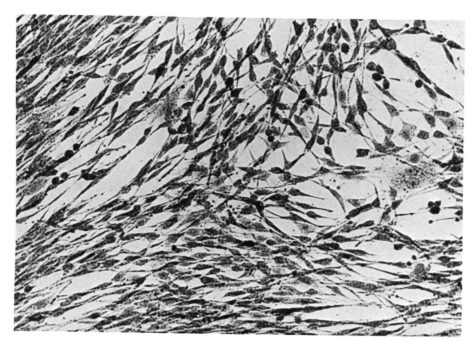

Fig. 4. Fibroblastic transformation of hamster lung cells; colony periphery with small spindle-shaped basophilic cells, showing "criss-crossing" and "piling-up". x 140

Table 2. Surviving colonies after 14 days of assay; 6×10^3 were plated in 50 mm Ø Petri dishes

DMSO (%)	DMSO (%)	+ PAH[a] (µg/ml)	Chrysene	Benzo(e)pyrene	Benz(a)anthracene
77.20 ± 10.08[b]	0.005	0.05	89.25 ± 1.50	83.20 ± 15.29	53.00 ± 26.30
44.80 ± 20.69	0.01	0.1	54.25 ± 7.23	56.80 ± 19.40	13.60 ± 4.36
42.40 ± 25.40	0.025	0.25	19.20 ± 16.12	15.00 ± 18.32	7.60 ± 3.91
34.10 ± 26.78	0.05	0.5	8.80 ± 4.21	4.80 ± 4.09	5.40 ± 2.51
30.60 ± 11.08	0.075	0.75	4.00 ± 4.32	4.80 ± 2.77	6.25 ± 6.18
13.60 ± 6.07	0.1	1.0	0.60 ± 0.89	1.40 ± 1.34	6.20 ± 7.76

[a] Polycyclic aromatic hydrocarbons
[b] Mean ± standard deviation of 5 dishes

Table 3. Colony-forming ability of fetal hamster lung cells in soft agar treatment with B(a)P or untreated

Cell clone no.	Treatment B(a)P <(µg/ml)> + DMSO <(%)>	Time in soft agar (days)	Size of colonies 0.1 mm	Size of colonies 0.2 mm
5-2/11 b	Untreated E[a]	42	–	–
4/153-6	Untreated F[b]	42	–	–
5-2/27 a	0.5 + 0.05 E	39	+	+
5-2/22 a	0.75 + 0.075 E	42	+	+
5-2/22 b	0.75 + 0.075 E	42	+	+
4-2/25 b	0.75 + 0.075 E	39	+	–
4-2/25 a	0.75 + 0.075 E	41	–	–
4-2/25 i	0.75 + 0.075 E	41	–	–

[a] Epithelial-like cells
[b] Fibroblastic cells

of fibroblasts and epithelial cells (9), results showing enhanced transformation rates could be expected. To what extent
the application of 200 µg/ml cis-hydroxyproline would be able
to change the morphology of a primary mixed lung cell population
is demonstrated in Fig. 5. The phase-contrast micrograph was
taken 10 days after the beginning of the amino-acid analogue
treatment, and an almost pure epithelial-like growth was
achieved.

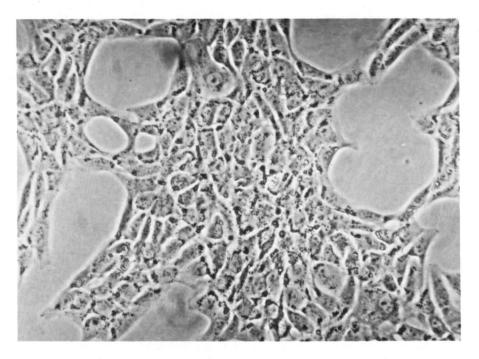

Fig. 5. Phase-contrast micrograph of epithelial-like cells selected from
mixed fetal hamster lung cell cultures after treatment with cis-hydroxyproline. x 140

In order to develop colonies with a relatively large diameter
and sufficient staining behavior, different serum concentrations
were tested as supplements to the growth medium. A supplement
of 20% FBS resulted in a constant colony growth with mean di-
ameters of more than 2 mm, while 16% was far less effective, as
Fig. 6 demonstrates. This is very important when an automatic
colony counter is routinely used for evaluating survival rates.
Although the automatic colony counter would probably leave out
many of the badly stained colonies and the ones which have grown
too close together, it is obviously far more accurate than the
human eye can ever be, particularly when dealing with the large
number of dishes used in just one experiment.

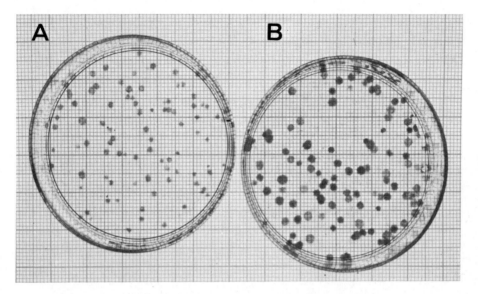

Fig. 6a and b. Different size of cell colonies after cultivation with 16% (a) or 20% (b) fetal bovine serum in the growth medium

The results obtained from the organ culture are listed in Table 4. Histopathologic alterations were observed in 50% of the explants treated with 0.75 µg/ml B(a)P and a somewhat lower percentage showed such changes after treatment with other dosages of this compound or with benz(a)anthracene. However, no alterations were observed in the explants which had been treated with chrysene.

By successfully cultivating fetal hamster tracheae and by paying particular attention to the synthetic function and development of the highly differentiated respiratory epithelium over a period of up to 2 months, we were able to demonstrate that in vitro added polycyclic aromatic hydrocarbons did indeed induce alterations in the epithelial tissue of the respiratory tract.

The principal alterations which we observed were loss of ciliated cells, focal hyperplasia of mucus-producing cells, and a slight tendency to reveal dysplasia as well as invasive growth (Fig. 7). Similar alterations, although more frequent and pathologically stronger, were recorded by Emura et al. (10) when diethylnitrosamine was administered transplacentally in high dosages and the fetal tracheae were kept in culture for up to 6 weeks. In order to shorten the evaluation time necessary for serial sections (longitude of an explant approx. 1.5-2.0 mm/90-150 sections of 3-5 µm), some explants in more recent experiments were fixed with 2% glutaraldehyde, cut longitudinally, and each half prepared for scanning electron microscopy by critical-point drying and with metal-dust contrast (Fig. 8). Ciliated cells as well as mucus-producing cells were detectable and showed the normal development of an explant after 4 weeks of cultivation. Since it is expected that results will be more easily and more rapidly

Table 4. Histologic changes induced by PAH[a] in fetal hamster tracheal explants

Carcinogen (μg/ml)	Day of gestation	Period of exposure (days)	Period of cultivation (days)	No changes				Changes			
				DMSO	B(a)P	B(a)A	Chrysene	DMSO	B(a)P	B(a)A	Chrysene
0	15	7	28	22				0			
0.75	15	7	28		9		4		9		0
1.5	15	7	28		8	3			2	1	
5.0	15	7	28		4				2		

[a] Polycyclic aromatic hydrocarbons

Fig. 7. Focal hyperplasia of mucus-producing cells with slightly infiltrating tendency. The tracheal explant was exposed to 1.5 μg/ml B(a)P for 7 days and cultivated for the total of 28 days. HE x 140

Fig. 8. Scanning electron micrograph showing the inner surface of a 6-week-cultured fetal hamster trachea; ciliated and mucus-producing cells. x 2500

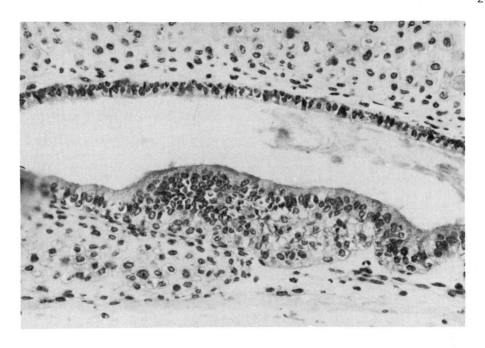

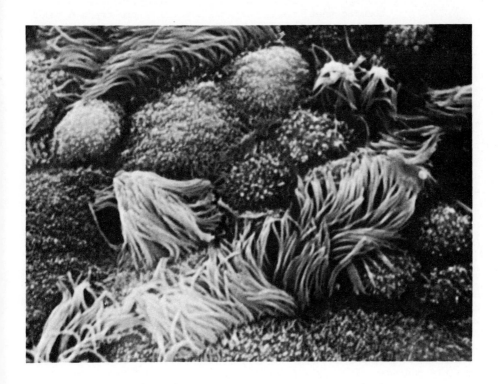

obtained by these techniques, investigations are now being carried out to see how such methods may be applied to routine examinations.

With regard to the time required for each of the described assays, although the optimal conditions must still be standardized and improved, it is expected that it would take about 3 months for results to become available (Table 5). Although the results so far obtained are somewhat preliminary, they do demonstrate that fetal hamster lung cells, when cultured in the short-term, can provide a sufficient amount of mixed-function oxidase capacity to reveal transformation with benzo(a)pyrene, without the use of any additional metabolizing system. At the same time, it was seen that the in vitro exposure of fetal hamster trachea to benzo(a)pyrene caused epithelial alterations. Although a great deal of work will be required before the system may be applied to the routine testing of unknown chemicals, it is hoped that, under similar conditions, cells and organ explants from human fetuses can be cultivated, which would perhaps further the understanding of the human situation.

Table 5. Comparison of time required for the evaluation of carcinogenicity of a substance in various test systems

	Colony-forming test	Soft agar test	Organ culture	Reimplantation of in vitro treated cell into compatible hosts
Evaluation after beginning of experiment	21 days	30–40 days	40–50 days	up to 90 days

Acknowledgments. These studies were performed in collaboration with the team "Inventory and biological impact of polycyclic carcinogens in the environment" and supported by the Bundesumweltamt, Berlin, FRG. (Contract ZJ6-50 424/11.) The authors would like to thank Rita Eichinger and Cornelia Schoch for excellent technical assistance, and Jenny Ross and Susan Hamilton for editorial help. The assistance of Prof. Dr. J. Althoff and Dorothee Kracke with the scanning electron microscope preparation is gratefully acknowledged.

References

1. Heidelberger C (1973) Chemical oncogenesis in culture. Adv Cancer Res 18:317-366
2. Ames AB, Durston WE, Yamasaki E, Lee FD (1973) Carcinogens are mutagens: a simple test system combining liver homogenates for activation and bacteria for detection. Proc Natl Acad Sci USA 70:2281-2285
3. Di Paolo JA, Nelson RL, Donovan PJ, Evans CH (1973) Host-mediated in vivo-in vitro assay for chemical carcinogenesis. Arch Pathol 95:380-385
4. Pienta RJ, Poiley JA, Leibherz WB (1977) Morphological transformation of early passage golden Syrian hamster embryo cells derived from cryopreserved primary cultures as reliable in vitro bioassay for identifying diverse carcinogens. Int J Cancer 19:642-655

5. Mohr U, Schmähl D, Tomatis L (eds) (1977) Air pollution and cancer in man. IARC Sci Publ 16:Lyon
6. Bartsch H, Sabadie N, Malaveille C, Camus A-M, Richter-Reichhelm H-B (1978) Carcinogen metabolism with human and experimental tissues: inter-individual and species differences. Proc XII Int Cancer Congr, Buenos Aires. Pergamon Press, Oxford
7. Emura M, Richter-Reichhelm H-B, Mohr U (1978) Epithelial alterations in fetal tracheal explants of Syrian golden hamsters exposed to di-ethylnitrosamine in utero. Cancer Lett 5:115-121
8. Emura M, Richter-Reichhelm H-B, Emura KM, Matthei S, Mohr U (1979) Tubular explant culture of fetal Syrian golden hamster tracheae. Exp Pathol 17:196-199
9. Huberman E, Sachs L (1973) Metabolism of the carcinogenic hydrocarbon benzo(a)pyrene in human fibroblasts and epithelial cells. Int J Cancer 11:412-418
10. Emura M, Richter-Reichhelm H-B, Mohr U (1978) Toxic and transforming effects of polycyclic hydrocarbons on fetal hamster lung cell cultures. I. Benzo(a)pyrene. Cancer Lett 4:343-348

Malignant Transformation of Mammalian Cells in Culture by Chemical Carcinogens

H. Marquardt[1]

The bioassay of the rapidly growing list of chemicals for mutagenic and carcinogenic properties by in vivo studies is an in-
surmountable task. It is, therefore, hoped that short-term in
vitro tests, especially those employing mammalian cells, may be
of predictive value in terms of human risk as prescreening
methods.

Perhaps the most promising new model systems for this in vitro
bioassay of chemical carcinogens and for the analysis of their
mechanism(s) of action are mammalian cell cultures in which
cells become tumorigenic following exposure to chemical carcinogens. The contributions of such malignant transformation
assays to the study of chemical carcinogenesis have recently
been reviewed (1). All of the presently available quantitative
systems employ rodent cell cultures: the hamster embryo system
utilizes diploid but heterogenous primary or secondary cultures
of hamster embryo fibroblasts, while the second highly quantitative system employs cloned long-term lines of aneuploid inbred-
mouse fibroblasts (for reference and methods, see 2,3). In addition, some attempts to chemically transform various epithelial
cells are being made now. A very interesting transformation
system, employing the in vitro carcinogen-induced conversion of
hematopoietic stem cells into leukemic cells and in which possibly transformation and differentiation could be studied con-
comitantly, has recently been described (for reference, see 3).

In our own studies we are using a cloned line of C3H mouse fibroblasts, M2, which is susceptible to malignant transformation by
chemicals (for methods and criteria of transformation, see 2,3).
To be able to compare different experiments, in all experiments
N-methyl-N'-nitro-N-nitrosoguanidine is used as a positive control.

Malignant Transformation — An Assay to Detect Oncogenic Potential of Chemicals

In general, a good correlation between in vivo carcinogenic
potential and in vitro transforming activity has been reported
for the direct-acting carcinogens and some indirect-acting

[1]Memorial Sloan-Kettering Cancer Center, New York, New York 10021/USA

Present address: Department of Toxicology, Universitäts-Krankenhaus Eppen-
dorf, University Hamburg Medical School, Martinistraße 20, D-2000 Hamburg 20/
FRG

carcinogens, such as polycyclic hydrocarbons. The most extensive survey of such carcinogens in a transformation assay, demonstrating a 91% positive correlation, has recently been published (4). Transformation assays for indirect-acting carcinogens can be improved qualitatively and quantitatively by addition of a metabolizing system, i.e., by addition of enzyme preparations (5,6) or by co-cultivation with metabolizing "feeder" cells (7,8).

The available data on another class of chemicals, the antitumor agents, indicate that a large number of them (i.e., alkylating agents, urethane, and antibiotics) are active in causing mammalian cell transformation in vitro and oncogenesis in vivo (9). Noteworthy exceptions are the antimetabolites, such as methotrexate and 5-fluorouracil. These latter compounds have been reported to induce malignant transformation in vitro, but in vivo carcinogenicity for these drugs has not yet been demonstrated (9).

In addition, transformation studies have also been useful to study the anticarcinogenic effect of chemicals, such as inhibitors of the activating metabolism or scavengers of free radicals (7,10).

It must, however, also be emphasized that in some instances poor correlations must be anticipated between in vivo tumorigenicity of chemicals and their activity in in vitro short-term tests as well as among different short-term tests (11). It is now generally agreed, therefore, that a battery of short-term tests must be used to detect the potential for carcinogenicity of chemicals.

Malignant Transformation — A Model System to Study Mechanism(s) of Action of Chemical Carcinogens

It appears that malignant transformation in vitro may indeed be an ideal model system for the study of chemical carcinogenesis. In many ways it seems to resemble the in vivo situation: it has been shown (a) that it does not involve the selection of pre-existing transformed cells, (b) that it does not involve an apparent switch-on of oncornaviruses, (c) that, as in in vivo carcinogenesis, it follows a two-stage mechanism (i.e., initiation and promotion), and (d) that clones transformed in vitro by exposure to chemicals exhibit non-cross-reacting, individual tumor-specific transplantation antigens.

Thus, transformation studies have been invaluable tools in studying the metabolic activation of chemical carcinogens. Particularly in the case of polycyclic hydrocarbons, in vitro results have led to the insight that oxides in general and particularly diol-epoxides of the bay-region type may be proximate carcinogens (see 2,3).

The cellular events, however, involved in chemical carcinogenesis and in chemically induced malignant transformation are
completely unknown. Two general mechanisms have been proposed
to explain the chemical induction of malignant transformation
in cultured mammalian cells (12).

On the one hand, transformation may be the result of a somatic
mutation, i.e., an alteration in gene structure. This "somatic
mutation theory" is supported by the observations: (a) that
genetic susceptibility to certain forms of cancer exists and
that some familial cancers appear to occur, (b) that covalent
binding to cellular DNA has been found for the ultimate electrophilic forms of almost all carcinogens, (c) that many, perhaps all, chemical carcinogens in their ultimate form are mutagens, and (d) that the induction of pyrimidine dimers in DNA
and their repair is apparently related to tumorigenesis (13). It
must be emphasized, however, that while qualitatively ultimate
carcinogens do react with DNA, quantitatively the capacity of
carcinogens to covalently interact with DNA does not correlate
well with their carcinogenic potency. Likewise, while qualitatively most ultimate carcinogens are mutagenic, quantitatively
a strong mutagen is not necessarily also a strong carcinogen
(for a review, see 12). In addition, inhibitors of reverse tran-
scriptase activity, polyriboinosinic-polyribocytidylic acid and
polyribocytidylic-oligodeoxyriboguanylic acid, inhibit the induction of malignant transformation but not mutagenesis by
chemicals (12,14). It should be noted in this context that Temin
visualizes RNA alterations and reverse transcription of these
as playing a role in chemical carcinogenesis (15).

Alternatively, malignant transformation in vitro may be the result of epigenetic changes in cellular transcription/translation.
Such changes are presumed to be responsible for much of normal
development, including the activation-inactivation of the mammalian X chromosome and the extinction and activation of differentiated functions which have been observed in cultured cells
(16). The ability of embryonic antigens to reappear in chemically induced tumor cells lends support to the idea that transformation results from a change in gene function rather than in
gene structure. Moreover, it seems evident that the frequency
of transformation is so much higher (100-1000-fold) than that
of mutation (12,17; Table 1) that it is probably more reasonable to consider transformation an event of the "epigenetic"
type (though these data could also be explained by assuming
multiplicity or abnormally large size of the genetic target or
mutational "hot spots"). It should also be noted in this regard
that human cells in culture, when compared to rodent cells, are
highly refractory to chemical transformation but show normal
frequencies and rates of mutation (18), an observation which also
suggests diverse mechanisms of action. Moreover, the numerous
observations that reversion of malignancy can be induced with
high frequencies in transformed cells in culture (for reference,
see 12) also lend strong support to the suggestion that fundamental differences between the nature of somatic mutation and
phenotypic transformation do exist. Since cellular differentiation is potentially reversible, the reversibility of malignant
transformation in vitro as well as the fact that its reversion

Table 1. Malignant transformation and mutagenesis by chemicals in M2 mouse fibroblasts

Compound	µg/ml	Plating efficiency (%)	Transformed foci/10^6 survivors	Ouabain-resistant colonies/10^6 survivors	Ratio transformants: ouabain-resistant colonies
Acetone	0.5%	50	0	0.7	
MNNG	0.25	41	2,700	90	30
	0.5	32	5,000	211	24
	1.0	21	19,760	618	32
7MBA-3,	1.0	39	3,800	3.4	1118
4-diol	5.0	15	14,000	17	859

MNNG, N-methyl-N'-nitro-N-nitrosoguanidine; 7MBA, 7-methylbenz(a)anthracene

is often induced by agents which also affect cellular differentiation suggest that malignant transformation in vitro may also arise from the action of epigenetic, cytoplasmic mechanisms. (It should be remembered that chemical carcinogens chemically interact as well with RNA and proteins as they do with DNA.)

Summary

The primary cellular event in chemically induced malignant transformation in vitro remains unknown. Though the observed interactions of carcinogens with DNA may not reflect the mutagenic nature of the events underlying their carcinogenicity but rather their almost universal electrophilic reactivity, assays for chemically induced malignant transformation as well as short-term mutagenicity tests appear to be invaluable tools in detecting the potential for carcinogenicity of chemicals.

References

1. Kuroki T (1975) Gann Monogr 17:69-85
2. Marquardt H (1976) IARC Sci Publ 12:389-410
3. Marquardt H (1978) Staub-Reinhaltung Luft 38:258-265
4. Pienta RJ, Poiley JA, Lebherz WB (1977) Int J Cancer 19:642-655
5. Krahn DF, Heidelberger C (1977) Mutat Res 46:27-44
6. Kuroki T, Montesano R (1977) Cancer Res 37:1044-1050
7. Marquardt H, Heidelberger C (1972) Cancer Res 32:721-725
8. Langenbach R, Freed HJ, Raveh D, Huberman E (1978) Nature 276:277-280
9. Marquardt H, Marquardt H (1977) Cancer 40:1930-1934
10. Marquardt H, Sapozink MD, Zedeck MS (1974) Cancer Res 34:3387-3390
11. Marquardt H, Philips FS, Marquardt H, Sternberg SS (1979) Proc Am Assoc Cancer Res 20:45
12. Marquardt H (to be published) In: Grover PL (ed) Chemical Carcinogens and DNA. CRC Press
13. Hart RW, Setlow RB, Woodhead AD (1977) Proc Natl Acad Sci USA 74:5574-5578

14. Marquardt H (1973) Nature - N Biol 246:228-229
15. Temin H (1971) J Natl Cancer Inst 46:III-V
16. Bouck N, Mayorca G di (1976) Nature 264:722-727
17. Parodi S, Brambilla G (1977) Mutat Res 47:53-74
18. Spandidos DA, Siminovitch L (1978) Cell 13:651-662

Section IV

Methodological Aspects with Emphasis on Standardisation of Test Procedures and Interpretation of Test Results

Metabolizing Systems Used for in Vitro Mutagenicity Testing

H. Greim, E. Deml, W. Göggelmann, G. Ludwig, L. Schwarz, and T. Wolff[1]

Introduction

In early 1977 a workshop was held to discuss the plate incorporation assay (Ames test) to detect mutagenic effects of chemicals (1-3). The aim of the workshop was to discuss a protocol and to identify those parts of the procedure which should be defined better. It turned out that the system for metabolic activation of the test compounds especially required better definition and standardization. All details were discussed and a revised test protocol has been elaborated (4). A consensus was reached that no rigid protocol should be prepared because the users of the Ames test are rather to be encouraged to vary the test procedure to adapt it to the special requirements of the different test compounds.

The participants of the workshop further agreed to evaluate the revised protocol in a ring test using three known carcinogens: benzo(a)pyrene, 2-aminoanthracene, and N-nitrosomorpholine. These three test compounds were purchased by one of the participants, who distributed them to the other participants.

Twenty of the participating laboratories submitted their data. Although all found the test compounds to be mutagenic, it turned out that only four laboratories performed the test in the same manner. It also became evident that most of the variations involved the metabolic activation system: The S-9 fraction has been isolated from noninduced mice or rats or from one of the two species after pretreatment with phenobarbital (PB) or polychlorinated biphenyls (PCB).

Moreover, different amounts of S-9 in the S-9 mix have been applied and different solvents have been used. This indicates that the essential aspects of the metabolizing system need to be discussed.

Metabolic Activation System

The S-9 fraction is the supernatant after centrifugation of a liver homogenate at 9000 g and includes cytoplasm and the microsomes which contain the enzmyes for metabolic activation of the test compounds (for review, see 5). These activating enzymes

[1]Abteilung für Toxikologie der Gesellschaft für Strahlen- und Umweltforschung München, Ingolstädter Landstraße 1, D-8042 Neuherberg/FRG

catalyze the primary oxidation steps called "phase I reactions," which include oxidation of aliphatic and aromatic hydrocarbons, epoxidation of alkenes, oxidative O-, S-, and N-dealkylations, and oxidative deaminations (6-8). Inactivation of the primarily formed metabolites by "phase II reactions" is mediated by enzymes located in the microsomal fraction as well as in the cytoplasm of the S-9. Typical examples of phase II reactions are the dihydrodiol formation from epoxides, formation of the glutathione-, glucuronic acid-, and sulphate-conjugates (9-12).

Several test compounds undergo only phase I reactions, whereas most test compounds are metabolized by both phase I and phase II enzymes. Dimethylnitrosamine (DMN) is a typical example of a compound which undergoes only a phase I reaction (13,14). It is oxidatively demethylated forming monomethylnitrosamine which is further degraded to alkylating species interacting with cellular macromolecules. Since no metabolic inactivation interferes with the reactive intermediates formed, a close correlation between enzyme activity and mutagenicity should occur.

This correlation is demonstrated in Fig. 1 when microsomes with low phase I activity, which is represented by the amount of microsomal cytochrome P-450 after feeding rats with diets of different protein content, are used for metabolic activation (15). This correlation also pertains to microsomes of high phase I activity after pretreatment with PB or PCB. A closely related increased mutation frequency is seen (16).

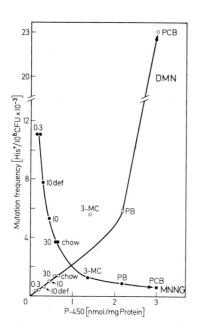

Fig. 1. The relationship between the cytochrome P-450 content of microsomal preparations and their ability to alter the mutagenicity of dimethylnitrosamine (DMN) and N-methyl-N'-nitro-N-nitrosoguanine (MNNG). Male Swiss-Webster mice were fed ad libitum either chow or semisynthetic diets containing 30%, 10%, 3%, or 0% protein (15). To induce the microsomal biotransformation system, others received 500 mg/kg Aroclor 1254 (PCB) given IP 4 days before sacrifice, 0.1% phenobarbital (PB) in the drinking water for 7 days or IP injections of 40 mg/kg 3-methylcholanthrene (MC) given days 2 and 1 before sacrifice. CFU = Colony Forming Units

Compounds such as methylnitronitrosoguanidine (MNNG), which only undergo inactivation by the microsomes, behave in an opposite way: increasing enzyme activities result in a decreased mutation frequency (Fig. 1). This correlation seems to apply to microsomes of other mammalian species tested, including man (17). Here again, a close correlation between cytochrome P-450 and activation of dimethylnitrosamine to a mutagen is observed (Fig. 2).

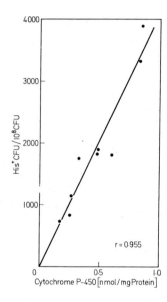

Fig. 2. Relationship between content of cytochrome P-450 of human liver microsomes and ability of these microsomes to activate the mutagenicity of dimethylnitrosamine. Liver tissue (0.2 g) was obtained during abdominal surgery from specimen taken for histologic examination (17)

Many examples, however, indicate that most of the test compounds undergo both phase I and phase II reactions. Benzo(a)pyrene (BP), for example, is activated to epoxides which are subsequently inactivated by microsomal hydratase activity to dihydrodiols which, again, may serve as a phase I substrate resulting in the formation of diol-epoxides (18,19).

Inactivation of BP oxides by hydratase activity has been evaluated by Oesch and his group (20), who demonstrated a close correlation between the activity of this phase II reaction and mutagenicity of compounds such as BP that are inactivated by diol formation. They also showed that hydratase activity, in relation to epoxide formation, was dependent on the species used and the inducer administered to enhance phase I reactions (21).

The metabolism of styrene further exemplifies different reactions involved in activation and inactivation. Styrene oxide, a product of styrene, formed in a phase I reaction, is the substrate of different phase II reactions such as conjugation with glutathione forming a mercapturic acid, hydration, glucuronidation, and others (22-25). Due to these potent phase II inactivations of styrene, such as hydration, only marginal mutagenic effects of styrene could be demonstrated (26) although styrene oxide is a known mutagen (27).

Thus, when a metabolizing system with high phase I activities is obtained after pretreatment of the animals with phenobarbital or polychlorinated biphenyls, altered inactivating capacities of phase II reactions must also be taken into account.

Modification of Phase I and Phase II Reactions by Inducing Agents

In Tables 1 and 2, the responses of rat and mouse liver micro-somal enzymes to pretreatment of the animals with commonly used inducers are given. In rats (Table 1), the BP hydroxylation re-action (= aryl hydrocarbon hydroxylase) is highly induced by PCB, less by PB or 3-MC. Moreover, addition of 7,8-benzoflavone (α-naphthoflavone), an inhibitor of a cytochrome P-448 type reaction (28,29), differently affects BP hydroxylation.

Table 1. Effect of pretreatment on hepatic microsomal enzymes of rats determined in the S-9 fraction

Enzyme activity	Untreated	PCBs	PB	3-MC
Aldrin- epoxidation	100	120	230	100
Ethylmorphine N-demethylation	100	360	360	120
Benzo(a)pyrene- hydroxylation	100	750	200	340
Its modification by 7,8-benzoflavone[a]	1.4	0.5	1.3	0.7
Styrene epoxide- hydratase	100	330	280	120

[a]Activity without modifier = 1

Activities in the S-9 fraction of untreated rats = 100%. Pretreatment: 1 × 500 mg/kg Clophen A50 (PCBs) by gavage 4 days before sacrifice; 0.1% phenobarbital-Na (PB) in the drinking water for 7 days; 40 mg/kg 3-methylcholanthrene (3-MC) intraperitoneally 2 and 1 days before sacrifice. Male Wistar rats, 190-210 g

Table 2. Effect of pretreatment on hepatice microsomal
enzymes of mice determined in the S-9 fraction

Enzyme activity	Untreated	PCBs	PB	3-MC
Aldrin epoxidation	100	380	520	70
Ethylmorphine N-demethylation	100	490	430	85
Benzo(a)pyrene-hydroxylation	100	950	630	990
Its modification by 7,8-benzoflavone[a]	3.3	1.4	1.4	0.5
Styrene epoxide-hydratase	100	240	180	190

[a]Activity without modifier = 1

Activities in the S-9 fraction of untreated mice = 100%.
Pretreatment: 1 × 50 mg/kg Clophen A50 (PCBs) by
gavage 4 days before sacrifice; 0.1% phenobarbital-Na
(PB) in the drinking water for 7 days; 40 mg/kg
3-methylcholanthrene (3-MC) daily intraperitoneally
2 and 1 before sacrifice. Male NMRJ mice, 11 weeks

This demonstrates that the inducers enhance qualitatively different microsomal phase I reactions. The greatest effects on the different enzymes are seen after pretreatment of rats with the PCB mixture Clophen A50, which is similar to Aroclor 1254. It also becomes apparent that styrene oxide hydratase activity is increased more than 3 fold after PCB application, whereas BP hydroxylase increased more than fourfold. The latter reactions are representative for the activation of benzpyrene and the hydratase activity for the inactivation of the epoxide. This explains why an increased mutagenicity of BP is observed after animal pretreatment with a PCB mixture (21).

Male NMRJ mice respond differently to the inducers (Table 2). PCB and PB enhance aldrin epoxidation and ethylmorphine demethylation fourfold whereas MC-treatment lowered these activities below the values detected in untreated mice. However, BP-hydroxylation activities increased 6-9fold after pretreatment with the three inducers while the deactivating styrene oxide hydratase activity increased only twofold. Thus, mutagenicity of the metabolically activated BP should be more pronounced in mice than in rats. This has been recently demonstrated by Oesch (43).

From the observations of Nebert et al. (30) and Wiebel et al. (31), it is apparent that mouse strains do respond differently to P-448 type inducers (Table 3); whereas, in the commonly used rat strains, such different responses to polycyclic aryl-hydrocarbon induction are not known. This indicates the advisability of using rats instead of mice for induction of microsomal enzymes unless the polycyclic aryl-hydrocarbon response of the mouse strain is known.

Table 3. Inducibility of hepatic benzo(a)pyrene hydroxylation in various mouse strains[a] (pmol/mg protein/30 min)

Species	Control	Benz(a)anthracene[b] IP
NZB	3080 + 1430	2500 + 470
NZW	2090 + 200	*2970* + 153
AKR	1810 + 560	*2808* + 241
SJL	2090 + 430	1790 + 370
DBA	920 + 90	995 + 155
C57	1550 ± 150	*5760* ± 500

[a] From Wiebel et al. (31)
[b] 1 × 100 mg/kg

The italic numbers indicate significant differences from the control experiment

Other inactivating phase II reactions are also enhanced after application of the inducing agents. Tables 4 and 5 show the effects on several glucuronidation reactions in rats and mice. Glucuronidation of BP, naphthol, and morphine has been deter-mined. In rat liver microsomes, glucuronidation of BP and naphthol is highly increased after PCB with little or no effect after PB or 3-methylcholanthrene, whereas conjugation of morphine is en-hanced by PCB and PB. In mouse liver microsomes after treatment with PCB, there is a slight increase in conjugation of 3-hydroxy-BP and of naphthol (Table 5). The effect of PB does not differ from that of the PCB, whereas pretreatment of the mice with 3-methylcholanthrene had no effect. Glucuronidation of morphine has not been enhanced after pretreatment with any of the three inducers; mice again respond differently than rats (Table 4).

Table 4. Effect of pretreatment on hepatic glucuronyltransferase activities in male Wistar rats, 220-250 g

Glucuronidation of	Untreated	PCBs	PB	3-MC
3-OH-Benzo(a)pyrene	100	590	120	110
Naphthol	100	380	135	110
Morphine	100	250	330	100

Activities in microsomes of untreated rats = 100%.
Pretreatment schedule, see Table 1.

Table 5. Effect of pretreatment on hepatic glucuronyltransferase
activities in male NMRJ mice, 11 weeks

Glucuronidation of	Untreated	PCBs	PB	3-MC
3-OH-Benzo(a)pyrene	100	120	60	55
Naphthol	100	140	145	110
Morphine	100	95	100	95

Activities with microsomes of untreated rats = 100%.
Pretreatment schedule, see Table 2.

The similar inducibility of BP and naphthol conjugation in rats
and mice indicates that both compounds are conjugated by the
same glucuronyltransferase. Morphine conjugation seems to be
catalyzed by a different transferase which is induced both by
the PCB and by PB (33). It also becomes apparent from the experiment that glucuronidation activities of NMRJ mice respond
less to the inducers than those of Wistar rats.

Following the Ames test protocol, glucuronidation reactions, as
well as sulfation, will not affect metabolic activation in mutagenicity test systems. Although the respective transferases are
microsomal or cytoplasmic enzymes being retained in the S-9 fraction, their cofactors are not available to support inactivation
reactions by glucuronidation or sulfation. However, epoxide
hydratase and glutathione transferase are active in the S-9
fraction. The epoxide hydratase requires water as cofactor (32)
and the glutathione transferase requires sufficient amounts of
glutathione, which is also present in the S-9 (41). To determine
the involvement of glucuronidation or sulfation in the metabolism of a test compound, one simply has to add the necessary
cofactors to the S-9 mix (11,42).

Conclusion. For routine testing, an enzyme preparation with high
phase I activities and relatively low phase II activities, especially hydratase activity, should be used. Moreover, because
of strain differences in the inducibility of polycyclic hydrocarbon hydroxylation in mice, rats pretreated with polychlorinated biphenyls should be used preferentially. Phenobarbital
does not sufficiently induce all phase I reactions in rats.

Amount of S-9 Protein

Another variable in many test protocols is the amount of S-9
used in the incubation mixture. According to Ames, 0.04 and
0.1 ml of S-9 per ml S-9 mix are used (3). This corresponds to
approximately 1.6 and 4.0 mg protein, respectively. Increasing
amounts of enzyme should increase metabolic activation of the
test compound with the consequence of increased mutation frequency. This is shown in the experiment with N-nitrosomorpholine
(Fig. 3). It should be noted, however, that relatively high concentrations of the test compounds are used.

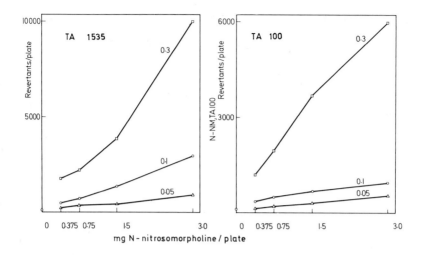

mg N - nitrosomorpholine / plate

Fig. 3. Relationship between mutation rate induced by N-nitrosomorpholine (N-NM) as determined with the *S. typhimurium* strains TA 1535 and T 100 and the amount of microsomal protein in the test system according to Ames et al. (1). The S-9 mix contained 0.05, 0.1, and 0.3 ml S-9/ml corresponding to 1.8, 4, and 12 mg microsomal protein/ml S-9 mix

In many cases, however, this correlation is not found. Using 2-aminoanthracene, the highest amount of S-9 induced the lowest mutation frequency (Fig. 4). Cytotoxicity of 2-aminoanthracene allowed only low concentrations of the test compound to be used.

These observations indicate that such seemingly paradoxical effects might especially occur when low concentrations of the test compounds are applied. This phenomenon may be explained by kinetic considerations. In the presence of a certain amount of enzyme protein, increasing substrate concentrations result in increasing metabolism leading to increasing mutation frequencies. This correlation is maintained until substrate saturation. On providing an unlimited supply of substrate, any increase in enzyme protein content will further increase metabolism resulting in increased mutation frequency.

This is pertinent to noncytotoxic compounds such as DMN or *N*-nitrosomorpholine which can be used at high concentrations. However, many test compounds are cytotoxic and can only be used at low concentrations. In consequence, only small amounts of reactive products are formed. Increasing concentration would reduce mutation frequency due to increased cytotoxic effects. It is also apparent that increasing amounts of S-9 can not result in an increased formation of reactive products. Moreover, it is known that reactive intermediates formed are inactivated by nonspecific binding to macromolecules such as microsomal protein (34,35). Increasing amounts of such proteins in the test system will increase nonspecific binding with the consequence of

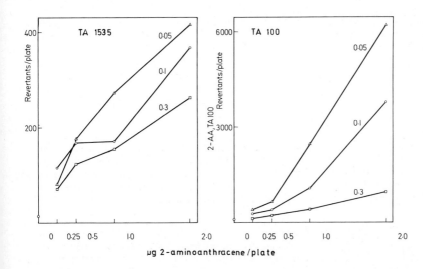

Fig. 4. Relationship between mutation frequency induced by 2-aminoanthracene (2-AA) as determined with the *S. typhimurium* strains TA 1535 and TA 100 and different amounts of microsomal protein in the test system according to Ames et al. (1). The S-9 mix contained 0.05, 0.1, and 0.3 ml S-9/ml corresponding to 1.8, 4, and 12 mg microsomal protein/ml S-9 mix

reduced mutagenicity, as demonstrated in Table 6. In the presence of unlimited concentrations of a test compound (100 μmol/ml), presumably 20% is metabolically activated during the experiment. If 90% of the reactive products formed are nonspecifically bound to microsomal protein, the remaining 2 μmol will reach the bacterial target cell. Increasing the amount of enzymes will increase the amount of reactive metabolites formed, resulting in an increased amount of metabolites reaching the target although more inactivation occurs. This represents the situation when a noncytotoxic compound is used.

Table 6. Hypothetic scheme of effects of substrate concentrations on mutation frequency at different amounts of S-9

ml S-9 per ml S-9 mix	Substrate μmol/ml	mol metabolized in 2h	Reactive intermediates bound (μmol)	Concentration of reactive intermediates at target (μmol)	Mutation frequency
0.05	100	20	18	2	+
0.3	100	100	90	10	+++
0.05	1	1	0.90	0.10	+
0.3	1	1	$\gg 0.90$	$\ll 0.10$	?

With a cytotoxic compound used at low concentrations, no such correlation can be expected. Most likely, all of the test compound is metabolized and only the portion which escapes inactivation due to nonspecific binding reaches the target. Increasing the concentration of microsomal protein will not increase metabolism but increase inactivation by unspecific binding. Less reactive intermediates will reach the target cells, resulting in reduced mutation frequency.

Conclusion. Thus, it is generally not sufficient to use only one or two amounts of S-9 in the test. Several low amounts of S-9 should be used when low amounts of test compounds can be applied; and a broad range from low to high amounts of S-9 when non-cytotoxic compounds at high concentrations are tested.

Effect of Solvents. Finally, concerning the use of solvents which potentially affect the metabolizing system, two points have to be considered: first, increasing lipophilicity of a solvent increasingly inhibits metabolism of a compound by microsomal enzymes (28,36,37) and, second, the more polar the test compound, the more its metabolism will be inhibited by lipophilic solvents (38).

Evidence for the first point is given in Fig. 5. The metabolism of aldrin has been determined in the presence of different solvents. Increasing lipophilicity of the solvents increasingly inhibits the enzyme reactions. Inhibition also depends on the concentration of the solvent.

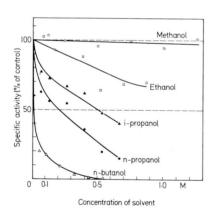

Fig. 5. Inhibitory effects of increasingly lipophilic aliphatic alcohols on aldrin epoxidase activity. The incubation mixture contained 0.5 mg microsomal protein/ml 0.1 M phosphate buffer, pH 7.4, 0.1 mM aldrin, a NADPH-generating system, and 0.2% to 5% (v/v) of a solvent (38)

Investigating the effects of other solvents frequently used in the incorporation assay in the presence of test compounds of different polarity extends this observation (Table 7). Metabolism of the highly lipophilic compounds aldrin and benzo(a)pyrene (BP) is little affected by the polar solvents acetone or methanol. Inhibition by ethanol and DMSO is modest. By contrast, metabolism of the highly polar DMN is already affected by 1/10 the concentration of methanol, ethanol, and DMSO concentration. At concentrations between 0.05 and 0.2 M these solvents inhibited the reactions by 50% (data not shown). Acetone was inactive at concentrations up to 1 M.

Table 7. Inhibition of hepatic microsomal enzymes by solvents

Solvent-Concentrations (1 M)	(% v/v)	Benzpyrene-hydroxylation	Aldrin-epoxidation	DMN-demethylation at 0.1 M of solvents
Methanol	3.2	90	100	70
Acetone	5.8	100	90	100
Ethanol	4.6	50	60	25
DMSO	7.8	20	80	50

Activity without inhibitor = 100.

These findings correspond to those of Sugimura et al. (39) and Norpoth et al. (40), and indicate that lipophilicity and the amount of a solvent affect mutation frequency in the plate incorporation assay, e.g., increasing amounts of DMSO increasingly inhibited mutation frequency induced by dimethylnitrosamine and diethylnitrosamine (39).

Conclusion. Thus, for solubilization of the test compounds, the most polar solvent possible should be chosen, preferentially buffer or the hydrophilic organic solvents methanol or acetone. If the test compounds are not sufficiently soluble in these solvents, ethanol or DMSO should be used. Furthermore, the quantity of all the solvents should be kept as small as possible.

General Conclusions

Being aware of several factors which affect the outcome of the test, one may become reluctant to accept that the plate incorporation assay is simple, rapid, and inexpensive. Nevertheless, it is one of the best understood in vitro systems for mutagenicity testing and there is urgent need to use it routinely. For routine application it is certainly acceptable to proceed according to a more or less rigid protocol initially. However, one has to be aware of the problems discussed in order to adapt experimental conditions to the special requirements of the test compound.

One has also to be aware that the test in general provides optimal conditions for metabolic activation of the test compound without interference of inactivating phase II reactions. Since these reactions do occur in mammals, the question of relevance, especially of the positive results, is raised. But here again, the test protocol can be modified to include cofactors for the inactivating reactions, if desired. This allows specific investigations on the inactivation mechanism of the test compound as well.

References

1. Ames BN, Gurney EG, Miller JA, Bartsch H (1972) Carcinogen as frameshift mutagens: metabolites and derivatives of 2-acetylaminofluorene and other aromatic amine carcinogens. Proc Natl Acad Sci USA 69:3128-3132
2. Ames BN, Durston WE, Yamasaki E, Lee DF (1973) Carcinogens are mutagens: a simple test system combining liver homogenates for activation and bacteria for detection. Proc Natl Acad Sci USA 8:2281-2285
3. Ames BN, McCann J, Yamasaki E (1975) Methods for detecting carcinogens and mutagens with the Salmonella/mammalian microsome mutagenicity test. Mutat Res 31:347-361
4. Mattern IE, Greim H (1978) Report of a workshop on bacterial in vitro mutagenicity test systems. Mutat Res 53:369-378
5. Serres FJ de, Fouts JR, Bend JR, Philpot RM (eds) (1976) In vitro metabolic activation in mutagenesis testing. North Holland, Amsterdam, New York, Oxford
6. Testa B, Jenner P (1976) Drug metabolism: chemical and biochemical aspects. Marcel Dekker, New York, Basel
7. William RT (1971) Introduction: pathways of drug metabolism. In: Brodie BB, Gillette JR, Ackerman HS (eds) Concepts in biochemical pharmacology. Springer, Berlin, Heidelberg, New York, pp 227-250
8. Hayaishi O (1969) Enzymic hydroxylation. Annu Rev Biochem 38:21-44
9. Oesch F, Kaubisch N, Jerina DM, Daly JW (1971) Hepatic epoxide hydratase: structure-activity relationship for substrates and inhibitors. Biochemistry 10:4858-4866
10. Roy AB (1971) Sulphate conjugation enzymes. In: Brodie BB, Gillette JR, Ackerman HS (eds) Concepts in biochemical pharmacology. Springer, Berlin, Heidelberg, New York, pp 536-563
11. Dutton GJ (1966) The biosynthesis of glucuronides. In: Dutton GH (ed) Glucuronic acid, free and combines. Academic Press, New York, London, pp 186-297
12. Boyland E, Chasseaud LF (1969) The role of glutathione and glutathione S-transferases in mercapturic acid biosynthesis. Adv Enzymol 32:173-219
13. Miller JA, Miller EC (1965) Metabolism of drugs in relation to carcinogenicity. Ann NY Acad Sci 123:125-140
14. Bartsch H, Malaveille C, Montesano R (1975) In vitro metabolism and microsome-mediated mutagenicity of dialkylnitrosamines in rat, hamster, and mouse tissues. Cancer Res 35:644-651
15. Czygan P, Greim H, Garro A, Schaffner F, Popper H (1974) The effect of dietary protein deficiency on the ability of isolated hepatic microsomes to alter the mutagenicity of a primary and a secondary carcinogen. Cancer Res 34:119-123
16. Czygan P, Greim H, Garro AJ, Hutterer F, Schaffner F, Popper H, Rosenthal O, Cooper DY (1973) Microsomal metabolism of dimethylnitrosamine and the cytochrome P-450 dependency of its activation to a mutagen. Cancer Res 33:2983-2986

17. Czygan P, Greim H, Garro AJ, Hutterer F, Rudick J, Schaffner F, Popper H (1973) Cytochrome P-450 content and the ability of liver microsomes from patients undergoing abdominal surgery to alter the mutagenicity of a primary and a secondary carcinogen. J Natl Cancer Inst 51:1761-1764

18. Yang SK, McCourt DW, Roller PP, Gelboin HY (1976) Enzymatic conversion of benzo(a)pyrene leading predominantly to the diol-epoxide r-7,t-8-dihydroxy-t-9,10-oxy-7,8,9,10-tetrahydrobenzo(a)pyrene through a single enantiomer of r-7,t-8-dihydroxy-7,8-dihydrobenzo(a)pyrene. Proc Natl Acad Sci USA 73/8:2594-2598

19. Thakker DR, Yagi H, Lu AYH, Levin W, Conney AH, Jerina DM (1976) Metabolism of benzo(a)pyrene: conversion of (+)-trans-7,8-dihydroxy-7,8-dihydrobenzo(a)pyrene to highly mutagenic 7,8-diol-9,10-epoxides. Proc Natl Acad Sci USA 73/10:3381-3385

20. Bentley P, Oesch F, Glatt H (1977) Dual role of epoxide hydratase in both activation and inactivation of benzo(a)pyrene. Arch Toxicol (Berl) 39:65-75

21. Oesch F, Raphael D, Schwind H, Glatt HR (1977) Species differences in activating and inactivating enzymes related to the control of mutagenic metabolites. Arch Toxicol (Berl) 39:97-108

22. Leibman KC, Ortiz E (1969) Oxidation of styrene in liver microsomes. Biochem Pharmacol 18:552-554

23. Ohtsuji H, Ikeda M (1971) The metabolism of styrene in the rat and the stimulatory effect of phenobarbital. Toxicol Appl Pharmacol 18:321-328

24. Leibman KC (1975) Metabolism and toxicity of styrene. Environ Health Perspect 11:115-119

25. Watabe R, Maynert EW (1968) Role of epoxides in the metabolism of olefins. Pharmacologist 10:203

26. Stoltz DR, Withey RJ (1977) Mutagenicity testing of styrene and styrene epoxide in Salmonella typhimurium. Bull Environ Contam Toxicol 17:739

27. Milvy P, Garro AJ (1976) Mutagenic activity of styrene oxide (1,2-epoxyethyl benzene), a presumed styrene metabolite. Mutat Res 40:15-18

28. Wiebel FJ, Lentz JC, Diamond L, Gelboin HV (1971) Aryl hydrocarbon [benzo(a)pyrene] hydroxylase in microsomes from rat tissues: differential inhibition and stimulation by benzoflavones and organic solvents. Arch Biochem Biophys 144:78-86

29. Poland AP, Glover E (1974) Genetic expression of aryl hydrocarbon hydroxylase activity. Induction of monooxygenase activities and cytochrome P_1-450 formation by 2, 3, 7, 8-tetrachlorodibenzo-p-dioxin in mice genetically "nonresponsive" to other aromatic hydrocarbons. J Biol Chem 249:5599-5606

30. Nebert DW, Goujon FM, Gielen JE (1972) Aryl hydrocarbon hydroxylase induction by polycyclic hydrocarbons: simple autosomal dominant trait in the mouse. Nature (New Biol) 236:107-110

31. Wiebel FH, Leutz JC, Gelboin HV (1973) Aryl hydrocarbon [benzo(a)pyrene] hydroxylase: inducible in extrahepatic tissues of mouse strains not inducible in liver. Arch Biochem Biophys 154:292-294

32. Bentley P, Oesch F (1975) Purification of epoxide hydratase to apparent homogenicity. FEBS Lett 59:291-295

33. Bock KW, Josting D, Lilienblum W, Pfeil H (1979) Purification of rat-liver microsomal UDP-glucuronyltransferase. Separation of two enzyme forms in ducible by 3-methylchlolanthrene or phenobarbital. Eur J Biochem 98:19-26

34. Gillette JR (1974) Commentary: A perspective on the role of chemically reactive metabolites of foreign compounds in toxicity. I. Correlation of changes in covalent binding of reactivity metabolites with changes in the incidence and severity of toxicity. Biochem Pharmacol 23:2785-2794

35. Uehleke H, Werner T, Greim H, Krämer M (1977) Metabolic activation of haloalkanes and tests in vitro for mutagenicity. Xenobiotica 7:393-400

36. Schüppel R (1969) Alkohole als Inhibitoren der mikrosomalen N-Demethyllierung in vitro. Naunyn Schmiedebergs Arch Pharmacol 264:302-303

37. Cohen GM, Mannering GJ (1972) Involvement of a hydrophobic site in the inhibition of the microsomal p-hydroxylation of aniline by alcohols. Mol Pharmacol 9:383-397

38. Wolff T (1978) In vitro inhibition of monooxygenase dependent reactions by organic solvents. In: Industrial and environmental xenobiotics. Excerpta Media Congress Series 440:196-198

39. Sugimura Ta, Yahagi T, Nagao M, Takeuchi M, Kawachi T, Hara K, Yamasaki E, Matsushima T, Hashimoto Y, Okada M (1976) Validity of mutagenicity tests using microbes as a rapid screening method for environmental carcinogens. IARC Sci Publ 12:81-89

40. Norpoth K, Djelani G, Gieselmann V (1980) Bacterial mutagenicity testing of polycyclic aromatic hydrocarbons

41. Summer KH, Göggelmann W, Greim H (1980) Glutathione and glutathione S-transferases in the Salmonella mammalian-microsome mutagenicity test. Mutat Res 70:269-278

42. Roy AB (1971) Sulphate conjugation enzymes. In: Handbook of Experimental Pharmacology. Vol XXVIII/2, Springer, Berlin, Heidelberg, New York pp 536-563

43. Oesch F (1979) Epoxide Hydratase. In: Progress in Drug Metabolism, Vol 3, Bridges JW, Chasseaud LF (eds) Wiley, Chichester

Factors Modulating Mutagenicity in Microbial Tests

T. Matsushima[1], T. Sugimura[2], M. Nagao[2], T. Yahagi[2], A. Shirai[1],
and M. Sawamura[1]

Summary

The preincubation of test compound, bacterial tester strain,
and S-9 mix or buffer before pouring a minimal-glucose agar
plate enhanced the sensitivity of mutation test and increased
the spectrum of mutagens detected. Addition of NADH and ATP in
S-9 mix enhanced the mutagenicity of some compounds. Addition
of norharman in the preincubation mixture made it possible to
detect a marginal or weak mutagenicity of certain types of mutagens. Addition of riboflavin revealed the mutagenicity of azo
compounds. Glycosidase was required to detect the mutagenicity
of glycosides or natural products.

Introduction

Environmental mutagens and carcinogens may cause mutation of
germ cells resulting in the accumulation of heritable abnormal
genes in the population and may also cause mutation of somatic
cells resulting in the formation of tumors in individuals. The
monitoring of environmental mutagens and carcinogens is extremely important. The most widely adopted short-term test to
detect chemical carcinogens in the environment is the method
developed by Ames et al. (1) which detects the mutagenicity of
chemicals by reverse mutation of an auxotroph for histidine of
Salmonella typhimurium. Many compounds have been tested by this
quick, simple, sensitive, and reliable method, and a good correlation between mutagenicity and carcinogenicity has been proved
(2-4). The *Salmonella* mutation test has two unique superior
points: one is the specially designed, sensitive tester strains
(5,6) and the other is the incorporation of the in vitro metabolic activation system of mammalian postmitochondrial supernatant to metabolize test compounds to their active proximate or
ultimate forms (7). However, several procarcinogens which require metabolic activation to exhibit their biologic activities
are negative in this assay method, and modifications and improvements of the in vitro metabolic activation system are required.
Factors improving the sensitivity and reliability of the *Salmonella* mutation test are described in this report.

---

[1]Department of Molecular Oncology, Institute of Medical Science, University
of Tokyo, Shirokane-dai, Minato-ku, Tokyo 108/Japan

[2]Biochemistry Division, National Cancer Center Research Institute, Tsukiji,
Chuo-ku, Tokyo 104/Japan

Preincubation Method

The pour-plate method of the *Salmonella* mutation test described by Ames et al. (1) was insensitive in detecting the mutagenicity of a potent hepatocarcinogen, dimethylnitrosamine (DMN), even in the presence of the metabolic activation system (S-9 mix) from rat liver. However, mutagenicity of DMN in *Salmonella* has been detected by the liquid method (8) or by the host-mediated method (8,9). The mutagenicity of DMN was clearly demonstrated by the preincubation method (10), which is a hybrid method combining the simplicity of the pour-plate method and the higher efficiency of metabolic activation of the liquid method. The procedure of the preincubation method is as follows: test compound, phosphate buffer (pH 7.4) or S-9 mix, and tester bacteria are mixed in a test tube and incubated with shaking for 20 min at 37°C or for 30 min at 30°C. After the preincubation, 2 ml of molten top agar is added and the mixture is poured onto a minimal-glucose agar plate and incubated for 2 days at 37°C. The procedure after the preincubation is the same as the pour-plate method of Ames et al. (1). Numbers of revertant colonies are scored and the bacterial growth of background-lawn is checked on every plate by a dissection microscope to monitor cell killing due to the toxicity of the test compound at the dose tested. Table 1 shows the numbers of revertant colonies of *S. typhimurium* TA 100 induced by DMN at 50 μmol/plate. The revertants increase with an increase of preincubation time at 30°C. In the pour-plate method, metabolic activation by S-9 mix is carried out in the agar, but in the preincubation method, metabolic activation is carried out efficiently in liquid at a higher concentration of S-9 mix and test compound than that in the pour-plate method.

Table 1. Mutagenicity of dimethylnitrosamine (DMN) by the preincubation method

Preincubation time (min)	His$^+$ revertants/plate	
0	111	120
10	213	218
20	508	532
30	1416	1636
40	2960	3040
50	3600	4480
60	5200	5240
Control	110	114

DMN (50 μmol) was incubated with *S. typhimurium* TA 100 and S-9 mix (PCB induced rat liver, 150 μl S-9 in 0.5 ml S-9 mix) at 30°C. Preincubation time (0 min) means the pour-plate method. Duplicate assay.

A comparison of the pour-plate method and the preincubation method was performed on procarcinogens, aflatoxin B₁ and benzidine, with S-9 mix. As shown in Fig. 1, the mutagenicity of aflatoxin was clearly detected by the preincubation method at a very low dose, when its mutagenicity was not detected by the pour-plate method. The mutagenicity of benzidine was also detected more sensitively by the preincubation method. o-Tolidine and dianisidine also showed higher mutagenic response by the preincubation method but β-naphthylamine and benzo(a)pyrene showed the same mutagenic response by both methods. Not only the promutagens, which require metabolic activation, but also direct-acting mutagens such as N-methyl-N'-nitro-N-nitrosoguanidine (MNNG) and ethylmethanesulfonate (EMS) showed a more sensitive response in the mutation assay by the preincubation method than by the pour-plate method.

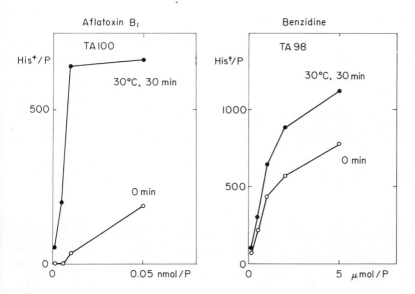

Fig. 1. Comparison of the pour-plate method and preincubation method. Aflatoxin B₁ was tested in S. typhimurium TA 100 and benzidine in S. typhimurium TA 98. Standard pour-plate method (———o———) of Ames et al. (1) or preincubation method (———•———) for 30 min at 30°C using 50 µl S-9 in 0.5 ml S-9 mix

Two different preincubation conditions, 30 min at 30°C or 20 min at 37°C, were compared using aflatoxin B₁ and benzo(a)pyrene on S. typhimurium TA 100 and acetylaminofluorene on S. typhimurium TA 98. As shown in Table 2, there is no big difference in the mutagenicity response by the two different preincubation conditions.

We recommend using 30-min preincubation at 30°C when one person is working. The preincubation of each test tube is started at 30-sec intervals and a total of 60 plates can be handled during a 30-min preincubation period. This means testing two chemicals

Table 2. Comparison of two different preincubation conditions, 30 min at 30°C and 20 min at 37°C

Compound[a]	Dose	His$^+$ revertants/plate	
		30 min at 30°C	20 min at 37°C
Aflatoxin B$_1$	20 nmol	700	742
	10	436	486
	5	329	345
	2	201	222
	1	195	197
	0.5	156	189
	0	135	160
Acetylaminofluorene	50 nmol	810	766
	40	708	580
	30	324	261
	20	236	207
	10	95	113
	0	28	27
Benzo(a)pyrene	10 μg	1142	1110
	5	1070	995
	2	412	638
	1	194	305
	0.5	102	172
	0	91	86

[a]Aflatoxin B$_1$ and benzo(a)pyrene were tested in *S. typhimurium* TA 100, and acetylaminofluorene was tested in *S. typhimurium* TA 98. S-9 amount in S-9 mix (0.5 ml) was 50 μl

at seven doses with and without S-9 mix by using two tester strains such as *S. typhimurium* TA 100 and TA 98. When two persons are doing the mutation test, 20 min preincubation at 37°C is suitable for handling many samples. The preincubation is started by one person and is stopped by the other.

Table 3 summarizes the preincubation method. Dimethylnitrosamine (10,11), diethylnitrosamine (10,11), and dimethylaminoazobenzene (11) are negative by the pour-plate method but become positive by the preincubation method. The mutagenicity of several carcino-genic pyrrolizidine alkaloids such as lasiocarpine, senkirkine, and heliotrine was recently found by the preincubation method (12). Many other chemicals such as aflatoxin B$_1$, benzidine, *o*-tolidine, dianisidine, *N*-methyl-*N*'-nitro-*N*-nitrosoguanidine, methylmethanesulfonate, and methylnitrosourea showed sensitive response in the mutation test by the preincubation method. Benzo-(a)pyrene, *o*-aminoazotoluene, β-naphthylamine, 2-nitrofluorene, and 4-nitro-*o*-phenylenediamine showed equal response in mutation tests by both methods. As far as we have tested, no compound showed a positive response by the pour-plate method but a nega-tive or less sensitive response in the mutation test by the pre-incubation method.

Table 3. Comparison of the pour-plate method and the preincubation method

Sensitivity of mutation test by		Compounds
Pour-plate method	Preincubation method	
-	+	Dimethylnitrosamine Diethylnitrosamine Dimethylaminoazobenzene Pyrrolizidine alkaloids
+	++	Aflatoxin B$_1$ Benzidine *o*-Tolidine Dianisidine MNNG Methylnitrosourea Ethylmethanesulfonate
+	+	Benzo(a)pyrene *o*-Aminoazotoluene β-Naphthylamine 2-Nitrofluorene 4-Nitro-*o*-phenylenediamine
++	+	None
+	-	None

Cofactors in S-9 Mix

Microsomes in the S-9 fraction (postmitochondrial supernatants) contain mixed-function oxygenases which require NADPH as a cofactor for metabolic activation of procarcinogens and promutagens. Glucose-6-phosphatase present in cytosol fraction produces NADPH from NADP and glucose-6-phosphate (G6P). NADP and G6P are used as the NADPH-generating system in S-9 mix (1). Additions of other fractors besides NADPH enhance the mutagenicity of some compounds.

Dimethylaminoazobenzene (DAB) is a potent hepatocarcinogen in rats. Its mutagenicity was scarcely detectable by the pour-plate method, but was clearly demonstrated by the preincubation method, as shown in the previous section. Addition of either NADH or ATP in the S-9 mix enhanced the mutagenicity of DAB as shown in Fig. 2. These enhancing effects of NADH and ATP were additive (13). The concentrations of NADH and ATP in S-9 mix were 4 mM and 5 mM, respectively. We recommend using NADH and ATP as cofactors in addition to NADPH in S-9 mix.

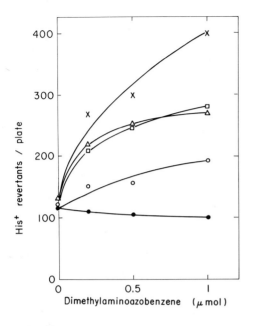

Fig. 2. Effect of NADH and ATP on mutagenicity of dimethylaminoazobenzene in *S. typhimurium* TA 100 by preincubation for 20 min at 37°C. Preincubation without S-9 mix (——●——), with S-9 mix (——○——), with S-9 mix + 2.5 µmol of ATP (——△——), with S-9 mix + 2 µmol NADH (——□——), and with S-9 mix + NADH + ATP (——x——)

Riboflavin

Azo and diazo dyes are widely used as dyestuffs for textiles, leathers, papers, and others. Although many diazo dyes contain benzidine, *o*-tolidine, and dianisidine, which are carcinogenic and mutagenic in *Salmonella*, these dyes were not mutagenic in *Salmonella* by the pour-plate method or even by the preincubation method. Addition of riboflavin, a cofactor for azo reductase present in microsomes, in S-9 mix revealed the mutagenicity of certain types of azo and diazo dyes by the preincubation method (14). The mutagenicity of carcinogenic trypan blue and ponceau R was demonstrated and that of carcinogenic ponceau 3R was enhanced by the addition of riboflavin in the preincubation mixture (Table 4). Although riboflavin was shown to be effective in exhibiting the mutagenicity of some azo and diazo dyes, the addition of riboflavin to the standard pour-plate method did not result in any enhancing effect.

The essential condition for exhibiting the mutagenicity of certain types of azo and diazo dyes is the preincubation of compounds with S-9 mix supplemented with riboflavin. Riboflavin was obligatory to detect the mutagenicity of some azo dyes, whereas the mutagenicity of some other azo dyes such as dimethylaminoazobenzene (DAB), 3'-methyl-dimethylaminoazobenzene (3'-Me-DAB) and *o*-aminoazotoluene (*o*-AT) decreased by the preincubation with riboflavin (Table 4). Therefore, we recommend that azo compounds should be tested first by the ordinary method and if the compound is not mutagenic then it should be retested by the preincubation method using S-9 mix supplemented with riboflavin. Ponceau SX, which is a none carcinogenic azo dye, was not mutagenic by the preincubation method with riboflavin. Amaranth (food color red no. 2) was tested by the preincubation method with and without riboflavin, but it showed no mutagenicity under either condition.

Table 4. Effect of riboflavin on the mutagenicities of azo and diazo dyes

Compound	Tester strain	His[+] revertants/nmol	
		−Riboflavin	+Riboflavin
Chlorazol violet N	TA 98	0	0.11
Congo red	TA 98	0	0.13
Benzopurpurine 4B	TA 98	0	0.13
Trypan blue	TA 98	0	0.36
Pontacyl sky blue 4BX	TA 98	0	0.55
Eriochrom blue black B	TA 98	0	0.10
Ponceau R	TA 100	0	0.15
Ponceau 3R	TA 100	0.11	1.0
Ponceau SX	TA 100, TA 98	0	0
Amaranth	TA 100, TA 98	0	0
DAB	TA 98	0.21	0.08
3'-Me-DAB	TA 98	0.70	0.34
o-AT	TA 98	5.8	1.2

The optimum concentration of riboflavin in S-9 mix depended on
the structure of the azo compound tested. The mutagenicity of
Congo red was increased with an increase of riboflavin from
0.1 µmol to 1 µmol per 0.5 ml S-9 mix (Table 5). However, the
mutagenicity of trypan blue was decreased with an increase of
riboflavin from 0.1 µmol to 0.5 µmol and it almost disappeared
at 1 µmol of riboflavin in 0.5 ml S-9 mix. It is recommended to
use 0.5 µmol of riboflavin in 0.5 ml S-9 mix for the testing of
azo compounds which are not mutagenic in the ordinary test.

Table 5. Effect of riboflavin concentration on mutagenicity
of diazo dyes

Riboflavin (µmol/0.5 ml S-9 mix)	His[+] revertants/plate	
	Trypan blue (0.2 µmol/plate)	Congo red (0.5 µmol/plate)
0	31	30
0.1	152	35
0.2	139	41
0.5	104	86
1.0	66	183

Diazo dyes were preincubated with various amount of riboflavin,
S-9 mix and S. typhimurium TA 98 for 30 min at 30°C.

Norharman

New potent mutagens were isolated from tryptophan pyrolysate
and identified as the γ-carboline derivatives, 3-amino-1,4-
dimethyl-5H-pyrido [4,3-b]indole (Trp-P-1) and 3-amino-1-methyl-
5H-pyrido [4,3-b]indole (Trp-P-2) (15) as shown in Fig. 3. Tryptophan pyrolysate also contained β-carboline derivatives, norharman and harman, but these compounds were not mutagenic (16).

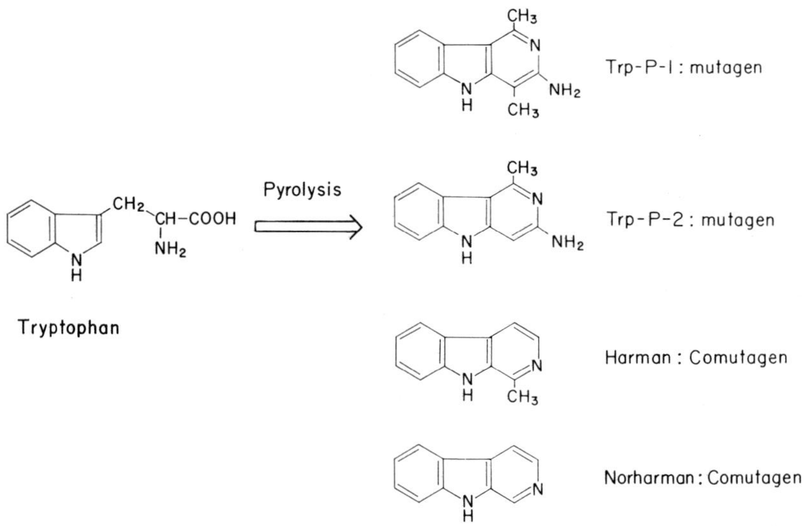

Fig. 3. Structure of mutagens and comutagens isolated from tryptophan pyrolysate

Norharman manifested a potential mutagenicity of aniline, *o*-toluidine and yellow OB (17,18). These compounds are carcinogenic, but not mutagenic in *S. typhimurium* TA 100 and TA 98 by the preincubation method with S-9 mix. However, they showed mutagenicity in *S. typhimurium* TA 98 by the addition of 200 µg of norharman in the preincubation mixture, as shown in Table 6. *o*-Toluidine was not mutagenic by itself, but it became mutagenic in the presence of norharman. However, *m*-toluidine and *p*-toluidine were not mutagenic with or without norharman (17).

The role of norharman is unknown. Norharman has been found to intercalate between base-pairs of double-stranded DNA (19) and this intercalation may increase the susceptibility of DNA to mutagens or active metabolites of mutagens. Norharman also modifies the metabolism of mutagens and may inhibit the inactivation or enhance the activation of mutagens (20).

Norharman enhanced the mutagenicity of dimethylaminoazobenzene (DAB) in *S. typhimurium* TA 98 as shown in Table 7. It also enhanced the mutagenicity of aminoazobenzene, *N*-methyl-aminoazobenzene and 3'-methyl-dimethylaminoazobenzene (13). The effect of norharman on the mutagenicity of azo dyes was demonstrated by *S. typhimurium* TA 98, but not by TA 100 (13). The enhancing effect or norharman on the mutagenicity of DAB increased with an increase of the amount of S-9 in S-9 mix (20).

Norharman also enhanced the mutagenicity of other types of mutagens such as benzo(a)pyrene, acetylaminofluorene, and Trp-P-1. These compounds had an optimum concentration of S-9 in S-9 mix to exhibit their maximum mutagenicity. The mutagenicity of these compounds was decreased in the presence of a large amount of S-9. Addition of norharman enhanced the mutagenicity of these

Table 6. Comutagenic activity of norharman

Compound	Dose (μg)	His[+] revertants/plate	
		−Norharman	+Norharman
Aniline	0	22	22
	40	25	1024
	120	22	4738
	200	20	5918
o-Toluidine	0	25	29
	40	26	1252
	80	15	3186
	120	17	4097
	200	21	5462
Yellow OB	0	20	21
	20	25	644
	50	26	1012
	100	31	1144

Test compound, *S. typhimurium* TA 98 and S-9 mix were preincubated with or without 200 μg of norharman.

Table 7. Effect of norharman on the mutagenicity of dimethylaminoazobenzene on *S. typhimurium* TA 98 and TA 100

Dose (μg)	His[+] revertants/plate			
	TA 98		TA 100	
	−Norharman	+Norharman	−Norharman	+Norharman
0	19	28	130	170
20	173	581	184	221
50	208	1180	207	370
100	243	1280	222	412

DAB, bacteria tester strain and S-9 mix were preincubated with or without norharman (200 μg).

compounds severalfold at the presence of a large amount of S-9 (20). However, norharman suppressed the mutagenicity of these compounds in the presence of a small amount of S-9 (20). This biphasic effect of norharman may be due to its modification of the metabolism and interference on the balance between the activation and inactivation of mutagens. The overall effect depended on the amount of S-9. Norharman has been reported to inhibit aryl hydrocarbon hydroxylase (21). Separation of the metabolites of benzo(a)pyrene by high-pressure liquid chromatography showed that norharman inhibited the conversion of hydrophobic to hydrophilic metabolites (22). 7,8-Dihydroxybenzo(a)pyrene, which is a strong mutagen and a precursor of the ultimate form of benzo(a)pyrene, 7,8-dihydroxy-9,10-oxy-7,8,9,10-tetrahydrobenzo(a)pyrene, was increased tenfold in the presence of norharman (22).

The effect of norharman on aniline, o-toluidine, and yellow OB
is called "comutagenic," because these carcinogens are mutagenic
only in the presence of norharman. The effect of norharman on
DAB can also be called comutagenic because its mutagenicity is
increased by norharman with all amounts of S-9 used (20).

We recommend to use norharman as comutagen or modulator of
metabolism for detecting a marginal or weak mutagenicity of certain types of mutagens. Norharman is contributing to the improvement and broadening of the short-term screening methods
for detecting environmental mutagens and carcinogens.

Glycosidase

Many naturally occurring compounds exist in conjugated form
such as glycosides. Cycasin, the carcinogenic principle present
in a cycad, is a β-glucoside of methylazoxymethanol (MAM).
Cycasin produced tumors in intestine and colon by oral administration to conventional animals, but not to germ-free animals.
Aglycon, MAM was produced from cycasin by the action of β-glucosidase of the gut microflora. Cycasin itself was not mutagenic,
but MAM was mutagenic in $S.$ $typhimurium$ (23). As shown in Table 8,
the mutagenicity of cycasin was demonstrated by the preincubation
of cycasin with almond β-glucosidase and $S.$ $typhimurium$ tester
strain at pH 6.5, but not by the pour-plate method with β-glucosidase (24). Although the optimum pH for the enzymic activity
of β-glucosidase was 5.5, pH 6.5 was selected to avoid decrease
in the survival of the bacteria below pH 5.5. About half of the
enzyme activity at pH 5.5 was present at pH 6.5.

Mutagenicity of several flavonols such as kaempferol and quercetin was detected by $S.$ $typhimurium$ TA 98 and TA 100 with S-9 mix
(25-28). These flavonols are naturally present as glycosides:
for instance, astragalin is a β-glucoside of kaempferol and
rutin is a rutinoside of quercetin. Mutagenicity of these glycosides could not be demonstrated by preincubation with S-9 mix.
However, the mutagenicity of astragalin was shown by preincubation with $S.$ $typhimurium$ TA 98, S-9 mix and almond β-glucosidase at pH 6.5 (Table 8). In this case, the phosphate buffer
solution used in S-9 mix was changed to pH 6.5 from pH 7.4. The
mutagenicity of rutin was also demonstrated by preincubation
with $S.$ $typhimurium$ TA 98, S-9 mix, and hesperidinase, a mixture
of hydrolases isolated from $Aspergillus$ $niger$ (Table 8).

For the screening of some naturally occurring mutagens and carcinogens, it is required to use glycosidase. This procedure was
also applied to study the mutagenicity of glucuronides using
$E.$ $coli$ β-glucuronidase.

In summary, we recommend to use these modulating factors as improved modifications of the standard method of bacterial mutation tests. The preincubation method and the addition of NADH
and ATP in S-9 mix should be used for general purposes. Norharman is used for compounds which are nonmutagenic by the standard
assay protocol. The use of riboflavin is restricted to azo com-

Table 8. Effects of glycosidase on the mutagenicity of cycasin, astragalin, and rutin

Compounds	Dose (µmol)	His$^+$ revertants/plate	Preincubation conditions
Cycasin	0	2	*S. typhimurium* HisG46
	2	30	30°, 90 min
	5	116	pH 6.5
	10	1508	30 unit β-glucosidase
	15	6478	
Astragalin	0	48	*S. typhimurium* TA 98
	0.02	100	30°, 30 min
	0.05	174	pH 6.5
	0.1	334	50 unit β-glucosidase
	0.2	475	S-9 mix
	0.5	681	
Rutin	0	21	*S. typhimurium* TA 98
	0.05	271	30°, 30 min
	0.1	536	pH 6.5
	0.2	756	2 mg hesperidinase
	0.5	1048	S-9 mix
	1	2700	

The compounds were preincubated with *Salmonella* tester strain at pH 6.5 for either 30 min or 90 min with or without S-9 mix.

pounds, which are negative by the standard test method. Glycosidase is used only for glycosides or natural products.

Acknowledgments. This work was supported in part by grant-in-aid for Cancer research from the Ministry of Education, Science and Culture and the Ministry of Health and Welfare, and grants from the Agency of Science and Technology, the Princess Takamatsu Cancer Research Fund, the Society for Promotion of Cancer Research, and the Japan Tobacco and Salt Public Corporation.

References

1. Ames BN, McCann J, Yamasaki E (1975) Method for detecting carcinogens and mutagens with *Salmonella*/mammalian microsome mutagenicity test. Mutat Res 31:347-363
2. McCann J, Choi E, Yamasaki E, Ames BN (1975) Detection of carcinogens as mutagens in the *Salmonella*/microsome test: assay of 300 chemicals. Proc Natl Acad Sci USA 72:5135-5139
3. Sugimura T, Sato S, Nagao M, Yahagi T, Matsushima T, Seino Y, Takeuchi M, Kawachi T (1976) Overlapping of carcinogens and mutagens. In: Magee PN, Takayama S, Sugimura T, Matsushima T (eds) Fundamentals in cancer prevention. University Park Press, Baltimore, pp 191-215
4. Purchase IFH, Longstaff E, Ashby J, Styles JA, Anderson D, Lefevre PA, Westwood FR (1978) An evaluation of 6 short-term tests for detecting organic chemical carcinogens. Br J Cancer 37:873-959

5. Ames BN, McCann J, Lee FD, Durston WE (1973) An improved bacterial test system for the detection and classification of mutagens and carcinogens. Proc Natl Acad Sci USA 70:782-786

6. McCann J, Spingarn NE, Kobori J, Ames BN (1975) Detection of carcinogens as mutagens: bacterial tester strains with R factor plasmids. Proc Natl Acad Sci USA 72:979-983

7. Ames BN, Durston WE, Yamasaki E, Lee FD (1973) Carcinogens are mutagens: a simple test system combining liver homogenates for activation and bacteria for detection. Proc Natl Acad Sci USA 70:2281-2285

8. Malling HV (1974) Mutagenic activation of dimethylnitrosamine and diethylnitrosamine in the host-mediated assay and the microsomal system. Mutat Res 26:465-472

9. Gabridge MG, Legator MS (1969) A host-mediated assay for the detection of mutagenic compounds. Proc Soc Exp Biol Med 130:831-834

10. Yahagi T, Nagao M, Seino Y, Matsushima T, Sugimura T, Okada M (1977) Mutagenicities of N-nitrosamines on *Salmonella*. Mutat Res 48:121-130

11. Sugimura T, Yahagi T, Nagao M, Takeuchi M, Kawachi T, Hara K, Yamasaki E, Matsushima T, Hashimoto Y, Okada M (1976) Validity of mutagenicity testing using microbes as a rapid screening method for environmental carcinogens. In: Montesano R, Bartsch H, Tomatis L (eds) Screening tests in chemical carcinogenesis. IARC, Lyon, pp 81-101

12. Yamanaka H, Nagao M, Sugimura T, Furuya T, Shirai A, Matsushima T (1979) Mutagenicity of pyrolizidine alkaloids in the *Salmonella*/mammalian-microsome test. Mutat Res 68:211-216

13. Nagao M, Yahagi T, Honda M, Seino Y, Kawachi T, Sugimura T, Wakabayashi K, Tsuji K, Kosuge T (1977) Comutagenic actions of norharman derivatives with 4-dimethylaminoazobenzene and related compounds. Cancer Lett 3:339-346

14. Sugimura T, Nagao M, Kawachi T, Honda M, Yahagi T, Seino Y, Sato S, Matsukura N, Matsushima T, Shirai A, Sawamura M, Matsumoto H (1977) Mutagen-carcinogens in food, with special reference to highly mutagenic pyrolytic products in broiled foods. In: Hiatt HH, Watson JD, Winsten JA (eds) Origins of human cancer. Cold Spring Harbor Lab. Cold Spring Harbor, New York, pp 1561-1577

15. Sugimura T, Kawachi T, Nagao M, Yahagi T, Seino Y, Okamoto T, Shudo K, Kosuge T, Tsuji K, Wakabayashi K. Iitaka Y, Itai A (1977) Mutagenic principle(s) in tryptophan and phenylalanine pyrolysis products. Proc Jpn Acad 53B:58-61

16. Nagao M, Yahagi T, Kawachi T, Sugimura T, Kosuge T, Tsuji K, Wakabayashi K, Mizusaki S, Matsumoto T (1977) Comutagenic action of norharman and harman. Proc Jpn Acad 53B:95-98

17. Nagao M, Yahagi T, Honda M, Seino Y, Matsushima T, Sugimura T (1977) Demonstration of mutagenicity of aniline and *o*-toluidine by norharman. Proc Jpn Acad 53B:34-37

18. Sugimura T, Nagao M, Matsushima T, Yahagi T, Hayashi K (1977) Recent findings on the relation between mutagenicity and carcinogenicity. Nucleic Acids Res special publ no 3:541-544

19. Hayashi K, Nagao M, Sugimura T (1977) Interactions of norharman and harman with DNA. Nucleic Acids Res 4:3679-3685

20. Nagao M, Yahagi T, Sugimura T (1978) Differences in effects of norharman with various classes of chemical mutagens and amounts of S-9. Biochem Biophys Res Commun 83:373-378

21. Levitt RC, Legraverend C, Nebert DW, Pelkonen O (1977) Effects of harman and norharman on the mutagenicity and binding to DNA of benzo(a)pyrene metabolites in vitro and on aryl hydrocarbon hydroxylase induction in cell culture. Biochem Biophys Res Commun 79:1167-1175

22. Fujino T, Fujiki H, Nagao M, Yahagi T, Seino Y, Sugimura T (1978) The effect of norharman on the metabolism of benzo(a)pyrene by rat-liver microsomes in vitro in relation to its enhancement of the mutagenicity of benzo(a)pyrene. Mutat Res 58:151-158

23. Smith DWE (1966) Mutagenicity of cycasin aglycone (methylazoxymethanol), a naturally occurring carcinogen. Science 152:1273-1274

24. Matsushima T, Matsumoto H, Shirai A, Sawamura M, Sugimura T (1979) Mutagenicity of the naturally occurring carcinogen cycasin and synthetic methylazoxymethanol conjugates in *Salmonella typhimurium*. Cancer Res 39:3780-3782

25. Sugimura T, Nagao M, Matsushima T, Yahagi T, Seino Y, Shirai A, Sawamura M, Natori S, Yoshihira K, Fukuoka M, Kuroyanagi M (1977) Mutagenicity of flavone derivatives. Proc Jpn Acad 53B:194-197

26. Bjeldanes LF, Chang GW (1977) Mutagenic activity of quercetin and related compounds. Science 197:577-578

27. Brown JP, Dietrich PS, Brown RJ (1977) Frameshift mutagenicity of certain naturally occurring phenolic compounds in the 'Salmonella/microsome' test: activation of anthraquinone and flavonol glycosides by gut bacterial enzymes. Biochem Soc Trans 5:1489-1492

28. MacGregor JT, Jurd L (1978) Mutagenicity of plant flavonoids: structural requirements for mutagenic activity in *Salmonella typhimurium*. Mutat Res 54:297-309

Oxygenase-Independent Activations of Carcinogens

U. Rannug[1]

In order to interpret experimental data and to extrapolate the results to man, one has to consider that the induction of mutations and cancer by chemicals implies a series of events. The common process can roughly be divided into three main levels — firstly the exposure, secondly the biotransformation, and thirdly the alteration of DNA and protein. An outline of the three levels can be seen in Fig. 1.

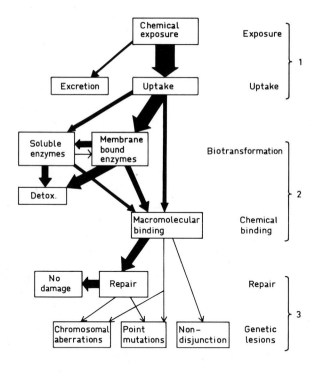

Fig. 1. An outline of the three main levels involved in the induction of genetic lesions in mammals by chemical carcinogens and mutagens. In the Ames test, levels two and three are taken into consideration and only point mutations can be detected by this test system

In this report, I will concentrate on the second level — biotransformation — and some problems related to it. It is known that a chemical often is altered in one way or another in the organism, and that in the mammalian body the liver constitutes the center for this biotransformation. Furthermore, these

[1]Environmental Toxicology Unit, Wallenberg Laboratory, University of Stockholm, S-10691 Stockholm/Sweden

chemical processes normally lead to products more water soluble, and therefore more readily excreted, than the original compound. Many different enzymes —both membrane bound and others — are involved in this detoxication. The important cytochrome P-450 enzymes, carrying out the mixed-function oxygenase reactions, belong to the membrane-bound enzymes.

Conjugations with different cellular constituents, such as glucuronic acid and glutathione, are other essential detoxication reactions catalyzed by enzymes outside the mixed-function oxygenase system. In contrast to this latter system, both the membrane-bound glucuronyl transferase and the soluble glutathione-S-transferases are NADPH-independent enzymes.

The detoxication system does not, however, operate without mistakes and many carcinogens are in fact activated by the enzymes involved. It is well known that strong eletrophilic metabolites, for instance, various epoxides, are produced by the mixed-function oxygenase system. Conjugation with glutathione, on the other hand, has been considered an efficient detoxication. In this report, however, examples of activation to potent carcinogens by this pathway will be given. Another oxygenase-independent and nonmicrosomal activation will also be discussed.

One general problem from the aspect of extrapolating mutagenicity data is, of course, that biotransformation pathways vary between species and individuals. Another essential question, especially when using short-term mutagenicity tests in vitro, is to what extent the metabolic system used in vitro mimics the situation in vivo.

In the following, I will base the discussion on results from tests carried out at our laboratory on *Salmonella typhimurium* with various metabolic systems (1,2).

When testing 1,2-dibromoethane (DBE) or 1,2-dichloroethane (DCE) in Ames' test, the following results were obtained. Both substances gave a weak direct mutagenic effect, DBE being the more potent. These effects on microorganisms have been reported earlier by other investigators (3,4). We found, however, that the direct mutagenic effect was enhanced by the addition of the metabolizing system (S-9 mix) and this has not been reported earlier. This enhancement was also dependent on the amount of S-9 added to the metabolizing system, as can be seen in Table 1. In order to test whether this activation was microsomal, the mutagenic effect with and without the addition of NADP to the NADPH-generating system was compared (Fig. 2). The results showed that this activation was NADPH-independent. In further experiments where the S-9 fraction was divided into a microsomal and a soluble fraction, the total activity was found in the soluble fraction (Fig. 3) and therefore microsomal enzmyes cannot be involved.

Another important observation was that an addition of glutathione (GSH) to the S-9 mix further enhanced the mutagenic effect (Fig. 4). Addition of other thiols like cystein, N-acetylcystein, or

Table 1. The mutagenic effect of 1,2-dichloroethane on *S. typhimurium* TA 1535 in the presence of different amounts of 9000 *g* supernatant from phenobarbital-induced rat livers (strains-R and SpD mixed)

Amount of S-9 per plate (μl)	Number of mutants per plate ± SE			
	Control Ethanol	1,2-Dichloroethane (μmol/plate)		
		20	40	60
25	7.0 ± 1.22[a]	11.6 ± 1.36*	16.6 ± 1.83**	16.6 ± 1.12***
75	10.0 ± 1.00[b]	22.2 ± 3.12*	44.0 ± 4.14***	57.6 ± 8.49***
150	10.6 ± 0.81	36.0 ± 3.86***	58.4 ± 4.18***	85.4 ± 6.50***

[a] 4 Plates
[b] 3 Plates

Statistical analyses were performed with Student's t-test with the following significance levels:
non-significant: $p > 0.05$
*: $0.01 < p < 0.05$
**: $0.001 < p < 0.01$
***: $p < 0.001$

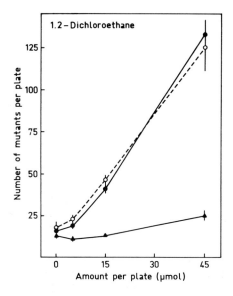

Fig. 2. The mutagenic effect on *S. typhimurium* TA 1535 of 1,2-dichloroethane in the presence of a postmitochondrial liver fraction (S-9) from phenobarbital-pretreated rats of strain R with (●) or without (O) NADP or in the absence of S-9 fraction (▲)

2-mercaptoethanol did not enhance the mutagenicity. It was also shown that no activation occurred with denatured S-9 fractions in the presence of GSH (Fig. 5).

These results indicated that glutathione-specific enzymes were involved. We therefore tested the mutagenic effect of DCE in the presence of glutathione and different glutathione-S-transferases,

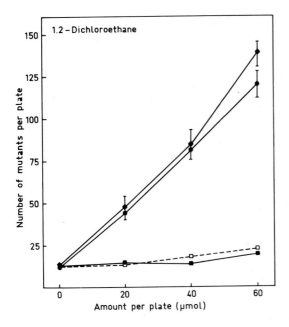

Fig. 3. The mutagenic effect on *S. typhimurium* TA 1535 of 1,2-dichloroethane in the presence of different liver fractions from rats of strain SpD pretreated with phenobarbitol. The following fractions were used: 9000 g supernatant (S-9) without NADP (●), 115,000 g supernatant without NADP (♦), and pure microsomal fraction with (■) or without (□) NADP

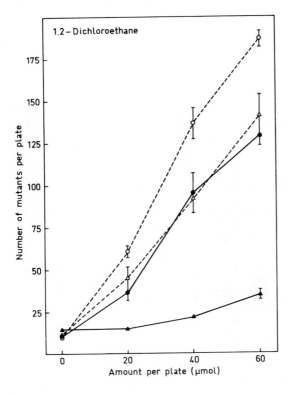

Fig. 4. The mutagenic effect on *S. typhimurium* TA 1535 of 1,2-dichloroethane in the presence of a postmitochondrial liver fraction (S-9) from phenobarbital-pretreated rats of strain SpD (▲;Δ) or strain R (●;O) with (*open symbols*) or without (*closed symbols*) addition of glutathione (1.6 μmol/ml S-9 mix)

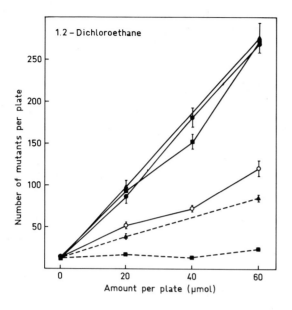

Fig. 5. The mutagenic effect on *S. typhimurium* TA 1535 of 1,2-dichloroethane in the presence of normal and denatured S-9 fractions from phenobarbital-pretreated rats of strain R. ○——○ S-9 mix without glutathione, ▲---▲ denatured S-9 mix (45°C, 150 min) with glutathione, ■---■ denatured S-9 mix (autoclaved 15 min) with glutathione, ●——●, ▲——▲, ■——■ experimental controls with S-9 mix and glutathione

and found that DCE can be activated by these enzymes (types A and C) in vitro (Fig. 6) and can therefore serve as a substrate for the enzymes in vitro.

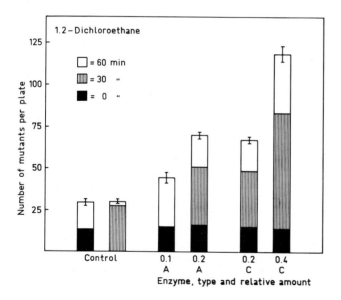

Fig. 6. The mutagenic effect on *S. typhimurium* TA 1535 of 1,2-dichloroethane (10 mM) after incubation (37°C) for different lengths of time (0, 30, and 60 min) in the presence of glutathione (5 mM) and glutathione S-transferase (0.1 mg of A, 0.2 mg of A, 0.2 mg of C, and 0.4 mg of C, respectively). In the control the enzyme was replaced with buffer

The next question was whether these reactive conjugates also are formed in a more complete in vitro system and in vivo. To answer this question, DBE and DCE were tested in a liver per- fusion system. The liver perfusion was performed in collab- oration with Dr. Brita Beije in our laboratory. She has deve- loped an in vitro perfusion system with rat liver, which is specially adapted to mutagenicity testing with bacteria and cell cultures (5). One advantage with the in vitro perfusion system is that the perfusate and the produced bile can be tested separately. The target cells can either be exposed continuously during the perfusion or exposed to samples of perfusate and bile taken at different times. In the latter case information about the rate of metabolism can also be obtained. DBE and DCE were both tested by this latter procedure. The results showed that the produced bile was highly mutagenic (Fig. 7), which also can be expected since glutathione conjugates are known to be excreted through the bile. Also with two additions of DCE the same results were obtained, i.e, the bile showed the highest mutagenic effect 15-30 min after each addition (Fig. 8).

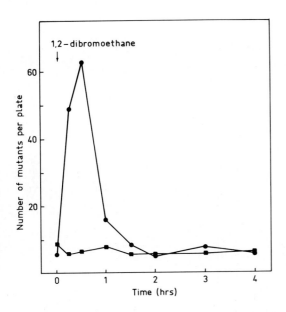

Fig. 7. The mutagenic effect on *S. typhimurium* TA 1535 of per- fusate (■) and bile (●) samples withdrawn from the perfusion system at different times. The erythrocytes in the perfusate were spun down and the superna- tant was filtered through a Millipore filter (0.45 μm) and 0.1 ml was tested per plate. The bile was diluted ten times and 0.1 ml was tested per plate. The *arrow* indicates the addition of 12 μmol 1,2-dibromoethane

1,2-Dichloroethane was also tested on mice in vivo and the bile produced was mutagenic also in this case. It can therefore be concluded that the activation first seen in Ames' test, in this case, is a reflection of a metabolism occurring in the intact liver.

Another compound — 2-chloroethanol — is also activated by the S-9 mix. In this case, however, the strain TA 1530 is more sen- sitive than TA 1535, as can be seen in Fig. 9. In this respect 2-chloroethanol differs from DCE but resembles vinyl chloride. Figure 10 shows that also the activation of 2-chloroethanol is

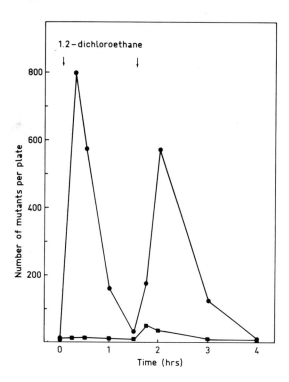

Fig. 8. The mutagenic effect on *S. typhimurium* TA 1535 of perfusate (■) and bile (●) samples withdrawn from the perfusion system at different times. The perfusate and bile was treated as in Fig. 7. The *arrows* indicate the addition of 360 μmol, 1,2-dichloroethane at 0 and 90 min, respectively

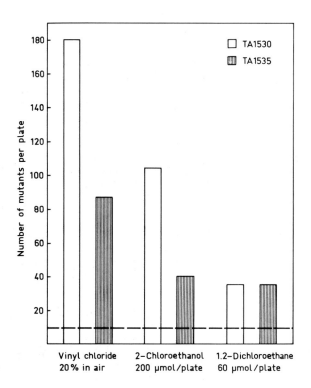

Fig. 9. A comparison of the relative mutagenic effects of vinyl chloride, 2-chloroethanol and 1,2-dichloroethane on the two different base substitution strains TA 1530 and TA 1535

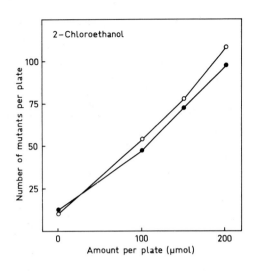

Fig. 10. The mutagenic effect on *S. typhimurium* TA 1530 of 2-chloroethanol in the presence of 9000 *g* supernatant (S-9) (●) or a 115,000 *g* supernatant (O)

mediated by the soluble fraction. Since alcohol dehydrogenase (ADH) is a soluble enzyme and known to oxidize different alcohols, we have carried out tests with 2-chloroethanol in the presence of ADH alone or in combination with the S-9 fraction (Table 2). These experiments show that 2-chloroethanol can act as a substrate for ADH. More experiments are needed, however, to clarify the significance of these reactions in vivo in regard to other competing metabolic pathways.

Table 2. The mutagenic effect of 2-chloroethanol on *S. typhimurium* TA 1530 in the presence of a postmitochondrial liver fraction (S-9) from rats pretreated with Aroclor 1254, alcohol dehydrogenase (ADH) from yeast, or a combination of both (S-9 + ADH)

Number of mutants per plate $\pm$ SE			
Control	2-Chloroethanol (100 µmol/plate)		
S-9	S-9	ADH	S-9 + ADH
7.4 $\pm$ 1.4	36.0 $\pm$ 3.1[***]	38.2 $\pm$ 4.7[***]	49.5 $\pm$ 5.8[***]

Statistical significance levels: see footnote to Table 1

The most likely interpretation of the results discussed is that nonmicrosomal enzymes play an essential role not only in the detoxication, but also in the activation of certain mutagens/carcinogens.

Although it is evident from the present results on DBE, DCE, and 2-chloroethanol that these activations can be detected by Ames test, it should be emphasized that the S-9 mix may not constitute the optimal system for the activation of compounds metabolized by other enzymes than the mixed-function oxygenase system. For instance, the cofactors required for an activation by such enzymes may not be present in sufficient concentrations. This is particularly true with the small amount of S-9 mix required when induced livers are used.

In conclusion it may be pointed out that the *Salmonella*/microsome test is specifically designed for mutagens and carcinogens, which are activated by the mixed-function oxygenase system, but this is evidently not the only one that has to be considered. Other activation enzyme systems, such as the ones dealt with in this work, may have other requirements in order to operate in an optimal way, and these requirements may not be fulfilled by the standard procedure in the Ames test. Detailed knowledge of the various activating mechanisms is of obvious importance in order to develop assay methods of optimum sensitivity to detect different kinds of environmental mutagens and carcinogens.

References

1. Rannug U, Sundvall A, Ramel C (1978) The mutagenic effect of 1,2-dichloroethane on Salmonella typhimurium. I. Activation through conjugation with glutathione in vitro. Chem Biol Interact 20:1-16
2. Rannug U, Beije B (1979) The mutagenic effect of 1,2-dichloroethane on Salmonella typhimurium. II. Activation by the isolated perfused rat liver. Chem Biol Interact 24:265-285
3. Brem H, Stein AB, Rosenkranz HS (1974) The mutagenicity and DNA-modifying effect of haloalkanes. Cancer Res 34:2576-2579
4. McCann J, Simmon V, Streitwieser D, Ames BN (1975) Mutagenicity of chloroacetaldehyde, a possible metabolic product of 1,2-dichloroethane (ethylene dichloride), chloroethanol (ethylene chlorohydrin), vinyl chloride, and cyclophosphamide. Proc Natl Acad Sci USA 72:3190-3193
5. Beije B, Jenssen D, Arrhenius E, Zetterqvist M-A (1979) Isolated liver perfusion—a tool in mutagenicity and carcinogenicity testing for the evaluation of carcinogens. Chem Biol Interact 27:41-57

Some Practical Problems Experienced in Attempts to Predict Carcinogenicity from Short-Term Tests

E. LONGSTAFF[1]

During the course of the last few years, a large variety of short-term predictive tests for carcinogenicity has been described. The majority of these are based on mutation as an end-point and have evolved substantially as a result of the notion that cancer is due to somatic cell mutation.

The Ames test (1), which is very extensively used for screening for carcinogens, is based on the induction of mutations in strains of *Salmonella typhimurium* using a system which incorporates liver enzymes to metabolise the chemical under test. It is this test in particular which, because of its early introduction into routine testing schemes, has now become the focus of most attention simply because we are becoming more experienced in the idiosyncracies of this test and aware of its short-comings than we are of any other test system. The performance of this test, in terms of its ability to discriminate between carcinogens and non-carcinogens, has been reported in several studies. McCann et al. (2), using data from a number of laboratories, found that 90% of carcinogens and 87% of non-carcinogens were correctly identified by the *Salmonella* assay. Purchase et al. (3,4), in a controlled blind study, and Sugimura et al. (5), reported similar results. Some chemicals have been tested twice in these studies and in a few cases inconsistencies between the results from the McCann et al. (2) and Purchase et al. (3,4), studies occur. Nevertheless, when viewed collectively, over 80% of the compounds were correctly identified as carcinogens or non-carcinogens in these reports.

However, in all of these validation studies, it is implied that all test results are generated from equivalent test protocols and procedures. It is the aim of this paper to present evidence to indicate that this is an erroneous assumption, and that it is possible to generate data which in the final analysis could be totally misleading. It is important to recognise that such technical variations can and do exist in the *Salmonella* reverse mutation test and presumably also in other tests, and that the advantages of using such tests may be inadvertently diluted if due care and attention is not paid to the practical details of the testing methodology.

The protocol we have used as a screen involved the use of four strains of histidine requiring mutants of *Salmonella typhimurium*. These were TA 1535, TA 1538, TA 98, and TA 100. Each test compound,

[1]ICI, Central Toxicology Laboratory, Alderley Park, Macclesfield/GB

usually dissolved in DMSO, was assayed in the plate incorporation assay over a wide dose-range (4-2500 µg/plate). Revertant colonies were counted using a Biotran electronic colony counter. A two-fold or more increase in the apparent reversion rate in any tester strain was taken as a positive response from the test. In keeping with the advice of Ames et al. (1), the tester strains were assessed at regular intervals (usually weekly) for main-tenance of the characteristics of deep rough, ampicillin resist-ance, DNA repair deficiency, etc.

During the course of the last 2-3 years, we have routinely screened about 500 compounds of unknown carcinogenicity, and of these compounds about 10% have revealed problems of one sort or another. Some of these can be categorised as follows:

1. Failure to Maintain the R-factor in Strains TA 98 and TA 100. The plasmid-induced characteristic of ampicillin resistance was found to be unstable, but eventually populations were stabilised by continuous culturing in the presence of ampicillin as the Ames group has recently recommended. We have not been able to maintain the tester strains by storage as stab cultures, on agar slopes, by lyophilisation, or by storage in DMSO in liquid nitrogen and we have had to depend very heavily on our colleagues in nearby laboratories to help us replace contaminated strains.

2. Variability in Spontaneous Mutation Rate and the Definition of a "Posi-tive". Stabilisation of the apparent spontaneous mutation rate was difficult if not impossible to achieve. Numerous claims that the rates should be fairly consistent from one laboratory to the other was unsubstantiated. The most stable background mutation frequency was the strain TA 1535. However, ranges between 0 and 3 times that published were often seen even when the positive controls gave normal responses. Obviously when no spontaneous mutants were seen, but when the background lawn was normal, the presence of one or more colonies on the test plates represented an infinite increase in the mutation rate and consequently by our own definition a positive response existed.

The value of these results was debatable and the experiments were always repeated but it left some doubt as to whether they re-presented real or artificial results when further experiments yielded contradictory data. Rules of thumb were eventually established using ranges of personally acceptable spontaneous background counts but the recommendation to see a dose-response was rapidly introduced to the protocol and applied.

3. Variation in Vogel-Bonner Medium: Effect of Sterilising Agents and Antifoam Agents on Test Results. The phenomenon which became known as the "Thursday effect" was both alarming and dramatic until recognised. The screening programme revealed, by following a rigid routine, almost any compound tested on a Thursday was found to be positive in the test. Eventually the cause was traced to an over-zealous ambition to follow the instructions of the pre-poured plate suppliers, that was, to store the plates

at 4°C and to take delivery of fresh plates every Wednesday.
Because our scheduling involved using newly arrived plates on
Thursdays and stored plates on Fridays through to the following Wednesday, one possible explanation could be that the fresh
plates were still contaminated with labile or volatile material
used in the packaging process or some sterilising agent such as
ethylene oxide which caused positive results to be generated.
We have since taken to storing the plates for at least 1 week
at room temperature before use and this procedure has apparently
solved the problem of generating some false positives. The
storage at room temperature has the added advantage of identifying microbially contaminated plates which can be rejected from
the batch as well as avoding the Thursday's "technical" false
positives.

In a carefully controlled experiment between our laboratory and
another, a false-positive result was established as occurring
in agar plates containing an antifoam agent (Table 1). This result was reproducible in each laboratory and it is assumed that
the "positive" result was obtained by the combined toxic action
of the chemical under test (paraquat dichloride) and the antifoam.

Table 1. Effect of antifoam in the medium (0.2% v/v) on the results
generated for paraquat dichloride. Results given as mean number of
revertant colonies per plate ($\pm$ SD) of 10 plates per dose level

Concentration paraquat/ plate (µg)	Strain TA 100 without S-9 mix	
	Plates without antifoam	Plates with antifoam
1000	2 $\pm$ 3	16 $\pm$ 18
500	5 $\pm$ 3	210 $\pm$ 312
100	18 $\pm$ 9 [a]	390 $\pm$ 471
20	29 $\pm$ 21 [a]	37 $\pm$ 28
2	48 $\pm$ 11	63 $\pm$ 25
0	47 $\pm$ 15	36 $\pm$ 36

[a] It should be noted that in addition to the colonies recorded here,
there were in the plates without antifoam only, 100-200 very small
colonies (i.e., less than 0.1 mm diameter) which were not recorded
by the colony counter but which could have been counted by hand if
necessary

In later studies the antifoam was shown to be mutagenic in its
own right producing several thousand colonies per plate but only
at the relatively high doses at which one would normally test
an "unknown" compound.

4. *Pseudo-revertants.* Perhaps the most surprising discovery to date
has been the finding that developed from the above exercise. It
was noted that in the absence of antifoam, as the concentration
of paraquat increased, the resulting revertant colony size

diminished, until at dose levels above 500 µg/plate, the material was quite clearly bacteriostatic. However, whilst the total numbers of all "revertant" colonies in both the absence and presence of antifoam was similar, only those on the anti-foam-containing plates were large enough to be counted and scored as positive in the normal manner. In order to assess whether these micro-colonies in the antifoam-less cultures were true revertants, 60 colonies were randomly transferred from these "positive" plates with a wire loop and streaked onto Vogel-Bonner medium. Identical replicate plates were prepared from "positive" antifoam-containing paraquat plates and also from colonies growing on plates incorporating antifoam alone as a test compound. Following incubation the numbers of streaks showing growth in the absence of histidine was determined and expressed as a percentage of the total number streaked. Table 2 shows the results from this experiment. It can be seen that neither of the paraquat-induced revertant colonies were histidine-independent whereas the antifoam-induced revertant colonies clearly were true revertants. Propane sultone-induced mutants in the positive controls also produced replicate revertant colonies as expected, as did the spontaneously derived negative control cultures in a ratio of about 80%. It must be concluded therefore that the appearance of an increase in the numbers of colonies in a test plate does not in itself necessarily indicate a positive response, but that experimental confirmation that the colonies are true revertants is also a necessary part of the protocol.

Table 2. Proportion of transferred *S. typhimurium* (TA 100) colonies appearing as revertants in apparent positive cultures which were subsequently identified as true revertants by replicate plating onto histidine-free Vogel-Bonner plates

Assay plate	Ratio real/apparent revertants	Percentage real/apparent revertants
Paraquat alone	8/60	13%
Paraquat + 0.02% antifoam	11/60	18%
Antifoam alone (0.2 µl/plate)	45/60	75%
1.3-Propane sultone	47/60	78%
DMSO	53/60	88%

In this particular case it is clear that paraquat dichloride did not induce true mutants either in the presence or absence of antifoam and therefore is not a mutagen to *Salmonella*.

Since this discovery it has become the practice at CTL to check for pseudo-reversion by replica plating and we have since found several compounds capable of producing such "technical false positives."

5. Exposure Methodology. The well-known carcinogen vinyl chloride, when incorporated into the test medium in the usual manner, was found to yield reproducibly negative results, but when seeded plates were exposed to gaseous VCM, a clear positive response was established (see also 4,6,7). The reason for this probably involves exposure-related phenomenon, but it is important, obviously, to check that volatile solvents of this type are negative both on plate and in "gas-phase" tests.

6. Exposure Time. In a recent study of the mutagenicity of the fluorocarbon refrigerant monochlorodifluoromethane (R-22) (8), it became apparent that the variation between laboratories in exposure time of a gas-phase study could readily result in the difference between a negative and positive result. When R-22 was incubated with the tester strains for less than 72 h, it frequently yielded a negative result and it is now established that a 3-day incubation/exposure time must be used to obtain a positive and reproducible response with this type of material.

7. Purity and Age of Test Compound. It is of paramount importance to establish the chemical composition of what is being tested. We have been able to demonstrate that in, for example, gas-phase studies on 1,1,1-trichloroethylene, traces of stabilisers such as epichlorhydrin (which is no longer used in the ICI product) or butylene oxide gave strong positive responses whereas unstabilised material is reproducibly negative. The degree of "positiveness" was not directly related to the absolute quantity of stabiliser present in the mixture but depended upon some unknown interactive effect to generate the positive result (see also 9,10). It is of added interest to recall that Henschler et al. (11) have suggested that the carcinogenicity of TCE could be ascribed to the impurities present in the product and not to the chemical itself.

We have also noted that a chemical originally thought to be chemically stable changed from negative to positive over a storage period of only 8 weeks. It is obviously important to detect "positiveness" in a sample, but if the result is taken by chemists to apply to their pure and unaged compound, considerable time and effort could be wasted in attempts to understand the structure/function relationships surrounding their product.

8. The Effect of Light. Some considerable confusion arose over the testing of the chemical Benzil (diphenylethanedione). Experiments conducted in several laboratories have shown that this material is negative if tested in subdued light conditions and positive if tested in bright light conditions (see also 12,13). It is interesting to note that this compound is negative in the Styles cell transformation test (14) if assayed in normal laboratory lighting conditions.

9. *Colony Counter Variation*. The considerable variation in spontaneous counts between laboratories can be more than adequately
accounted for by the erratic behaviour of colony counters. A
simple comparison of two similar models in the same laboratory
using the same standard plates illustrates the problem.

For the purposes of our own routine work and these experiments,
I have arbitrarily defined a revertant colony to be counted as
one which reaches a minimum diameter of 0.1 mm. This option can
readily be elected for by adjusting the discriminators on the
counting machines.

Hand counts were made for several plates and then the same plates
were counted with two Biotran colony counters, each standardised
to the standard "1000 colony" plate. The variation between the
hand counts and the two machines is recorded in Table 3.

Table 3. Comparison of accuracy of two automatic colony counters

"Real" number of colonies	Machine A		Machine B	
	Display	% Error	Display	% Error
Std 1000	1004	+ 0.4	1052	+ 5.2
84	94	+ 12	165	+ 96
120	73	- 39	215	+ 79
137	164	- 20	242	+ 77
250	383	+ 53	753	+ 201
400	460	+ 15	1615	+ 303

Also, because in our experience plates rarely produce colonies
which are randomly distributed in size and position, the effect
on the revertant count of rotating the position of a plate which
obviously has non-random distributed colonies in size and position was investigated. These data are presented in Table 4. A
count variation of almost 30% can be obtained simply by changing
the counting field.

Table 4. Effect of rotating the position of the Petri
dish culture on the colony count displayed by an
automatic colony counter

Position of plate	Count displayed	% Variation
0°	127	0
90°	107	- 16
180°	92	- 28
270°	97	- 24

In summary then, it should be noted that short-term predictive
tests such as that of Ames et al. demand great care in their
execution and that, whilst in principle they are simple and

rapid to conduct, in practice, as demonstrated here, one can occasionally be mislead into believing a product is "positive" when in fact alternative explanations can, and sometimes do, exist. In conclusion, however, I would wish to re-emphasise that it is our experience that these tests are extremely valuable and useful to the industrial toxicologist and research chemist and that they have helped us considerably in working through planned projects to identify structure/function correlations. The purpose of this paper is merely to draw your attention to the fact that results from simple predictive tests are not always simple to interpret. Paradoxically, perhaps, the more we learn about the mistakes that these tests can make, the more confident we become in predicting carcinogenicity from results we have generated from up-dated protocols which take into account each idiosyncracy as and when it is identified.

References

1. Ames BN, McCann J, Yamasaki E (1975) Mutat Res 31:347-364
2. McCann J, Choi E, Yamasaki E, Ames BN (1975) Proc Natl Acad Sci USA 72:5135-5139
3. Purchase IFH, Longstaff E, Ashby J, Styles JA, Anderson D, Lefevre PA, Westwood FR (1976) Nature 264:624-627
4. Purchase IFH, Longstaff E, Ashby J, Styles JA, Anderson D, Lefevre PA, Westwood FR (1978) Br J Cancer 37:873-903
5. Sugimura T, Kawachi T, Matsushima R, Nagao M, Sato S, Yahagi T (1977) Progress in genetic toxicology. In: Scott D, Bridges BA, Sobels FH (eds) Elsevier/North Holland, Amsterdam, pp 125-154
6. Rannug U, Johansson A, Ramel C, Wachmeister CA (1974) Ambio 3:194-197
7. Bartsch H, Malaveille C, Montesano R (1975) Int J Cancer 15:429-437
8. Longstaff E, McGregor D (1978) Toxicol Lett 2:1-4
9. Donahue EV, McCann J, Ames BN (1978) Cancer Res 38:431-438
10. Henschler D (1977) Environ Health Perspect 21:61-64
11. Henschler D, Eder E, Neudecker T, Metzler M (1977) Arch Toxicol (Berl) 37:233-236
12. Davis MJ, Green PN (1978) Paint Manufacture 48:32
13. McGregor DB (1977) Mutagenicity Testing of Benzil
14. Styles JA (1977) Br J Cancer 36:558-563

Interlaboratory Variations of Test Results

J. C. TOPHAM

The generation of different results in different laboratories apparently conducting similar experiments is not new. Indeed it has been a source of debate and confusion for many years in many disciplines. Short-term tests for carcinogenicity are no exception. Brief inspection of the literature finds numerous examples of conflicting and often apparently contradictory data. These differences occur to a lesser or greater extent in the mutation-based tests that have been widely used as short-term tests for carcinogenicity.

A few examples will serve to illustrate the problem. TCDD has been tested in the *Salmonella typhimurium* system in three laboratories (1) (Table 1). Two laboratories reported positive results in strain TA 1532 but the third could not obtain positive results in this strain or the related strains TA 1537 and TA 1538.

Table 1. Published differences in results: TCDD (2,3,7,8-tetrachlorodibenzo-*p*-dioxin; *S. typhimurium* (frameshift-detecting strains)

Laboratory	Method	TA 1531	TA 1532	TA 1534	TA 1537	TA 1538
1	Liquid	NT	+	NT	NT	NT
2	Plate	$\pm$	++	+	NT	NT
3	Plate	$\overline{\text{NT}}$	−	$\overline{\text{NT}}$	−	−

NT, not tested; + positive result; − negative result; $\pm$ equivocal result.

There have been five studies on the effect of LSD on cultured human lymphocytes (2) (Table 2). Two laboratories reported mitotic inhibition only, three laboratories found single chromosome breaks, but only one observed chromosome rearrangements.

The problem is not restricted to in vitro techniques. There have been three published interlaboratory comparisons of the dominant lethal test (3-5). In these studies a qualitative similarity of the data was achieved. The major variation between the laboratories was in preimplantation losses. Least variation was found in the numbers of dead implants and total implants. Some of these variations were considered to be due to strain differences in the animals used.

---

[1] Imperial Chemical Industries Limited, Pharmaceuticals Division Mutagenicity and Carcinogenicity Unit, Safety of Medicines Department, Mereside, Alderley Park, Macclesfield, Cheshire SK 10, 4TG United Kingdom

Table 2. Published differences in results; LSD (lysergic acid diethylamide);
in vitro studies with normal human lymphocytes

| Laboratory | Mitotic inhibition | Chromosome damage | |
		Single breaks	Rearrangements/double breaks
1	+	+	+
2	NT	+	−
3	+	+	−
4	+	−	−
5	+	−	−

NT, not tested; + positive result; − negative result.

16 compounds have been tested in the micronucleus test in more
than one laboratory, (6-10) (Table 3). Only three compounds,
EMS, mitomycin C and cyclophosphamide gave consistently positive results. Five compounds, diethylnitrosamine, 2-napthylamine,
MNNG, caffeine and acetylsalicyclic acid gave consistently negative results. Conflicting results were obtained with the remaining eight compounds (i.e., 4-nitroquinoline-1-oxide, aflatoxin, dimethylnitrosamine, 3-methylcholanthrene, 2-AAF, dimethylbenzanthracene, urethane and colchicine).

Table 3. Comparison of published data on the micronucleus test

| Compound | Laboratory | | | | |
	A	B	C	D	E
EMS	+		+	+	
Cyclophosphamide	+		+	+	+
Mitomycin C			+	+	
MNNG			−	−	
Caffeine			−	−	
Acetylsalicyclic acid			−	−	
2-Naphthylamine	−			−	
DEN	−				−
4-NQO	+			−	
Aflatoxin B_1	$\pm$	+		−	
DMN	$\pm$	+		−	+
3-Methylcholanthrene		+		−	
2-AAF	−	+			
9,10-Dimethylbenzanthracene	−			+	
Urethane	−			+	
Colchicine			+	−	

Space, not tested; + positive result; − negative result; $\pm$ equivocal
result.

What then, are the origins of these interlaboratory variations? Historically detailed examination of a specific compound or lesion by a specific technique in a specialised laboratory has been most usual. However, with the enormous rapidly increasing demand for early information on carcinogenic potential, numerous laboratories with a range of dissimilar skills and experience are attempting to apply a range of published techniques to an assortment of chemicals. This has undoubtedly been an important factor in the development of different results with apparently the same procedure in different laboratories.

ABPI Collaborative Study with *S. typhimurium*

In 1974, the ABPI (Association of the British Pharmaceutical Industry) recognised this problem and initiated a programme of collaborative work. The objectives were to establish the reproducibility of the test results with standard compounds in several laboratories in order to gain confidence in laboratory methodology and also in the robustness of the tests. This required that each laboratory should work from the same defined protocol and use test compounds from the same central supply. The protocol used was similar to that described by Ames et al. (11), with and without metabolic activation. Strains TA 1535, TA 1537, and TA 1538 only were used. The liver activation system was prepared from rats that had been pre-treated with phenobarbitone. The concentrations of each compound tested were selected on the basis of toxicity studies conducted in each laboratory (Table 4). It is apparent that this resulted in some considerable differences in the concentrations tested. However, the results obtained by the four laboratories were in very close agreement (Table 5). In some laboratories toxic effects caused the appearance of pseudorevertants (12) (microcolonies due to bacterial killing) with safrole, nitrofurantoin and 5-fluorouracil. However, no false "positives" or false "negatives" were found with the compounds tested. This, admittedly limited, collaborative study showed that the *S. typhimurium* test was robust and produced reproducible results when used in four laboratories with widely different experience with the technique. However, the results highlighted the need to (a) test a standard range of concentrations of unknown compounds, and (b) define the limits of detection and the sensitivity of the method. A second ABPI collaborative study looked at the sensitivity of TA 1538 and TA 98 to 2-nitrofluorene. The amount of 2-nitrofluorene required to double the spontaneous colony count is shown in Table 6. It is apparent that there is at least a fourfold range in sensitivity among the laboratories and that is not related to the considerable variations in spontaneous colony count per plate.

Between 1974 and 1978, it had become apparent that a large range of variations are possible within (or very close to) a published technique. Because the *S. typhimurium* test is most widely used, variations in this technique have been most widely recognised (Table 7). Longstaff (12) describes some examples of differences that can be attributed to some of these variations and I will briefly discuss some problems that we have encountered in our laboratory.

Table 4. *S. typhimurium* test (ABPI): range of concentrations tested (µg/plate)

Compound/Laboratory	A	B Maximum	D	E
Cyclophosphamide	1.0 – 1,000	5,000	10 – 100	250 – 1,000
Ethanol	1.0 – 1,000	50,000	0.1 – 100	250 – 1,000
Penicillin	1.0 – 1,000	1.0	NT	3 – 12.5
Safrole	1.0 – 1,000	3.2	0.1 – 100	62.5 – 250
Glucose	1.0 – 1,000	5,000	0.1 – 1,000	250 – 1,000
Adrenalin	100 – 2,000	500	0.1 – 100	250 – 1,000
Chlordiazepoxide	100 – 2,000	500	0.1 – 100	250 – 1,000
Nitrofurantoin	1.0 – 1,000	0.5	0.1 – 1.0	1.25 – 3.1
5-Fluorouracil	1.0 – 1,000	100	> 1.0	0.2 – 3.1
2-AAF	1.0 – 1,000	20	10 – 100	250 – 1,000

NT, not tested.

Table 5. Results of *S. typhimurium* test (ABPI)

Compound/Laboratory	A	B	D	E
Cyclophosphamide	1535 + S-9	1535 + S-9	1535 + S-9[a]	1535 + S-9
Ethanol	–	–	–	–
Penicillin	–	–	NT	–
Safrole	–	–	–	–
Glucose	–	–	–	–
Adrenalin	–	–	–	–
Chlordiazepoxide	–	–	–	–
Nitrofurantoin	–	–	–	–
5-Fluorouracil	–	–	–	–
2-AAF	1538 + S-9	1538 + S-9	1538 + S-9	1538 + S-9

+ S-9, with S-9 mix; ± S-9, with or without S-9 mix; NT, not tested; – negative result.

[a] Failure to detect activity in the absence of the S-9 mix may be due to the low concentration tested (maximum 100 µg/plate)

Table 6. Sensitivity of TA 1538 and TA 98 to 2-nitrofluorene (ABPI)

Laboratory	µg NF/plate to double spontaneous colony count[a] TA 1538	TA 98
A	0.016 (17)	0.016 (16)
B	0.016 (8)	0.031 (17)
C	0.063 (6)	1.0 (169)
D	0.063 (10)	0.016 (9)
	0.016 (10)	

[a] Numbers in parenthesis are spontaneous colony count/plate

Table 7. Problems in protocol definition. A large range of variations are possible within (or very close to) a published technique

Examples of variations in the standard *S. typhimurium* test

1. Strain
2. Plate, liquid, host-mediated assay, fluctuation
3. Organ/species for S-9
4. Induction agent
5. Cofactors: quantity and ratio
6. Addition of other enzymes (e.g., glucuronidase)
7. Addition of competitors to assay medium (e.g., harman)
8. Duration of incubation/oxygen/other gas tension
9. Content of media (e.g., tap or distilled water to prepare agar)
10. Presentation of compound (extracts/concentrates/solvent)
11. Method of colony counting
12. pH of media

We have noticed that the number of spontaneous revertants appearing on the plates varies with the supplier of minimal media (P.A. Watkins, unpublished work) (Table 8). This is important as the lower limit of sensitivity is often defined as twice the spontaneous colony count. Another more dramatic effect was seen when tap water was substituted with distilled water in the "top agar". This resulted in the complete loss of sensitivity of TA 1535 and TA 1538 to each of our standard positive controls for these strains (P.A. Watkins, unpublished work) (Table 9).

Table 8. Effect of minimal media plates on spontaneous colony count in *S. typhimurium* test (no "activation")

| | TA 1538 No. colonies/plate | |
	Supplier 1	Supplier 2
Experiment 1	4	24
water controls	6	24
	11	27
Experiment 2		
water controls	7	25

We have collected data from four laboratories on the activity of pronethalol with TA 1535 (Table 10). Two laboratories reported negative results and two positive results. The negative results may be due to the use of phenobarbitone as an induction agent or to an unfortunate choice of dose levels of pronethalol. Aroclor is not invariably the "best" inducer of "positive" results. Experiments with substituted anilines (P.A. Watkins, unpublished work) (Table 11) show that for this class of compound either positive or negative results can be easily obtained by manipulation of the test system.

Table 9. Effect of water in "top agar" on response of *S. typhimurium*

	No. colonies/plate TA 1535 + S-9		Spot test TA 1538	
	Tap water	Distilled water	Tap water	Distilled water
Vehicle control	30;19	23;15	3;7	7;6
10 µg ICI 42464 per plate	39;27	346;278	NT	NT
100 µg spot 2-nitro-fluorene	NT	NT	No response	+++

NT, not tested; +++ strong positive effect.

Table 10. Effect of dose levels (µg pronethalol/plate) and activation system in *S. typhimurium* TA 1535

Activation	Laboratory			
	A	B	C	D
Phenobarbitone	2.5			
	25 −			50 −
	250 −			100 −
	2500 −			
Aroclor			33 −	
		100 −	100 +	
		500 +	500 +	
		750 +		
		1000 +	1000 +	
		1500 +	1500 +	
		2000 + (Toxic)	2000 +	
			2500 +	

− negative result; + positive result; ± equivocal result.

Table 11. Effect of inducing agent on response of TA 1535

	Inducing agent		
	No S-9	Aroclor	Phenobarbitone
P-Phenylenediamine	−	+	+
P-Nitroaniline	+	−	+
4-Aminothiophenol	−	++	+
4-Fluoroaniline	−	−	+

ABPI Collaborative Study of the Dominant Lethal Test

The ABPI also organised a collaborative study of the dominant lethal test using five compounds in four laboratories. The results of one compound (cyclophosphamide) are available.

The protocol used for this work is shown in Table 12 and the results are summarised in Fig. 1. The most important similarities between the laboratories are:

1. a positive effect in weeks 1 and 2 for pre- and post-implantation deaths, and
2. the occurrence of a dose response in weeks 1 and 2 for pre- and post-implantation deaths.

The most important differences between the laboratories were:

1. a positive effect on post-implantation deaths was seen in week 3 for laboratories A and B (high dose only).
2. an increase in pre-implantation losses was seen for the high dose in weeks 5 and 6 for laboratory A only,
3. a low dose only increase in post-implantation deaths in week 5 for laboratory C only, and
4. control mean % deaths/week varies between 7.6 and 11.8.

The dominant lethal test gave reproducible responses in the predicted area of activity but the sporadic "positive effects" seen in unexpected areas require further investigation and understanding if "false positives" are to be avoided.

Table 12. ABPI Dominant lethal test

Common protocol outline	
Mice	AP, laboratory A CFLP, laboratories B, C, and D
Group size	15 ♂/Group
Groups	1. Vehicle control 2. 20 mg/kg Cyclophosphamide (1/4 MTD) 3. 80 mg/kg Cyclophosphamide (MTD)
Dosage	Once daily for 5 days by gavage
Sperm sampling	2 ♀/♂/Week for 8 weeks after the last dose
Statistics	Trial of various methods

The Relationship Between Mutation Tests and Carcinogenic Activity

The techniques used in the ABPI collaborative studies and other widely used short-term tests for carcinogenicity are basically reproducible and robust when using high levels of potent positive controls and bland negative controls. At low levels of positive controls variations in sensitivity may be seen. With chemically or biologically active negative controls, system-specific effects may appear. Some examples and the consequences of these effects are reported by Ashby (13).

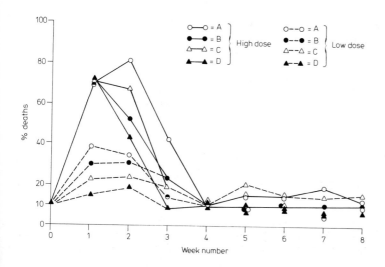

Fig. 1. Dominant lethal test cyclophosphamide (ABPI)

So far I have been considering variables which may account for
interlaboratory differences in results obtained with mutation
tests. However, when these results are used to predict carcinogenic activity additional variables and difficulties are introduced. Probably the most important of these is the difficulty in the definition of carcinogenicity and the great
variations in the quality of the data on which classification
of carcinogens and non-carcinogens is based (14). All correlations between mutagenesis and carcinogenesis are limited by
this uncertainty in the classification of carcinogens. Other
important factors are:

1. the chemical quality and identity used for both the carcinogenic and mutagenic tests (they should be equivalent if
   the tests are to be comparable (12), and
2. compound selection (i.e., classes of carcinogen detected and
   discrimination between positives and negatives within a class
   by a particular short-term test (13).

The importance of compound selection in correlations with carcinogenic activity is illustrated by comparison of results
published with polycyclic hydrocarbons by three laboratories
using *S. typhimurium* (15,17) (Table 13). The most striking discrepancy is the identification of eight non-carcinogens as
"positive" in the test by laboratory 1 whereas the other laboratories identified almost all of the non-carcinogens tested
correctly. The reasons for this discrepancy lay in the selection
and classification of the non-carcinogens:

1. benzo(e)pyrene was classed as non-carcinogenic by laboratory
   1 but as a carcinogen by laboratory 3,
2. none of the other seven non-carcinogens tested by laboratory
   1 were tested by either of the other laboratories, and

Table 13. Differences in published results correlation
of results in *S. typhimurium* with carcinogenic activity:
Hydrocarbons

Laboratory	Carcinogens Tested	Positive	Non-carcinogens Tested	Negative
1	16	14	8	O
2	11	11	9	8
3	26	26	7	6

3. three non-carcinogens were tested and found negative in both
   laboratories 2 and 3.

A similar difference in correlation with carcinogenic activity
was seen with a group of nitrosoureas and nitrosamines that have
been tested in three laboratories (16,18) (Table 14). Laboratories 2 and 3 correctly identified all the agents they tested.
However, the five compounds incorrectly identified by laboratory
1 were not tested in the other laboratories. Considering all
the data it seems that the correlation with carcinogenic activity is good for the 17 cyclic nitrosamines (including only
two non-carcinogens) tested, but is less good for aliphatic
nitrosamines and nitrosoureas.

Table 14. Differences in published results correlation of
results in *S. typhimurium* with carcinogenic activity:
Nitrosoureas and nitrosamines

Laboratory	Carcinogens Tested	Positive	Non-carcinogens Tested	Negative
1	22	19	4	2
2	5	4(5[a])	2	2
3	17	17	O	O

[a]When DMN tested in liquid culture

Optimum Use of Short-Term Tests

In order to obtain the best from short-term tests for carcinogenicity it is essential that (a) each laboratory at a specific
time calibrates for sensitivity to a particular class of compounds, and (b) if no related compounds of known carcinogenicity
are available, then it should be recognised that the value of
the test is much more limited.

It is apparent that short-term tests can be "tuned" to detect
almost any agent as either "positive" or "negative" (e.g., the
addition of Harman to *S. typhimurium* cultures will result in
aniline being identified as a positive (19). An understanding
of the factors modifying the action of compounds in rapid-test

systems may give important insights into the mode of action of
carcinogens and also a better understanding of the predictive
potential of short-term tests. There may in fact be no clear
distinction between positive and negative results in short-term
tests but this in no way limits their usefulness as aids in the
determining of carcinogenic potential. Paradoxically, the more
we learn of the limitations of short-term tests the more power-
ful they become.

Abbreviations: TCCD (Dioxin): 2,3,7,8-tetrachlorodibenzo-*p*-dioxin; LSD:
lysergic acid diethylamide; EMS: ethyl methane sulphonate; MNNG: N-methyl-
N'-nitro-N-nitrosoguanidine; 2-AAF: N-2-fluorenyl acetamide; 2-NF: 2-nitro-
fluorene; 4-NQO: 4-nitroquinoline-N-oxide; DMN: dimethylnitrosamine; DEN:
diethylnitrosamine; ICI 42,464: 2-(α-chloro-β-isopropylamino)ethylnaphthylene
hydrochloride; pronethalol: 2(α-hydroxy-β-isopropylaminoethyl)naphthylene.

References

1. Wassom JS, Huf JE, Loprieno N (1977) Mutat Res 47:141-160
2. Cohen MM, Shiloh Y (1977) Mutat Res 47:183-209
3. Anderson D, McGregor DB, Purchase IFH, Hodge MCE, Cuthbert JA (1977)
   Mutat Res 43:231-246
4. Ehling UH, Fröhberg H, Schülze-Schencking M, Lang R, Lörke D, Machemer
   L, Matter BE, Muller D, Röhrborn G, Buselmaier W, Roll R (1975) Mutat
   Res 29:261
5. Moreland F, Kiliand DJ, Palmer KA, Sprinker A, Green S (1976) Toxicol
   Appl Pharmacol 37:107-108
6. Heddle JA, Bruce WR (1977) In: Scott D, Bridges BA, Sobels FH (eds)
   "Progress in genetic toxicology". Elsevier/North-Holland, Amsterdam,
   pp 265-274
7. Wild D (1976) Mutat Res 38:105
8. Matter BE, Grauwiler J (1974) Mutat Res 23:239-249
9. Trzos RJ, Petzold GL, Brunden MN, Swenberg JA (1978) Mutat Res 58:79-86
10. Friedman MA, Staub J (1977) Mutat Res 43:255-262
11. Ames BN, Durston WE, Yamasaki E, Lee FD (1973) Proc Natl Acad Sci USA
    70:2281-2285
12. Longstaff E (1980) In: Norpoth K, Garner RC (eds) Short-term muta-
    genicity test systems for detecting carcinogens. Springer, Berlin,
    Heidelberg, New York
13. Ashby J (1980) In: Norpoth K, Garner RC (eds) Short-term mutagenicity
    test systems for detecting carcinogens. Springer, Berlin, Heidelberg,
    New York
14. Shubrik P, Hartwell JL (1969) Survey of compounds which have been
    tested for carcinogenic activity, PHS Publication No 149. Springer,
    Berlin, Heidelberg, New York, reprinted 1969
15. Andrews AW, Thibault LH, Lijinsky W (1978) Mutat Res 51:311-318
16. McCann J, Choi E, Yamasaki E, Ames BN (1975) Proc Natl Acad Sci USA
    72:5135-5139
17. Purchase IFH, Longstaff E, Ashby J, Styles JA, Anderson D, Lefèvre PA,
    Westwood FR (1978) Br J Cancer 37:873-959
18. Andrews AW, Thibault LH, Lijinsky W (1978) Mutat Res 51:319-326
19. Sugimura T, Kawachi T, Matsushima T, Nagao M, Sato S, Yahagi T (1977)
    In: Scott D, Bridges BA, Sobels FH (eds) "Progress in genetic toxicology".
    Elsevier/North-Holland, Amsterdam, pp 125-140

Biostatistics of Ames-Test Data

K. Norpoth[1], A. Reisch[2], and A. Heinecke[2]

In 1976, Matter stated with regard to the problem of interpreting mutagenicity test results: "Although most environmental compounds can be expected to produce either negative or 'weak' effects, there seems to be no scientific work available today that deals with the statistical handling of such results. In consideration of this, it is no wonder that interpretations made by different scientists may be subjective, often contradicting each other" (1). Two years later, this statement still draws our attention to a most critical point of short-term mutagenicity testing. Statistical evaluation of Ames-test data seems to be one of the main topics which requires more attention and research work. Numerous proposals made during the last two years to solve the problem from a theoretical viewpoint (2,3) give rise to the question of whether the empirical basis of biostatistics in this field has been adequately considered.

Frequency Distributions of Mutant Colonies per Plate

To obtain more information on this empirical basis, we studied frequency distributions of the number of back mutations in histidine-dependent *Salmonella typhimurium* cells. Since back mutations can be considered as rare events one should expect Poisson distributions on each plate and the values of different plates should be distributed in a negative binominal fashion. In the case of mutation frequencies which are usually found in the Ames-test procedure, normal distribution should be considered as a good approximation. This is indeed what we found in experiments with treated as well as with nontreated cells of *S. typhimurium* tester strains using large numbers of plates. As shown in Fig. 1, in six cases the probits of cumulative frequencies of back mutations found with *S. typhimurium* TA 98 and *S. typhimurium* TA 100, respectively, increased nearly linearly with increasing back mutation numbers.

In five of these cases, testing showed that normal distribution cannot be rejected at the level of $p < 0.05$. In a further experiment (see D in Fig. 1), the data obtained are in accordance with a normal distribution pattern, if one postulates the significance level of $p < 0.01$ for rejection. On the other hand,

---

[1] Institut für Staublungenforschung und Arbeitsmedizin der Universität Münster, D-4400 Münster/FRG

[2] Institut für Medizinische Informatik und Biomathematik der Universität Münster, D-4400 Münster/FRG

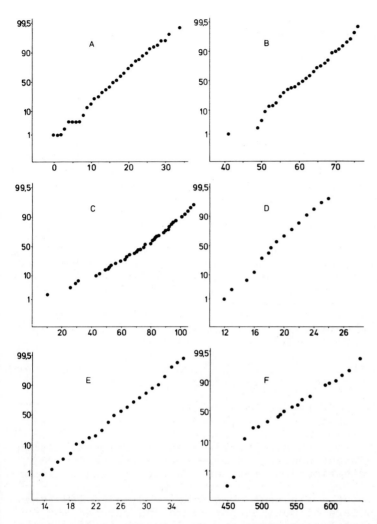

Fig. 1A-F. Cumulating frequencies of reverting numbers (expressed in % of the final value; see *ordinate*) found in six experiments with *S. typhimurium* TA 100 and TA 98 and plotted against their increasing values. (A) TA 100 grown without activating system; n = 100; $\bar{x}$ = 25.2; s = 5.2. (B) TA 98 grown in the presence of mouse liver S-9 mix (obtained after Aroclor pretreatment) and 30 μg/plate cyclophosphamide; n = 100; $\bar{x}$ = 61.5; s = 7.3. (C) TA 98 grown in the presence of activating system (see B) and 2 μg/plate benzo(a)-pyrene; n = 60; $\bar{x}$ = 274; s = 22.9. (D) TA 98 grown without activating system; n = 100; $\bar{x}$ = 19.4; s = 3.0. (E) TA 98 grown in the presence of activating system (see B) n = 100; $\bar{x}$ = 25.2; s = 5.2. (F) TA 100 grown under the influence of 0.025 ml 3-chloropropene in 1000 ml air; n = 22; $\bar{x}$ = 537; s = 56.6. Normal distribution could not be excluded by means of χ^2 testing at the level of $p < 0.05$ with the exception of D (no exclusion possible at the level of $p < 0.01$)

striking deviations from a symmetric distribution pattern were
found in two further (hundred plates) experiments carried out
with *Escherichia coli* WP2 uvrA (incubated with mouse liver S-9 mix
in plates for detecting trp$^+$ back mutants) and with *E. coli* K12
(343/113) (incubated without activating system in plates for detecting gal$^+$ mutants). In these experiments, however, unusually
small mutation frequencies were found (the mean was about 5/plate
in each). To obtain indirect evidence on the distribution pattern of mutants per plate in experiments with smaller numbers of
plates we looked at a series of two sample experiments which
conformed to the following conditions:

1. The mutant frequencies should have been increased by a test
   compound to less than 100%.
2. Five plates should be used in each experiment.
3. The effect should be proven significant by means of further
   dose-response investigations.

As shown in Table 1, we tested the deviations caused by the
test compound in 12 such experiments using Student's t-test and
Wilcoxon's (4) distribution-free two-sample rank test, respectively.

The following conclusions can be drawn from the data given in
Table 1.

1. Student's t-test is in general the more efficient test. Therefore, the distribution of mutant frequencies can in no case
   deviate dramatically from a symmetric pattern.
2. The less marked differences between the significance levels
   found with both tests refer to experiments leading to small
   mean revertant numbers. In accordance with theoretical considerations (2), one should postulate an experimental design
   leading to revertant numbers of more than 25/plate. In all
   other cases a distribution-free test should be used addition-
   ally.
3. Even in experiments with test compounds leading to less than
   doubling in numbers of mutants per plate and carried out
   using five plates for controls (as well as for treated cells),
   mutagenic effects can often be proven significant at the
   level of $p < 0.01$. Therefore it cannot be accepted as a rule
   to consider only doubled mutation frequencies as indications
   of true mutagenic effects (see 2). By this approach weak mutagens may be overlooked frequently.

Critical Considerations on the Use of Two-Sample Tests

Although small differences in mutation frequencies of two samples
can often be proven significant by correct statistical evaluation,
there is some doubt as regards the usefulness of designing Ames-
test experiments with respect to the requirements of statistical two-sample tests. The efficiency of such experiments should
be considered sceptically for the following reasons.

Table 1. Significance levels obtained by using Student's *t*-test and Wilcoxon's distribution-free two-sample rank test (4) for calculating the significance of enhanced revertant numbers with low doses of 12 mutagens in the Ames assay

No.	Method	Test compound	Tester strain	Mean value ± standard deviation		Significance of the difference B-A	
				A) Without test compound	B) With test compound	Student's *t*-test	Wilcoxon's test
1	PIT AS	Benzo(a)pyrene (0.3 µg/plate)	*S. typhimurium* TA 100	64.8 ± 13.3	89.4 ± 11.1	p < 0.01	p < 0.01
2	PIT AS	7,12-Dimethyl-benzanthracene (10 µg/plate)	*S. typhimurium* TA 98	22.2 ± 5.1	35.6 ± 5.1	p < 0.005	p < 0.01
3	PIT AS	Benzo(k)-fluoranthene (1 µg/plate)	*S. typhimurium* TA 100	39.6 ± 9.7	65.2 ± 3.8	p < 0.001	p < 0.01
4	DES	Bis(chloromethyl) ether (0.5 µl/ 2000 ccm)	*S. typhimurium* TA 1535	8.4 ± 3.4	15.2 ± 3.8	p < 0.01	p < 0.025
5	DES	Chloromethyl methyl ether (1.0 µl/ 2000 ccm)	*S. typhimurium* TA 98	12.2 ± 2.5	22.4 ± 6.4	p < 0.01	p < 0.015
6	PIT AS	Di-2-ethylhexyl-phthalate (5 µg/plate)	*E. coli* WP2 uvrA	4.6 ± 1.3	8.6 ± 2.7	p < 0.01	p < 0.01
7	DES AS	Chloroform (0.2 ml/2000 ccm)	*S. typhimurium* TA 98	21.0 ± 4.7	33.0 ± 3.5	p < 0.005	p < 0.01
8	DES AS	Trichloroethylene (0.2 ml/2000 ccm)	*S. typhimurium* TA 98	39.2 ± 3.0	50.6 ± 3.6	p < 0.001	p < 0.01

Table 1 (continued)

9	PIT AS	Chloroethanol (10 μg/plate)	*E. coli* WP2 uvrA	52.4 ± 4.1	75.0 ± 9.3	p < 0.01
10	DES AS	1,1,1-Trichloro-ethane (0.4 ml/2000 ccm)	*E. coli* WP2 uvrA	14.6 ± 3.6	23.4 ± 2.9	p < 0.005
11	DES AS	Carbon tetrachloride (0.2 ml/2000 ccm)	*E. coli* WP2 uvrA	42.4 ± 4.1	54.2 ± 3.8	p < 0.005
12.	DES AS	Acetonitrile (0.4 ml/2000 ccm)	*S. typhimurium* TA 98	41.8 ± 3.6	58.0 ± 7.4	p < 0.005

PIT, plate incorporation test; DES, test carried out by means of a desiccator to evaluate the mutagenicity of volatile compounds; AS, activating system added (liver oxigenase of Aroclor-treated mice); five plates were used in each investigation with as well as without test compound; p = α in each case

The application of two-sample tests including the use of tables published by Kastenbaum and Bowman (5) is limited by well-known restrictions (6). There is no empirical evidence that mutant frequencies are always proportional to the number of cells inoculated. Furthermore, while populations compared must be of equal size, they are not, if the test compound or other experimental conditions can influence the colony-forming ability of a tester strain. As shown in Table 2, examples can be given for significantly lower numbers of mutant colonies found in the presence of some test compounds. These deviations cannot be explained by altered survivor numbers. Regardless of whether the results indicate true effects of the compounds tested, the possibility must be considered that weak mutagenic effects can be overlooked, as well as falsely accepted, due to unavoidable variances in test results.

In this context it should be emphasized that statistical evidence for dose-dependent increases in revertant numbers is of essentially higher value than evidence drawn from one-dose experiments.

Statistical Evaluation of Dose-Response Relationships

As discussed in the field of radiation biology, mutation frequency of cell populations depends on mutagenic as well as on lethal effects of a given mutagen. Haynes and Eckhardt proposed that these interfering phenomena may lead to similar-dose response functions in testing chemical mutagens (F. Eckhardt, 1978, personal communication). By our results with several directly acting mutagens together with those of other groups kindly provided for statistical analysis, one of the conclusions of Haynes and Eckhardt can be confirmed mostly by empirical data. The data, given in Table 3, suggest that indeed the highest number of back mutations can be seen at the dose level of 63% cell killing. Hence, it follows that, for evaluating dose-dependent increases of back mutations caused by directly acting mutagens, Jonckheere's distribution-free rank variation test (7) is an appropriate procedure, provided that no revertant numbers are considered which belong to a higher than the 63% lethal dose.

The rank test examines data collectives which should be equal in size, according to their central tendencies. The required number of plates is minimal if the mutagenic effect is striking. 3-Chloropropene, for example, which was tested by V.F. Simmon (1978, personal communication) using the desiccator method (8), caused markedly increasing revertant numbers in *S. typhimurium* TA 100 (Table 4). If only the two lower values of each collective are calculated, the first eight values are sufficient for a resulting probability level of $p < 0.0004$. The procedure is very simple. The rank sum of all values which are higher than each value of lower dose collectives can be judged by Jonckheere's tables (7). A second example (Fig. 2), namely, results with bis(chloroethyl) ether tested in our laboratory using the same tester strain, demonstrates that weak effects may also be detected

Table 2. Lowered mutant frequencies of *S. typhimurium* TA 98 and TA 100 found in five experiments with low doses of test compounds. Mouse liver S-9 mix was added as activating system in experiments 1, 2, 3, and 5

No.	Tester strain	Compound tested (concentration)	Mean revertant number per plate ± standard deviation				Significance of the difference A - B (Student's t-test) ($p = \alpha$)
			n_1	A) Without test compound	n_2	B) With test compound	
1	*S. typhimurium* TA 100	Dibutylphthalate (0.1 µg/plate)	5	52.4 ± 13.1	5	37.2 ± 8.0	$p < 0.05$
2	*S. typhimurium* TA 100	Di-2-ethylhexyl-phthalate (1.0 µg/plate)	5	60.2 ± 5.2	5	53.2 ± 5.6	$p < 0.05$
3	*S. typhimurium* TA 98	Benzo(a)pyrene (0.1 µg/plate)	3	41.3 ± 3.1	3	35.0 ± 2.7	$p < 0.005$
4	*S. typhimurium* TA 98	1,1,1 Trichloro-ethane (0.1 ml/1000 cm^3 air in a desic-cator)	5	54.2 ± 5.4	5	37.2 ± 2.2	$p < 0.0005$
5	*S. typhimurium* TA 98	Chloroethanol (0.3 ml/1000 cm^3 air in a desic-cator)	5	38.8 ± 3.1	5	20.2 ± 7.3	$p < 0.0005$

Table 3. Comparison of dose-dependent increases of mutant frequencies and dose-dependent cell killing in 4 desiccator experiments with 3 direct-acting mutagens

E. coli WP2 uvr A (desiccator)
Ethylenimine (μl/2500 cm^3)

Revertants/plate	0.0	5.0	10	20	40	80
Revertants/plate	22	410	560	596	21	4
Revertants/plate	23	420	564	618	21	40
Revertants/plate	23	436	580	620	106	52
Revertants/plate	30	468	600	626	146	87
Revertants/plate	31	472	614	680	212	102

% Growth with histidine:

	100	100	100	67	11	0

S. typhimurium TA 100 (desiccator)
3-Chloro-propene (μl/2500 cm^3)

Revertants/plate	0.0	0.05	0.1	0.2	0.3
Revertants/plate	45	724	1004	121	3
Revertants/plate	49	816	1009	139	5
Revertants/plate	51	820	1124	145	5
Revertants/plate	52	864	1236	166	6
Revertants/plate	56	888	1320	168	8

% Growth with histidine:

	100	52	49	0	0

S. typhimurium TA 98 (desiccator)
Dichlorodimethyl ether (μl/2500 cm^3)

Revertants/plate	0.0	0.5	1.0	1.5	2.0
Revertants/plate	4	11	36	88	0
Revertants/plate	7	13	86	92	0
Revertants/plate	8	15	94	118	0
Revertants/plate	10	16	106	120	0
Revertants/plate	13	21	112	126	0

% Growth with histidine:

	100	100	93	60	0

E. coli WP2 uvr A (desiccator)
Dichlorodimethyl ether (μl/2500 cm^3)

Revertants/plate	0.0	0.3	0.5	1.0	1.5
Revertants/plate	2	3	6	11	15
Revertants/plate	2	5	8	13	16
Revertants/plate	4	7	10	14	19
Revertants/plate	5	7	13	14	19
Revertants/plate	6	8	18	16	21

% Growth with tryptophan:

	100	100	100	100	31

Table 4. Revertant numbers found in a desiccator experiment with 3-chloropropene and *S. typhimurium* TA 100 as the tester strain. The data were kindly provided by Dr. V. Simmon (1978, personal communication). Regarding the significance of the dose-dependent effect, see text

	3-Chloropropene (μl/9000 cm^3)					
Revertants/plate	0.0	0.1	0.2	0.3	0.4	0.5
Revertants/plate	117	359	640	910	730	970
Revertants/plate	130	374	780	990	850	1000
Revertants/plate	147	394	820	1050	940	1140

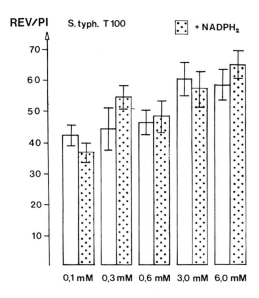

Fig. 2. Revertant numbers obtained with bis-(2-chloroethyl) ether in a plate incorporation test with *S. typhimurium* TA 100. Liver S-9 of Aroclor-treated mice was added and for each dose tested 4 plates were incubated with and without additional NADPH

at reasonable cost. The significance level calculated is $p < 0.001$.

Apparently different from the dose-response curves seen with directly acting mutagens are often dose-effect functions which result from the action of mutagens requiring metabolic activation. Relatively rare events are linear regression functions as described after treatment of *S. typhimurium* TA 98 strain with metabolically activated aflatoxin B_1 (9,10). If linearity cannot be refused on an adequate probability level, regression coefficients can be calculated and dose-related revertant numbers can be compared.

Another type of dose-response function seems to reflect more the enzyme-catalyzed transformation of an indirect mutagen which depends on the substrate concentration. Investigating benzo(k)-fluoranthene which is considered as a noncarcinogenic polycyclic hydrocarbon, we found a characteristic increase of revertant numbers using only one plate per dose (Fig. 3). This experimental

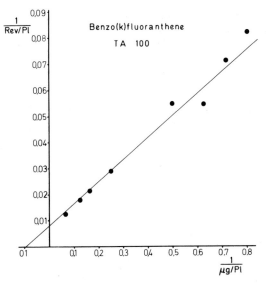

Fig. 3. Lineweaver-Burk plot of values obtained in a plate incorporation test with benzo(k)fluoranthene and *S. typhimurium* TA 100 as the tester strain. Liver S-9 of Aroclor-treated mice was added and single plates were incubated at each dose tested

design allows to test the dose-dependent increase of back mutations by means of Spearman's rank correlation coefficient. The significance level found was $p < 0.01$. Plotting the values according to a Lineweaver-Burk plot after subtraction of the control level led to an K_m value of 5×10^{-6}.

In summary, it is noted that different distribution-free test procedures can be considered as adequate for different types of dose-response functions. In general, the choice of an appropriate test requires prior information on the respective type of dose-response relationship. To use the right test means to enhance the probability of a correct interpretation of test results. On the other hand, working at the lowest level of cost is only possible by designing each experiment with regard to the requirements of statistical data evaluation.

References

1. Matter BE (1976) Problems of testing drugs for potential mutagenicity. Mutat Res 38:243-258
2. Ehrenberg L (1977) Aspects of statistical interference in testing for genetic toxicity. In: Kilbey BJ, Legator M, Nichols W, Ramel C (eds) Handbook of mutagenicity test procedures. Elsevier Scientific Publishing, Amsterdam, New York, Oxford, pp 419-459
3. Weinstein D, Lewinson TM (1978) A statistical treatment of the Ames mutagenicity assay. Mutat Res 51:433-434
4. Documenta Geigy (1968) Wissenschaftliche Tabellen, 7. Aufl Geigy AG, Pharma, Basel, pp 124-127, 139
5. Kastenbaum MA, Bowman KO (1970) Tables for determining the statistical significance of mutation frequencies. Mutat Res 9:527-549
6. Auerbach C (1970) Remark on the "tables for determining the statistical significance of mutation frequencies". Mutat Res 10:256

7. Jonckheere AR (1954) A distribution free k-sample test against ordered alternatives. Biometrica 41:133-145
8. Simmon VF, Kauhanen K, Tardiff RG (1977) Mutagenic activity of chemicals identified in drinking water. In: Scott D, Bridges BA, Sobels FH (eds) Progress in genetic toxicology. Proceedings of the Second International Conference on Environmental Mutagens, Edinburgh, July 11-15, 1977. Elsevier/North-Holland, Amsterdam, New York, Oxford, pp 249-258
9. Wong JJ, Hsieh DPH (1976) Mutagenicity of aflatoxins related to their metabolism and carcinogenic potential. Proc Natl Acad Sci USA 73:2241-2244
10. Norpoth K, Großmeyer R, Bösenberg H, Themann H, Fleischer H (1979) Mutagenicity of aflatoxin B_1, activated by S-9 fractions of human, rat, mouse, rabbit and monkey liver, towards S. typhimurium TA 98. Int Arch Occup Environ Health 42:333-339

Section V

New Experiences with Short-Term Tests –
Response of Some Environmental Carcinogens

Mutagenic Effects of Chlorinated Aliphatic Hydrocarbons; Influence of Metabolic Activation and Inactivation

D. Henschler[1]

Chlorinated aliphatic hydrocarbons are extensively used as systemic anaesthetic agents, as organic solvents for degreasing and dry-cleaning processes, as aerosol propellants and pesticides, for organic syntheses, and especially as monomers for plastics. Central nervous system depressant effects and damage to parenchymal tissues, e.g., liver and kidney, have been known for a long time. However, no significant attention was paid to genetic effects until 1974 when it became evident that one of the most extensively produced compounds, vinyl chloride, induced cancer in humans, (1,2) as well as in a variety of experimental animals (3,4). With this evidence, considerable concern arose in the public as well as in the scientific community as to whether this carcinogenic potential is encountered in other, if not in the majority of the chlorinated compounds, and which parts of the molecular structure were responsible for activity. Recent findings of the formation of such compounds as a consequence of chlorination of drinking water (5) have posed the urgent question to determine which chlorinated aliphatics may be hazardous and more important, whether safe alternative processes exist.

At an early stage, we initiated a systematic study of structure-activity relationships in short-chain chlorinated aliphatic compounds (6). Until recently, it seemed to be well established that these compounds are not genotoxic per se, but need metabolic conversion to reactive intermediates which are capable of interacting with nucleophilic sites of DNA to interfere with vital processes of replication. This view is no longer tenable since some types of chlorinated aliphatics have been described which react directly with nucleophiles. These will be dealt with later in this presentation. As a first step, it seems reasonable to look at the chemical reactivity of the molecules to predict possible pathways of enzymatic bioactivation.

Chemical Stability Versus Biological Reactivity

In general, the chemical behaviour of chlorinated aliphatic compounds is governed by the peculiarities of the C-Cl bond. This is characterized by an interplay of the -I effect of the chlorine substituent with the mesomeric donor effect of the involved C. The result of the dominating electron withdrawal effect upon the adjoining C-C bond, which then determines the

---

[1]Institut für Toxicologie, Universität Würzburg, Versbacher Straße 9, D-8700 Würzburg/FRG

stability of the whole molecule, is completely different in alkanes and alkenes. In alkanes, the electron deprivation induces
a loss of stability. Typical reactions, chemically as well as
metabolically, are (a) formation of free radicals, or (b) elimination of HCl or Cl_2, respectively, with the formation of an
olefin.

A quite different situation prevails in olefinic compounds with
chlorine substitution of hybridized C atoms in which the decrease in electron density in the C=C double bond exerts a
stabilizing effect. Therefore, formation of free radicals becomes very improbable, and other pathways of bioactivation
should be anticipated. So far, epoxidation of the olefinic bond
has been demonstrated as the prevailing, if not the exclusive,
mechanism. These highly electrophilic epoxides may undergo a
variety of reactions within biological systems which constitute
activation and deactivation mechanisms as well, and which can
explain most of the differences of various members of this class
of compounds with regard to their toxic potential.

Finally, a special type of reactivity is encountered in intermediate structures in which a chlorine substitution is located
at the C atom next to the olefinic C=C system: These are allyl
or allylogenic chlorides. Here, the destabilizing effect of the
chlorine favours the formation of a cation (7) which renders
direct S_N1- and S_N2-alkylating properties; these might compete
with metabolic epoxide formation (8) and result in a combination
of toxic mechanisms.

Chlorinated Alkanes

With chlorinated methanes, negative or inconclusive mutagenic
results have been obtained. The reason for this lack of genotoxic activity may in part be sought in the prevailing activation
mechanisms through insertion of oxygen into C-H bonds; geminal
substitution of carbon atoms with Cl and OH tends towards elimination of HCl. In the case of methyl chloride this results in
the formation of formaldehyde and subsequently formate, whereas,
with methylene chloride, carbon monoxide is the end product of
the reaction (9). Chloroform is converted to phosgene (10), an
acylating agent which might be responsible for the carcinogenic
potential. Carbon tetrachloride is oxidatively converted to
trichloromethyl radicals which induce lipid peroxidation (11).
The lack of mutagenic potential with CCl_4 and $CHCl_3$ is explained
by the very low or non-existent amount of covalent binding of
activated metabolites to DNA (12).

At least one chlorinated ethane derivative, 1,2-dichloroethane,
reveals significant mutagenic (13) and carcinogenic (14) effects. An enzymatic bioactivation mechanism has been proposed
which finally results in the formation of S-(2-chloroethyl)-
cysteine (13), the alkylating properties of which are common
knowledge. One could, however, also envisage a dehydrochlorin-
ation of 1,2-dichloroethane to vinyl chloride, and subsequent
addition to cysteine. The latter mechanism has been considered

by Green and Hathway (15). With other chlorinated ethanes or homologues, no convincing metabolic activation mechanisms have been described thus far.

Chlorinated Ethylenes

It has been suggested that all chlorinated ethylenes are metabolically transformed to epoxides (16). The rate of this oxidative step is determined by the number of chlorine substituents. It decreases with increasing chlorine substitution on account of their stabilizing effect in conjunction with a steric protection of the involved C atoms. The rather unstable epoxides may react in different ways: (a) they may alkylate nucleophilic sites in cellular macromolecules; this is regarded as the basis for acutely toxic and mutagenic and/or carcinogenic effects; (b) they may bind to soluble low-molecular nucleophiles like glutathione, cysteine, and others; (c) they may hydrolyze, enzymatically or non-enzymatically, to non-reactive diols; or (d) they may rearrange to less reactive or non-reactive acyl chlorides or chlorinated aldehydes, respectively (Fig. 1). Reactions (b)-(d) constitute deactivation mechanisms. The genotoxic potential is expected to depend on the relative rates of reactions (a) versus (b)-(d). At first glance, it seems impossible to predict which pathways might prevail. Since rearrangement might play an important role, we have studied the thermal rearrangement mechanisms and compared these to the metabolites detected in vitro and in vivo.

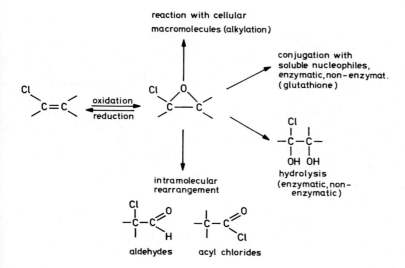

Fig. 1. Formation and possible reactions of chlorinated aliphatic epoxides in biological systems

As can be seen from experiments depicted in Fig. 2, the products of rearrangement represent either acid chlorides (tetra-, tri- and vinylidene chlorides) or aldehydes (1.2-dichloroethylenes cis- and trans-, vinyl chloride). The metabolites detected in vivo (or in the isolated rat liver preparation) are consistent with these in vitro rearrangement products (16), with one important exception: this is trichloroethylene. With this compound, the in vivo rearrangement goes entirely to trichloroacetaldehyde whereas the thermal rearrangement renders dichloroacetyl chloride. We have found an explanation for the unexpected behaviour in vivo: Lewis acids can induce rearrangement to chloral, and this mechanism might occur in the hydrophobic pocket of the oxidizing enzyme, cytochrome P-450, the trivalent iron of which could function as a Lewis acid (6,17).

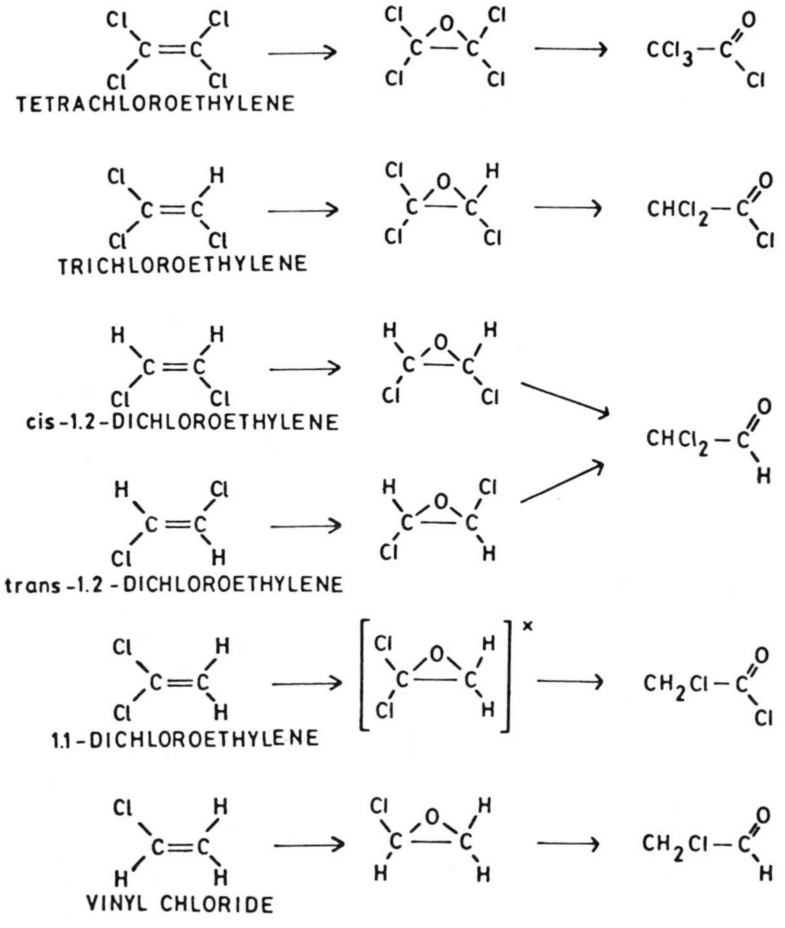

Fig. 2. Formation and thermal rearrangement mechanisms of epoxides of chlorinated ethylenes. The epoxide of vinylidene chloride has not been obtained by conventional methods of synthesis; instead of the epoxide, the anticipated rearrangement product, chloroacetyl chloride, has been isolated

The mutagenicity of chlorinated ethylenes has been tested by several authors. The first study involving all six members of the family of compounds employing an Ames-like test system, revealed (18) inactivity when no microsomes were added. With addition of S-9 mix, three chlorinated olefins gave positive results (Fig. 3): vinyl chloride, vinylidene chloride, and trichloroethylene. These results have been confirmed, with single compounds, by several other investigators. From this result we have concluded that the common feature of the mutagenic compounds is an asymmetric chlorine substitution which renders the respective epoxides, due to the unbalanced electron withdrawing effect of the chlorine atoms, highly electrophilic and reactive to nucleophilic macromolecules compared with the relatively stable symmetrically substituted ones in which deactivation mechanisms may prevail (19).

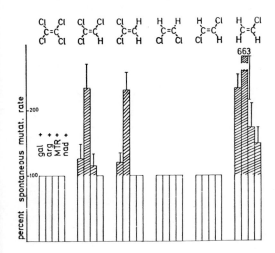

Fig. 3. Mutagenicity of chlorinated ethylenes in *Escherichia coli* K_{12} after incubation with phenobarbital-stimulated rat liver microsomes in aerophobic media as indicated (18)

Trichloroethylene is an exception which deserves special mention. The mutagenic activity of this compound is only marginal. A report on the carcinogenic activity of trichloroethylene (20) has been questioned since the sample used in the test had been stabilized with mutagenic and carcinogenic epoxides such as epichlorohydrin and epoxybutane (21). We have shown recently that in aequous systems adjusted to physiological pH, the trichloroethylene epoxide decomposes rapidly to carbon monoxide, formic acid, hydrochloric acid, and dichloroacetic acid and glyoxylic acid (22). None of these compounds are detected as metabolites in vivo. These findings strongly confirm the above outlined hypothesis that the highly reactive trichloroethylene oxide is completely converted, by P-450 to the non-reactive chloral immediately after its formation. Thus it escapes hydrolysis as well as reaction with essential nucleophilic macromolecules. This assumption would explain the low or missing mutagenic and carcinogenic potential of trichloroethylene.

Allyl and Allylogenic Chlorides

Allyl chloride, as well as some other substituted allyl compounds, have been shown to be mutagenic in microbial test systems without enzymatic activation (7,8,23). Figure 4 represents
a summary of these findings. This direct mutagenic effect correlates with the alkylating properties of allylic structures as
characterized by positive nitrobenzylpyridine tests. This alkylating potential can be explained by at least four different
mechanisms (6): (a) S_N1 reactivity by formation of an allyl
cation which is stabilized by resonance; (b) radical formation,
again favoured by resonance stabilization; (c) S_N2 and (d) S_N2'
mechanisms due to a special bimolecular nucleophilic displacement reaction which takes place at the unsaturated γ-carbon
atom. Whether and to what extent this direct alkylating mechanism
interferes or combines with an oxidation of the olefinic double
bond in vivo cannot be clearly predicted at present, and is open
to further investigations.

Compound	NBP-Test	TA 100
CH$_2$=CH—CH$_2$—Cl Allyl chloride	+	+
Cl—CH$_2$—CH=CH—CH$_3$ 1-Chlorobutene-2	+	+
Cl, CH$_3$—CH$_2$—C=CH$_2$ 1-Chloro-2-methyl-propene-2	+	+
Cl, Cl—CH$_2$—CH=CH$_2$ 1,3-Dichloropropene (cis- & trans-)	+	+
Cl, Cl—CH$_2$—CH=CH—CH$_2$ 1,4-Dichlorobutene-2	+	+
CH$_2$=C—CH=CH$_2$ (Cl) 2-Chlorobutadiene	+	+
Cl—CH=CH—CH=CH$_2$ 1-Chlorobutadiene	+	+
CH$_2$=CH—C=CH (Cl Cl) 3,4-Dichlorobutene-1	+	+

Fig. 4. Alkylating and direct mutagenic properties in *Salmonella
typhimurium* TA 100 of allyl and
allylogenic chlorides

Summary

Chlorinated aliphatic compounds may be mutagenic and/or carcinogenic with and without enzymatic activation in mammalian
and microbial organisms. Direct alkylating properties are found
in several allyl or allylogenic compounds. Alkanes may be activated by oxidative radical formation, or by hydroxylation of
C-H bonds; a special activation mechanism to produce an ethylating intermediate has been suggested for 1.2-dichloroethane.
Olefins may be activated by epoxidation, resulting in highly
electrophilic oxiranes in which the potential for direct alkylation of nucleophilic sites in macromolecules competes with deactivation mechanisms such as hydrolysis, conjugation with soluble nucleophiles, and intramolecular rearrangement to less
reactive acid chlorides or aldehydes. A molecular rule is proposed for the series of chlorinated ethylenes which explains,
by virtue of the unbalanced electron withdrawal effects of
chlorine substituents in the oxiranes, the high chemical and
biological reactivity of asymmetric molecules like vinyl and
vinylidene chloride.

References

1. IARC Int Technical Report 75/001, Lyon 1975
2. Brady J, Liberatore F, Harper P, Greenwald P, Burnett W, Davies JNP,
    Bishop M, Polan A, Viana N (1977) J Nat Cancer Inst 59:1383-1385
3. Viola PL, Bigotti A, Caputo A (1971) Cancer Res 31:516-519
4. Maltonic C, Lefemine G (1974) Environ Res 7:387-405
5. Bellar TA, Lichtenberg JJ, Croner RC (1974) J Am Waterworks Assoc 66:
    703-706
6. Bonse G, Henschler D (1976) CRC Crit Rev Toxicol 4:395-409
7. Eder E, Neudecker T (1978) Naunyn Schmiedebergs Arch Pharmacol [Suppl]
    302:83
8. Barbin A, Planche G, Croisy A, Malaveille C, Bartsch H (1977) Abstr,
    2nd Int Conf on Environm Mutag, Abstract p 59 Edinburgh July 1977
9. Kubic VL, Anders MW (1975) Drug Metab Dispos 3:104-112
10. Pohl LR, Bhooshan B, Whittaker NF, Krishna G (1977) Biochem Biophys
    Res Commun 79:684-691
11. Recknagel RO, Glende EA (1973) CRC Crit Rev Toxicol 2:263-297
12. Uehleke H, Werner T, Greim H, Krämer M (1977) Xenobiotica 7:393-400
13. Rannug U, Sundwall A, Ramel C (1978) Chem Biol Interact 20:1-16
14. D.H.E.W., USA, Techn Backgr Inform, Sept 26, 1978
15. Green T, Hathway DE (1975) Chem Biol Interact 11:545-562
16. Bonse G, Urban T, Reichert D, Henschler D (1975) Biochem Pharmacol 24:
    1829-1834
17. Henschler D, Bonse G (1978) 7th Int Congr Pharmacol, July 17, Paris
    1978. Advances in Pharmacology and Therapeutics Vol 9 Toxicology.
    Pergamon Press Oxford, New York 1978
18. Greim H, Bonse G, Radwan Z, Reichert D, Henschler D (1975) Biochem
    Pharmacol 24:2013-2017
19. Henschler D, Bonse G, Greim H (1976) IARC Sci Publ 13, Inserm Symp
    Series Vol 52 171, Environmental Pollution and Carcinogenic Risk
20. D.H.E.W., USA Techn Backgr Inform, May 1975

21. Henschler D, Eder E, Neudecker T, Metzler M (1977) Arch Toxicol (Berl) 37:233-236
22. Henschler D, Hoos WR, Fetz H, Dallmeier E, Metzler M (to be published) Biochem Pharmacol
23. McCoy EC, Burrows L, Rosenkranz HS (1978) Mutat Res 57:11-15
24. Neudecker T, Stefani A, Henschler D (1977) Experientia 33:1084-1085

Comparative Mutagenic Evaluation of Some Industrial Compounds

N. Loprieno[1] and A. Abbondandolo[2]

In the past few years, a number of compounds of industrial relevance have been tested by our group, using test systems for the detection of genetic effects in bacteria, yeasts, cultured mammalian cells, and laboratory animals. Essentially, the aim of such studies is to collect data which allow an evaluation of the possible genotoxic activity of chemicals produced on an industrial scale, molecules to which human exposure is unique with respect to intensity, duration, or possibility of synergistic effects.

There are some considerations which are implicit in a study of this kind:

1. Mutagenicity testing should be considered as a part of the general toxicologic evaluation of chemicals.
2. Mutagenicity tests essentially tell us whether a compound is able to modify the genetic material. They may also tell us *how potent* a chemical is as a mutagen in comparison with reference mutagens (e.g., X-rays). Most mutagenicity tests are, however, of very little or no value for the prediction, in quantitative terms, of the genetic risk for the human population. Calculation of human risk is best based on the very laborious animal tests, such as the dominant lethal test or the specific locus assay, and may also be attempted using data from in vitro experiments, but we are still far from a completely satisfactory recipe for the estimation of human genetic risk.
3. The results of mutagenicity tests can be used for predicting the potential carcinogenicity of chemicals. The limits of such an extrapolation are a matter of discussion at this meeting.
4. Our confidence in the use of mutagenicity data, either for the estimation of genetic risk or for the prediction of carcinogenicity, will be greater if such data come from more than just one test system. Any experimental investigator is aware that every single test has its own pitfalls and limitations, but coherent results obtained from several test systems cannot be due to chance. This will be particularly true for compounds showing a low genetic activity in a given test: the demonstration of an equally low, but consistent, activity in a range of test systems will increase our confidence in that result.

[1]Laboratorio di Genetica dell'Università di Pisa, I-56100 Pisa/Italy

[2]Laboratorio di Mutagenesi e Differenziamento CNR, Istituto di Antropologia e Paleontologia Umana dell'Università Degli Studie, I-56100 Pisa/Italy

In our study, we have used six different assays for the detection of:

1. base-pair substitutions or frameshift mutations in *Salmonella typhimurium* (the "Ames test"),
2. forward mutation at five loci in the yeast *Schizosaccharomyces pombe*,
3. mitotic gene conversion in the yeast *Saccharomyces cerevisiae*,
4. mutation to 6-thioguanine resistance in V79 Chinese hamster cells,
5. unscheduled DNA synthesis in EUE human cells, and
6. chromosome aberrations in mouse bone marrow cells.

Using these test systems, a number of industrial compounds were studied, including vinyl chloride and its metabolites, styrene, trichloroethylene, 1,4-dichlorobutene and their epoxides, chlorodifluoromethane and atrazine. Not all compounds were submitted to all tests, since this work was developed through a number of years and only recently the whole battery of test systems was set up.

Vinyl chloride has been in the past few years the object of many investigations. Extensive epidemiologic studies have shown that it has to be considered a human carcinogen; tumors were induced in laboratory animals to which vinyl chloride had been given by inhalation. The mutagenicity of vinyl chloride has been assessed on *Salmonella typhimurium*, yeasts, cultured mammalian cells, *Drosophila*, and lymphocytes of humans exposed to this compound (1).

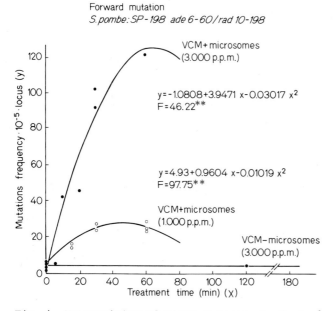

Fig. 1. Mutagenicity of vinyl chloride in *S. pombe* (P$_1$ strain; SP 198 *ade6-60/rad 10-198/h$^-$*) in the presence of purified mouse liver microsomes (12)

The mutagenicity of vinyl chloride in *Schizosaccharomyces pombe* is shown in Fig. 1. There was no activity in the absence of metabolic activation and a dose-dependent increase was found when liver microsomes from mice were added to the yeast cells.

Figure 2 shows the mutagenic effect of vinyl chloride in the host-mediated assay. Yeast cells were injected into the peritoneal cavity of mice and an oil solution of vinyl chloride was administered by gavage.

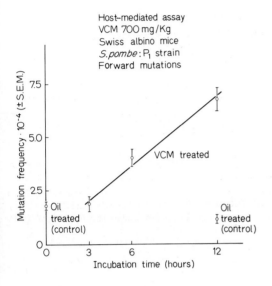

Fig. 2. Mutagenicity of vinyl chloride in *S. pombe* (P$_1$ strain) in the host-mediated assay: mice (Swiss albino) were treated by gavage with 1 ml of oil solution of VCM, with a dose corresponding to 700 mg/kg (13)

A comparison of the results obtained after in vitro or in vivo treatments is shown in Fig. 3. The slow response in the host-mediated assay is probably due to the short half-life of the metabolite, which makes it unlikely that a mutagenic concentration builds up in the peritoneal cavity early after administration.

Three metabolites of vinyl chloride have been tested for mutagenicity. 2-Chloroethylene oxide, as shown in Fig. 4, proved highly mutagenic per se. In Fig. 5, a comparison between this metabolite and microsome-activated vinyl chloride is reported.

Results obtained with 2-chloroacetaldehyde are shown in the next figures. This metabolite did not increase the mutation frequency after in vitro treatment both without and with metabolic activation (Fig. 6). Neither was it able to induce gene conversion in the yeast (Fig. 7). In the last figure, the induction of both forward mutation and gene conversion by 2-chloroethylene oxide are reported for comparison.

2-Chloroethanol was unable to induce gene mutation, as shown in Fig. 8, or gene conversion.

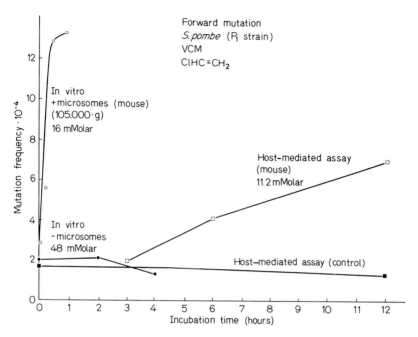

Fig. 3. A comparison of the effects produced in vitro by 16-mM (in the presence of mouse liver microsomes) and in vivo by 11.2-mM solutions of VCM (14)

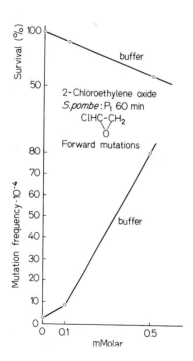

Fig. 4. Mutagenicity of 2-chloroethylene oxide on P_1 strain of *S. pombe* (13)

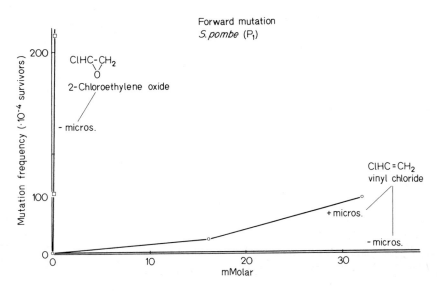

Fig. 5. Mutagenicity of VCM and its metabolite 2-chloroethylene oxide on P_1 strain of *S. pombe*

Table 1 shows a comparison between the results obtained with yeasts and those observed in *S. typhimurium*. In this organism, some direct effect of vinyl chloride was observed whereas the two yeast species were sensitive only if the microsomal enzymes were present. Moreover, 2-chloroethanol and 2-chloroacetaldehyde showed some mutagenic activity toward *Salmonella*.

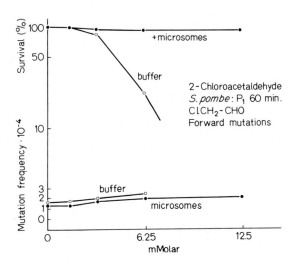

Fig. 6. Mutagenicity of 2-chloroacetaldehyde on P_1 strain of *S. pombe* (13)

338

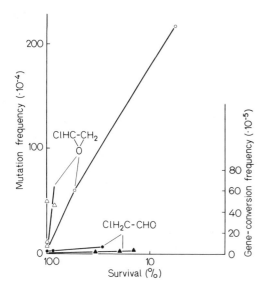

Fig. 7. Frequency of genetic effects produced by chloroethylene oxide (*open symbols*) and 2-chloroacetaldehyde (*closed symbols*) in yeasts. *Circles*, forward mutation in *S. pombe*; *triangles*, gene conversion in *S. cerevisiae* (1)

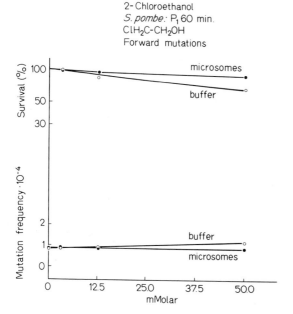

Fig. 8. Mutagenicity of 2-chloroethanol on P_1 strain of *S. pombe* (13)

Styrene has been produced commercially since 1940 and at present is among the top 50 chemicals in production volume. Some 440,000 tons per year is made in Italy and this represents the fifth largest producer after the USA, Japan, the Federal Republic of Germany, and the Netherlands. The main use of styrene is in the production of plastics and resins. A derivative of styrene, styrene oxide, is an intermediate in the preparation of cosmetics

Table 1. Comparative response of *S. typhimurium* and yeasts to vinyl chloride and its metabolites (13)

| | Salmonella | | | | | | Yeasts | | | |
| | Malaveille et al. 1975 (1530) | | Rannug et al. 1975 (1535) | | McCann et al. 1975 (100) | | Forward mutations (P_1) | | Gene-conversions D_4 | |
	+ micros.	-	+ micros.	-	+ micros.	-	+ micros.	-	+ micros.	-
Vinyl chloride	+++	+	+++	+	+	+	+++	-	++	-
Chloroethylene oxide	n.t.	+++	n.t.	+++	n.t.	+++	n.t.	n.t.	+++	+++
Chloroethanol	++	+	n.t.	-	++	+	-	-	-	-
Chloroacetaldehyde	++	+	n.t.	(+)	n.t.	++	(+)	(+)	(+)	(+)

and other chemicals of agricultural or biological interest. According to Leibman (2), styrene is metabolically converted to styrene oxide and subsequently to styrene glycol. Hippuric acid is known to be excreted in urine.

When tested in *Salmonella*, styrene was unable to induce reverse mutations both in the absence and in the presence of microsomes. Styrene epoxide was active per se and microsomes showed some protective effect. Also in the yeast *S. pombe* (Fig. 9), the metabolite was mutagenic whereas the parent molecule was inactive, even in the presence of microsomal enzymes. Styrene oxide was also able to induce gene conversion, as shown in Fig. 10. In the host-mediated assay, both styrene and styrene oxide slightly increased the frequency of gene conversion. They were, however, unable to induce mutations in this assay. In Fig. 11, the mutagenic effect of styrene oxide on cultured Chinese hamster cells is reported. Styrene was inactive in this test system, both in the presence and absence of microsomes.

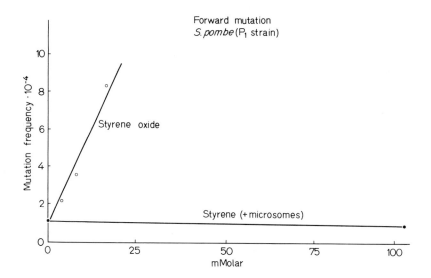

Fig. 9. Mutagenicity of styrene and styrene oxide on P_1 strain of *S. pombe*

Figure 12 shows the results of in vivo experiments in the mouse for the induction of chromosome aberrations in bone marrow cells. An increased number of cells with chromosomal breaks was observed. However, statistical treatment of data showed that the difference between treated and control animals was not significant. Styrene oxide, as shown in Figs. 13 and 14, caused a dose-dependent linear increase in cells with chromosome aberrations.

The results obtained with styrene oxide are summarized in Fig. 15, where the relative increase of genetic effects in the treated over the control series is plotted against the dose.

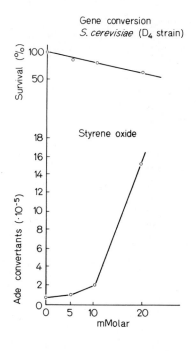

Gene conversion
S. cerevisiae (D$_4$ strain)

Styrene oxide

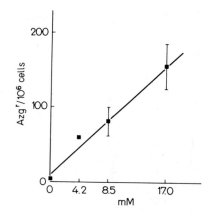

▲
Fig. 11. Dose-response curve for styrene-oxide-induced mutants in V79 Chinese hamster cells (16)

◀Fig. 10. Mitotic gene conversion induced by styrene oxide in *S. cerevisiae*, D$_4$ strain (*ade* locus) (15)

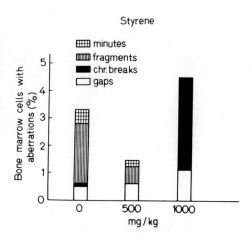

Styrene

⊞ minutes
▥ fragments
■ chr. breaks
□ gaps

Fig. 12. Induction of chromosome aberrations in bone marrow cells of CD-1 mice treated by gavage with styrene

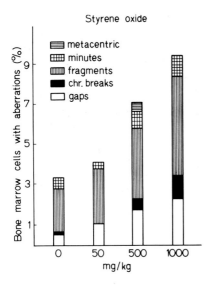

Styrene oxide

Fig. 13. Induction of chromosome aberrations in bone marrow cells of CD-1 mice treated by gavage with styrene oxide

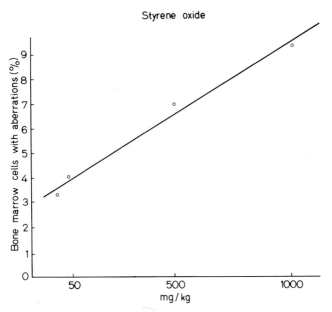

Fig. 14. Dose-response curve for styrene-oxide-induced chromosome aberrations in CD-1 mice

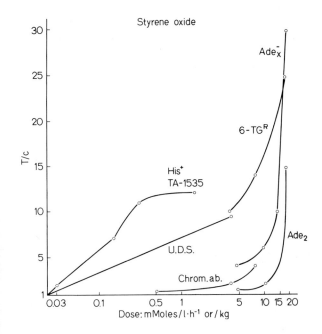

Fig. 15. Summary of genetic effects observed in different test systems, after treatment with styrene oxide: reverse mutations in *Salmonella* (*his*+), forward mutation in *S. pombe* (*ade*$_x$⁻) and V79 Chinese hamster cells (*6-TG*^{R}), gene conversion in *S. cerevisiae* (*ade*$_2$), unscheduled DNA synthesis in human cells (UDS), chromosome aberrations in CD-1 mice (*chrom.ab.*)

The different curves represent the induction of reverse mutation in *Salmonella*, unscheduled DNA synthesis in cultured human cells, chromosome aberrations in bone marrow cells of mice, gene conversion at the adenine-2 locus in *S. cerevisiae*, and forward mutation in *S. pombe* and in Chinese hamster cells.

In summary, only in the host-mediated assay did styrene show some genetic activity. It is possible that only in this test a sufficient concentration of the active metabolite is reached. It should be noted also (Fig. 16) that styrene oxide does not seem to be a very strong mutagen when compared with the active metabolite of vinyl chloride, at least in yeast.

Trichloroethylene, an organic solvent used in many industrial processes, has also been the subject of many recent studies. This compound can be metabolically converted to epoxy-1,1,2-trichloroethane, which is subsequently transformed to further metabolites (3). Trichloroethylene has been reported to be carcinogenic in mice (4) and mutagenic in different test systems (see below).

In our experiments, trichloroethylene did not increase the mutation frequency in *S. pombe* either in the absence or in the presence of microsomal activation; negative results were also obtained in the host-mediated assay when rats were used as hosts (Fig. 17). A weak mutagenic effect was observed using mice. The increase in mutation frequency was dependent both on the length of time the yeast cells remained in the peritoneal cavity (Fig. 18) and on the dose applied (Fig. 19).

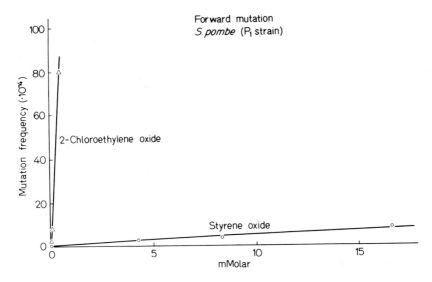

Fig. 16. A comparison of the mutagenic effect of styrene oxide and 2-chloro-ethylene oxide on P_1 strain of *S. pombe*

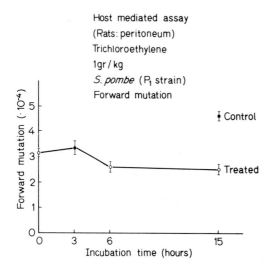

Fig. 17. Mutagenicity of trichloroethylene in *S. pombe*. Yeast cells were incubated in the peritoneum of rats (Sprague-Dawley) treated by gavage with an oil solution of TCE

As shown in Table 2, the intrasanguineous host-mediated assay using mice as hosts gave a negative result after recovering the yeast cells from kidney and lung and only a slight increase was observed in cells recovered from the liver. Negative results were obtained in in vivo experiments for the detection of chromosome aberrations in the mouse (Fig. 20). The slight increase in chromosome breaks was not significant by a chi-square test.

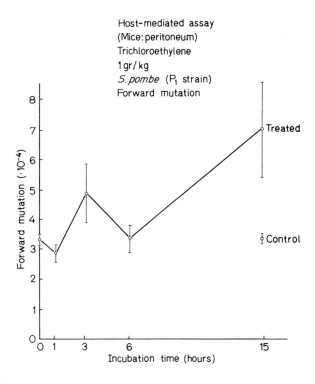

Host-mediated assay
(Mice:peritoneum)
Trichloroethylene
1 gr/kg
S. pombe (P$_1$ strain)
Forward mutation

Fig. 18. Mutagenicity of trichloroethylene in *S. pombe*. Yeast cells were incubated up to 15 h in the peritoneum of mice (CD-1) treated by gavage with an oil solution of TCE

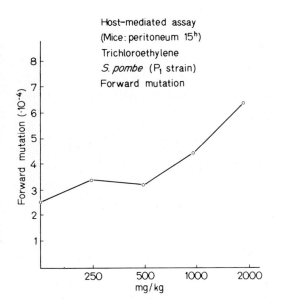

Host-mediated assay
(Mice: peritoneum 15^h)
Trichloroethylene
S. pombe (P$_1$ strain)
Forward mutation

Fig. 19. Mutagenicity of trichloroethylene in *S. pombe*. Yeast cells were incubated for 15 h in the peritoneum of mice (CD-1) treated by gavage with an oil solution of TCE

Table 2. Mutagenic activity of trichloroethylene on yeast (forward point mutation) incubated in vivo in different organs of mouse treated with 2000 mg/kg for 5 h

Treatment	Mutation frequency $\times 10^{-4} \pm SD$[a]		
	Liver	Kidney	Lung
Control	1.38 ± 0.62 (5)	NT	NT
Treated	4.68 ± 2.65 (4)	2.31 ± 1.37 (2)	1.32 ± 0.99 (2)

[a]In parentheses, the number of animals treated and evaluated; NT, not tested

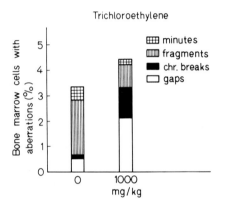

Fig. 20. Induction of chromosome aberrations in bone marrow cells of CD-1 mice treated by gavage with trichloroethylene

Epoxy-1,1,2-trichloroethane, a presumed metabolite of trichloroethylene, was highly mutagenic in cultured mammalian cells and also increased the forward mutation frequency in *S. pombe* (Fig. 21).

Trichloroethylene has been found weakly mutagenic in *Escherichia coli* (5), *Salmonella* (6), and *Saccharomyces cerevisiae* (7-9). It has been reported that trichloroethylene was able to induce somatic mutations in *Tradescantia* (A. Sparrow 1978, personal communication) and in mouse (7).

Henschler et al. (10) have raised the question of the purity of the samples of trichloroethylene used in the biological assays. According to these authors, epichlorohydrin and diepoxybutane, two known mutagens, are normally present as stabilizers in commercial trichloroethylene. They have also demonstrated that a pure sample of trichloroethylene was not mutagenic in *Salmonella*, whereas the two stabilizers were both active. Given the

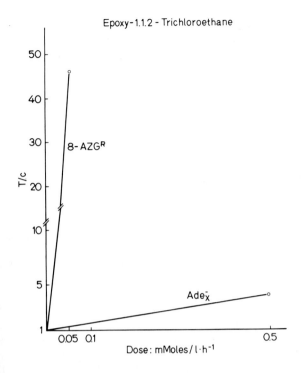

Fig. 21. Forward mutations induced in *S. pombe* (ade_x^-) and V79 Chinese hamster cells ($8-AZG^R$) by epoxy-1,1,2-trichloroethane

difficulty of checking the purity of all the samples used in the experimentation carried out so far, the mutagenicity of trichloroethylene is still an open question. Experiments with pure versus commercial samples are at present in progress in our laboratory.

In Fig. 22, a summary of data obtained with four epoxides and their parent molecules is shown. In addition to vinyl chloride, styrene and trichloroethylene, 1,4-dichlorobutene is also reported: this molecule was active per se in the yeast.

Chlorodifluoromethane is a fluorinated hydrocarbon gas used as an aerosol propellant. The possible mutagenicity of this compound was evaluated by means of a battery of test systems: forward mutation and gene conversion in yeasts, forward mutation and unscheduled DNA synthesis in mammalian cells, in vivo chromosome aberrations in the mouse. The results were negative in all tests as shown in Tables 3-10 and Fig. 23.

From this consistent pattern of results it seems reasonable to conclude that chlorodifluoromethane is not genetically active. This conclusion should, however, be confirmed in experiments with chronic treatments in which the route of human exposure (inhalation) should be reproduced. A result in contrast with our data has recently been published by Longstaff and McGregor (11): in this study, an increase in reverse mutations in the

Compounds		Yeast	Mutagenic	Activity (*)
Oxirame	Epoxide	In vitro buffer	In vitro met.act.	In vivo H.M.A.
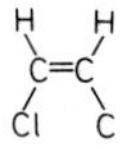 Vinyl chloride		−	+	+
	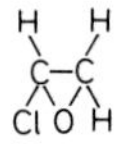 (chloroethylene epoxide)	+		
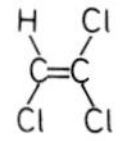 Trichloro-ethylene		−	−	(+)
	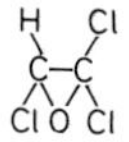 (trichloro epoxide)	+		
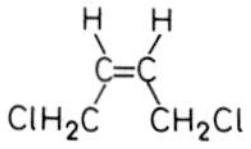 1.4-Dichloro-butene-2		+	+	+
	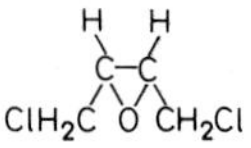 (dichlorobutene epoxide)	+		
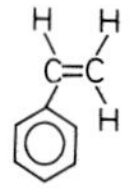 Styrene		−	−	(+)
	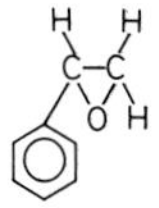 (styrene epoxide)	+		(+)

*Forward mutation *S. pombe* P₁ strain

Fig. 22. Mutagenicity of olefins and their epoxides in the yeast *S. pombe*

Table 3. In vitro forward mutations induced by chlorodifluoromethane (FL-22) on yeast *S. pombe* (P_J strain) treated in buffer pH 7.4

Time[a]	Survival (%)	Mutation frequency ($\times 10^{-4}$ survivors)
0	100	0.75 ± 0.04 (4/53593)
1	95	0.79 ± 0.01 (4/50479)
2	85	0.65 ± 0.003 (3/46440)
4	80	0.61 ± 0.005 (3/49113)

[a] $CHClF_2$ = 500 ml/min (1:1 air); a 20-mM concentration has been used during treatments

Table 4. In vitro forward mutations induced by chlorodifluoromethane (FC-22) on yeast *S. pombe* (P_J strain) · metabolic activation (S-10 mouse liver microsomal preparation)

Time (min)[a]	10.7 mM[b]	+ (S-10) 19.2 mM[b]
0	0.49 ± 10^{-4} (0/20400)	0.45 ± 10^{-4} (1/22280)
30	0.40 ± 10^{-4} (1/24840)	0.74 ± 10^{-4} (2/27040)
60	0.93 ± 10^{-4} (2/21416)	2.38 ± 10^{-4} (5/20982)
120	0.46 ± 10^{-4} (1/21824)	1.04 ± 10^{-4} (2/19257)

[a] $CHClF_2$ = 500 ml/min (1:1 air)
[b] Survival 100% in all treatments

Table 5. In vitro gene conversions induced by chlorodifluoromethane (FC-22) on yeast *S. cerevisiae* (D_4 strain) treated in buffer pH 7.4

Time (h)[a]	Survival (%)	Gene conversions ($\times 10^{-5}$)	
		Ade	*Trp*
0	100	1.2 ± 0.5	1.2 ± 0.6
1	83	0.9 ± 0.3	0.7 ± 0.1
2	62	0.6 ± 0.2	0.8 ± 0.2
4	80	1.1 ± 0.2	1.2 ± 0.3

[a] $CHClF_2$ = 500 ml/min (1:1 air); a 20 mM concentration has been used during treatments

Table 6. In vitro gene conversions induced by chlorodifluoromethane (FC-22) on yeast *S. cerevisiae* (D_4 strain) + metabolic activation (S-10 mouse liver microsomal preparation)

Time (min)[a]	Microsomes omitted			Microsomes added		
	Survival (%)	Gene conversions ($\times 10^{-5}$)		Survival (%)	Gene conversions ($\times 10^{-5}$)	
		Ade	*Trp*		*Ade*	*Trp*
0	100	1.5 ± 1.0	1.7 ± 0.1	100	1.6 ± 0.1	1.4 ± 0.1
30	91	1.5 ± 0.0	1.9 ± 0.1	103	1.3 ± 0.0	1.4 ± 0.0
60	96	1.5 ± 0.1	1.4 ± 0.1	100	1.4 ± 0.1	1.3 ± 0.0
120	97	1.6 ± 0.1	1.6 ± 0.2	95	1.4 ± 0.1	1.2 ± 0.0

[a] $CHClF_2$ = 500 ml/min (1:1 air) a 20 mM concentration has been used during treatments

Table 7. In vivo forward mutations induced by chlorodifluoromethane (FC-22) on yeast *S. pombe* (P_1 strain); host-mediated assay: intrasanguineous test CD-1 mice 5 h of incubation

Treatment	Mice		Mutation Frequency ($\times 10^{-4}$)
Control	1	0/8565	
	2	1/11913	
(oil)	3	1/12916	0.51 ± 0.19
	4	1/21766	
FC-22	1	1/9859	
816 mg/kg	2	0/3960	
(oil)	3	1/10720	0.70 ± 0.23
	4	1/11574	
Positive		Control	
Control	1	4/20613	
	2	4/18300	
(water)	3	1/13053	2.14 ± 1.19
	4	3/8173	
DMNA	1	47/19428	
2.5 mg/kg	2	37/10368	33.45 ± 4.83
(water)	3	49/12100	

Table 8. In vivo gene conversions induced by chlorodifluoromethane (FC-22) on yeast *S. cerevisiae* (D_4 strain); host-mediated assay: intrasanguineous test CD-1 mice 15 h of incubation

Treatment		Gene conversions ($\times 10^{-5}$)	
		Ade	*Trp*
Control	1	12.74 ± 1.36	2.44 ± 1.52
(oil)	2	3.23 ± 0.45	2.16 ± 0.30
	3	4.52 ± 0.72	4.62 ± 0.48
Pooled data		6.83 ± 2.97	3.07 ± 0.80
Treated	1	6.57 ± 0.44	1.89 ± 0.40
816 mg/kg	2	5.32 ± 0.70	1.83 ± 0.87
(oil)	3	6.08 ± 1.18	2.30 ± 0.24
Pooled data		5.99 ± 0.36	2.00 ± 0.15

Positive control; styrene oxide; 1,4-dichlorobutene-2; methylmethanesulfonate; ethylmethanesulfonate

Table 9. In vitro forward mutations induced by chlorodifluoromethane (FC-22) on Chinese hamster cell line V79 grown in vitro

Treatment time[a]	Survival		Cell population evaluated $\times 10^6$	Mutations	
	0 h	114 h[b]		n	$\times 10^{-6}$
Control	100.0	100.0	1.26	45	35.75
30 min	32.5	81.30	1.02	50	49.02
60 min	6.7	100.0	1.27	49	38.58

[a] Cells treated in monolayer with $CHClF_2$ at a flux intensity = 500 ml/min (1:1 air)

[b] Expression time

Table 10. Unscheduled DNA synthesis
induced by chlorodifluoromethane (FC-22)
on human heteroploid cell line grown
in vitro (EUE line)

Treatment (1 h)	S-10	^{3}H-TdR HU-resistant % incorporation
Untreated	−	5.06
FC-22	−	3.33
Untreated	+	5.14
FC-22	+	3.90

Cells treated in buffer with $CHClF_2$ at
a flux intensity of 500 ml/min (1:1
air); a 20 mM solution was obtained
during treatment

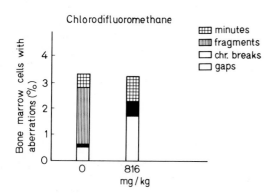

Fig. 23. Induction of chromosome aberrations in bone marrow cells of CD-1 mice treated
by gavage with an oil solution
of chlorodifluoromethane

S. typhimurium strain 1535 was demonstrated. There is clearly a
need for further investigations to come to a conclusion as to
the possible genetic activity of this compound.

Atrazine is a herbicide largely used in Italy for the protection
of crops. In Fig. 24 a summary of data obtained in different
test systems is reported. All the positive results (induction of
6-thioguanine resistance in Chinese hamster cells, forward mutation in the yeast, unscheduled DNA synthesis in human cells)
obtained with in vitro systems employed plant microsomes as a
metabolizing system. Atrazine was not mutagenic per se, nor was

it activated by mouse microsomes. The compound was also active
in the intrasanguineous host-mediated assay using yeast cells
and mice. The study of atrazine is at an early stage and further
work is required to define the precise metabolic requirements
to convert this compound to mutagenic intermediates.

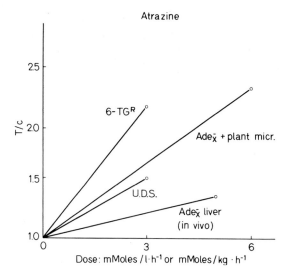

Fig. 24. Summary of genetic effects observed in different test systems after treatment with atrazine. Symbols as in Fig. 15

Comparative results obtained with known mutagens are shown in Figs. 25-27.

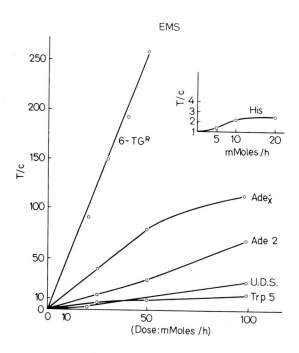

Fig. 25. Summary of genetic effects observed in different test systems after treatment with ethyl-methanesulfonate. Symbols as in Fig. 15

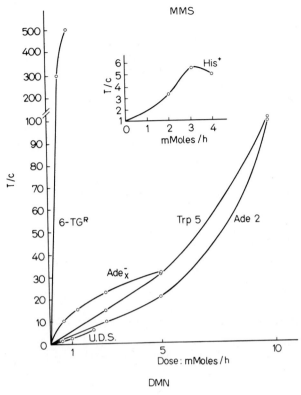

MMS

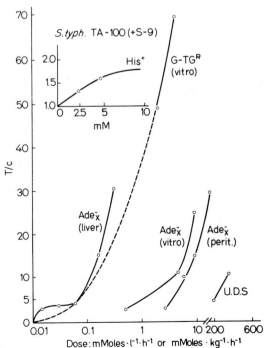

DMN

Fig. 26. Summary of genetic effects observed in different test systems after treatment with methylmethanesulfonate. Symbols as in Fig. 15

Fig. 27. Summary of genetic effects observed in different test systems after treatment with dimethylnitrosoamine (mouse liver microsomes were present in the in vitro tests). Symbols as in Fig. 15

Table 11. Comparative response of six different test systems to reference mutagens and environmental compounds

Chemicals	Bacteria S. typhimurium gene mutation in vitro	Yeast S. pombe gene mutation in vitro in vivo	Mamm. cells CH-V79 gene mutation in vitro	Mammal Mouse cytogenetic effects in vivo	Yeast S. cerevisiae gene convers. in vitro in vivo	Human cel. E.U.E. U.D.S. in vitro
EMS	M	M	M		M	M
MMS	M	M	M		M	M
DMN	M	M	M		M[3]	(M)
Mitomycin	M		M	M		(M)
Hycanthone	M	M	M	M	M	M
Atrazine	inactive[1]	M[2] inactive[1]	M[2] inactive[1]	M	inactive[1]	M[2] inactive[1]
Styrene	inactive	inactive	inactive	inactive	inactive	inactive
Styrene oxide	M	M	M	M	M	M
Trichloroethylene	(?)[3]	inactive	inactive	inactive	inactive	inactive
Epoxy,1,1,2-trich-loroethane		M	M		M	inactive
Chlorodifluoro--methane	(?)[3]	inactive	inactive	inactive	inactive	inactive
Praziquantel-embay 8440	inactive[3]	inactive	inactive	inactive	inactive	inactive

[1] + liver S-9
[2] + plant S-9
[3] data from the literature

Table 11 summarizes the results obtained with a number of chemical compounds, including some which were the object of this communication.

The results from the few examples that are presented in this paper show that there are compounds for which a knowledge of biological effects such as mutagenicity or carcinogenicity would be essential, given the large exposure of the human population to them, but which still oppose a strong resistance to be easily classified as mutagens or nonmutagens, despite large experimental efforts. Clearly we are facing here the limits which are inherent in most experimental assays. For such compounds, other relevant biological information, such as knowledge of human metabolism and of the interindividual variations in critical metabolic steps, might be essential. Direct studies on exposed people, such as the detection of chromosomal aberrations in lymphocytes, may play an important role in so far as they may indicate the presence, in humans, of the metabolites which have been identified as genetically active in experimental systems.

This may help to overcome the problem of the existence of contrasting results obtained with different biological systems: epidemiological data are not particularly difficult in these cases, since human exposure has occurred for many years during the production of these types of chemicals.

References

1. Loprieno N, Barale R, Baroncelli S, Bartsch H, Bronzetti G, Cammellini A, Corsi C, Frezza D, Nieri R, Leporini C, Rosellini D, Rossi AM (1977) Induction of gene mutations and gene conversions by vinyl chloride metabolites in yeasts. Cancer Res 36:253-257
2. Leibman KC (1975) Metabolism and toxicity of styrene. Environ Health Perspect 11:115-119
3. Duren BL van (1977) Chemical structure, reactivity, and carcinogenicity of halohydrocarbons. Environ Health Perspect 21:17-23
4. NCI Carcinogenesis Technical Report Series No 2 (1976). Carcinogenesis bioassay of trichloroethylene CAS No 79-01-6. US Dept of Health Education and Welfare, DHEW Publ No 76-802, pp 197
5. Greim H, Bonse G, Radwan Z, Reichert D, Henschler D (1975) Mutagenicity in vitro and potential carcinogenicity of chlorinated ethylenes as a function of metabolic oxirane formation. Biochem Pharmacol 24:2013-2017
6. Simmons VF, Kauhanen K, Tardiff RG (1977) Mutagenic activity of chemicals identified in drinking water. In: Scott D, Bridges BA, Sobels FH (eds) Progress in genetic toxicology. Elsevier, Amsterdam, p 249-258
7. Fahrig R (1977) The mammalian spot test (Fellfleckentest) with mice. Arch Toxicol (Berl) 38:87-98
8. Shahin MM, Borstel RC von (1977) Mutagenic and lethal effects of α-benzene hexachloride, dibutyl phtalate and trichloroethylene in Saccharomyces cerevisiae. Mutat Res 18:173-180
9. Bronzetti G, Zeiger E, Frezza D (1978) Genetic activity of trichloroethylene in yeast. J Environ Pathol Toxicol 1:411-418
10. Henschler R, Eder E, Neudecker T, Metzer M (1977) Carcinogenicity of trichloroethylene: facts or artifacts? Arch Toxicol (Berl) 37:233-236

356

11. Longstaff E, McGregor DB (1978) Mutagenicity of α-halocarbon refrigerant monochlorodifluoromethane (R-22) in Salmonella typhimurium. Toxicology 2:1–4
12. Loprieno N, Barale R, Baroncelli S, Bronzetti G, Cammellini A, Corsi G, Leporini C, Nieri R, Rossi AM (1976) Screening tests in chemical carcinogenesis. IARC Sci Publ 12:505–516
13. Loprieno N (1977) Colloques internationaux du CNRS no 256. Cancerogen Chim 256:315–331
14. Loprieno N, Barale R, Baroncelli S et al. (1976) Evaluation of the genetic effect induced by vinyl chloride monomer (VCM) under mammalian metabolic activation: studies in vitro and in vivo. Mutat Res 40:85–96
15. Loprieno N, Abbondandolo A, Barale R et al. (1976) Mutagenicity of industrial compounds: styrene and its possible metabolite styrene oxide. Mutat Res 40:317–324
16. Bonatti S, Abbondandolo A, Corti G, Ficrio R, Mazzaccaro A (1978) The expression curve of mutants induced by styrene oxide at the HGPRT locus in V79 cells. Mutat Res 52:295–300

Test Systems for Detection
of Mutagenic Activity of Environmental Pollutants

N. P. Dubinin and L. M. Kalinina[1]

A negative result of scientific and technological progress is the increasing pollution of the environment by physical, chemical, and biological factors. Of particular hazard are factors possessing mutagenic properties, since they can cause hereditary diseases in people and either significant changes in the structure of natural populations or even the extinction of certain species.

The last years have seen the rapid increase of environmental pollution by industrial products and wastes containing significant amounts of heavy metals. These include cadmium, zinc, and chromium. Cadmium and zinc are known to be involved in main metabolic processes because their ions are a part of vitally important enzymes (1). During chronic exposure, these metals can accumulate in the organs of man and cause toxic reactions (2,3). It has been experimentally shown that carcinogenesis in the hamster depends on the amount of zinc in the organism although the mechanism of this process is unknown (4). Chromium and its compounds also possess toxic, allergic, and carcinogenic properties (5).

A series of test systems to determine the genetic effects of environmental pollutants have been described by various laboratories all over the world. Many of these are well studied (6-10). It should be noted, however, that none of the known test systems permits one to make a final conclusion about the genetic risk of this or that substance to man.

Different testing schemes are suggested for use in progressive stages. Preliminary screening should be regarded as one of the stages. We suggest three tests to be used as methods of preliminary screening: a gene mutation test in the system with metabolic activation in vitro and in vivo using microbial indicator strains, a chromosome aberration test in the culture of human leukocytes and in mammalian bone marrow cells, and the dominant lethal test in mice.

We shall present experimental data obtained at the Institute of General Genetics of the USSR Academy of Sciences, Moscow, and at the Medical Institute of the Kazakh SSR, Aktyubinsk, regarding the mutagenic effect of cadmium, zinc, and chromium compounds observed by using the earlier mentioned test systems.

---

[1]Institute of General Genetics, USSR Academy of Sciences, Profsoyuznaya 7(I) Moscow 117312/USSR

The ability of heavy metal salts to induce gene mutations was determined in the system in vitro without metabolic activation, in vitro with metabolic activation , and in vivo with the use of a host-mediated assay and indicator *Salmonella* strains (11, 12). The results obtained in this series of experiments are shown in Table 1. Thus, in the system in vitro without metabolic activation, heavy metal salts displayed a low mutagenic effect. The frequency of cadmium-induced back mutations on strain TA 1535 was higher than on strain TA 1537 and, depending on the dose, it was 2.5-5 times as high as the frequency of spontaneous mutations. The mutagenic effect of zinc chloride was more pronounced on strain TA 1537. It was 1.2-6.4 times higher than the spontaneous level of reversions. An analogous effect on this strain was also displayed by sodium dichromate (1.8-6 times).

In the system in vitro with metabolic activation, zinc chloride and sodium dichromate displayed a significant mutagenic effect. The frequency of induced reversion increased with the dose and exceeded the control level 7- to 40-fold and 2- to 22-fold for zinc chloride and sodium dichromate, respectively. The activity of cadmium chloride in this system was analogous to that in vitro without metabolic activation. This result may probably be explained by the known fact that cadmium can inhibit the activity of many enzymes containing sulfhydryl groups (13) as well as of certain liver enzymes (14). In studying the genetic effect of zinc chloride in the system in vitro with metabolic activation, a comparative analysis of the effect of liver homogenates of different mammals (mouse, two rat species, and man) on the induction of back mutations in *Salmonella* was carried out. It was found that the highest mutagenic effect was observed when using mouse liver homogenates (15).

The mutagenic activity of heavy metal salts in the host-mediated assay was determined using strains TA 1950 and TA 1534. All the compounds under study displayed a considerable mutagenic effect. Thus, as compared with the control, cadmium chloride increased the frequency of mutations on TA 1950 strain 17- to 40-fold depending on the dose, zinc chloride on TA 1534 14- to 22-fold, and sodium dichromate 4- to 12-fold.

The results obtained suggest that the heavy metal salts under study can induce gene mutations in *Salmonella* in systems with metabolic activation. The genetic construction of Ames' strains makes it possible to conclude that cadmium chloride induces base-pair substitutions, and zinc chloride and sodium dichromate induce frameshift mutations.

Experiments on the induction of dominant lethals by zinc chloride and cadmium chloride in mice showed an absence of an effect at the genetic level. However, a toxic effect of cadmium chloride on mouse testes resulting in decrease of the weight of the organ and complete sterility of males was established. The chromosome aberration test in bone marrow cells did not reveal a mutagenic effect of cadmium and zinc salts (16,17).

Table 1. Mutagenic effect of heavy metal salts on *Salmonella*

Metal compounds	in vitro without metabolic activation		in vitro with metabolic activation		in vivo host-mediated assay	
	TA 1535	TA 1537	TA 1535	TA 1537	TA 1950	TA 1534
$CdCl_2$	2.5 – 5[a]	1.2 – 1.6	2.1 – 6.2	1.2 – 2	17 – 40	2.4 – 5.3
$ZnCl_2$	1.4 – 2.5	1.2 – 6.4	2.6 – 3.8	7 – 40	2 – 4.5	14 – 22
$Na_2Cr_2O_7$	1.2 – 3	1.8 – 6	1.6 – 4.3	2 – 22	3.6	4 – 12

[a]Excess of the frequency of induced back mutations over the spontaneous background

Table 2. Frequency of chromosome aberrations in bone marrow of rats exposed to potassium dichromate

Experimental conditions	Time of fixation	Number of analysed metaphases Total	Cells with aberrations Total	%
Control	–	566	11	1.97
Chronic intoxication	1 year	969	125	12.89
Acute intoxication	2 hours	334	18	5.37
	4 hours	311	20	6.43
	6 hours	353	26	6.81
	12 hours	305	22	7.21

Experiments with potassium dichromate were carried out on white mongrel rats which were exposed for an year to chronic intoxication at a dose of 15 mg/kg. In acute intoxication studies the animals were killed 2, 4, 6, 8, and 12 h after treatment. As seen from Table 2, the percentage of cells with chromosome aberrations in the control (nontreated) animals was 1.97. In chronic intoxication, the number of cells with different chromosome aberrations markedly increased (12.89%) as compared with the control. With acute intoxication, the frequency of cells with chromosome aberrations significantly increased as compared with the control. As the term of fixation was prolonged, the frequency of structural chromosome aberrations increased and in 12 h reached the maximum (7.21%). Chromatid aberrations were observed during both chronic and acute intoxication.

Of particular interest is the investigation of the effect of chromium compounds on the human organism under industrial conditions. Studies were conducted on the peripheral blood leukocyte culture of persons who were exposed to chromium compounds (19). Blood samples were drawn from persons of both sexes aged from 20 to 40 years. The following groups were composed according to the working period: I, up to 3 years; II, 3-5 years; III, 5-8 years; IV, 8 years and more. Blood of clinically normal donors served as the control. The metaphase analysis of chromosomes was performed following the recommendations suggested by the Institute of General Genetics of the USSR Academy of Sciences (20). The data presented in Table 3 indicate that the frequency of cells with chromosome aberrations in the groups studied is higher than in the control. The mutagenic effect exhibits a tendency to increase in direct relationship to the duration of exposure and reaches a maximum in group IV (7.9%). Analysis of chromosome aberrations has shown that the actions of chromium compounds give rise mainly to chromatid aberrations in human blood cells. Thus, the data presented suggest that chromium compounds are potential mutagens that can induce both gene mutations and chromosome aberrations.

It should be noted that such complex studies will permit to solve the problems connected with estimating the risk of environmental pollution to the health of man.

Table 3. Frequency of chromosome aberrations in human leucocytes as a function of exposure duration

Experimental groups	Group size	% Aberrant cells		$M \pm m$	P
		Total of analysed metaphases	Metaphases with aberrations		
I-up to 3 years	34	1806	117	6.42 ± 0.85	0.01
II-3 to 5 years	23	1498	55	3.00 ± 0.49	0.01
III-5 to 8 years	34	1722	97	5.63 ± 0.57	0.01
IV-8 years and more	35	2216	177	7.98 ± 0.48	0.01
Control	7	383	7	1.82 ± 0.68	

References

1. Williams SD (1975) Metals of life. "Mir", Moscow
2. Foulkes E (1974) In: Center for the study of the human environment. Annual report, p 56
3. McDonald Foulkes E (1974) In: Center for the study of the human environment. Annual report, p 52
4. Wys W de, Porties WJ, Richter MC, Strain W (1970) Proc Soc Exp Biol Med 135:17-22
5. Raffetto G, Parodi S, Parodi C, Ferrari M de, Troiano R, Brambilla G (1977) Tumori 63 6:503-512
6. McCann J, Choi E, Yamasaki E, Ames BN (1975) Proc Natl Acad Sci USA 72:5135-5139
7. Mohn GR (1977) Arch Toxicol (Berl) 38(1-2): 109-133
8. Sobels FH, Vogel E (1976) Mutat Res 41:95-106
9. Bateman A, Epstein S (1971) In: Hollaender A (ed) Chemical mutagens: principles and methods for their detection, Vol I. Plenum Press, New York, p 54
10. Dubinina LG (1977) Leucocytes of human blood - test system for detection of environmental mutagens. "Nauka", Moscow
11. Kalinina LM, Polukhina GN, Lukasheva LI (1977) Genetika 13:1089-1092
12. Polukhina GN, Kalinina LM, Lukasheva LI (1977) Genetika 13:1492-1494
13. Granata A, Barbaro M, Maturo L (1970) Arch Mal Prof 31:357-363
14. Schroeder LA, Whanger PD, Weswing PH (1973) Fed Proc 32:3967
15. Polukhina GN, Kalinina LM, Lukashova LI (1977) Abstracts of III sezda VOGIS, p 164
16. Ramaiia LK, Pomerantseva MD (1977) Genetika 13:59-63
17. Pomerantseva MD, Ramaiia LK, Vilkina GA (1976) Genetika 12(7):56-63
18. Bigaliev AB, Turebaev MN, Elemesova MS (1977) In: Genetic consequences of environmental pollution. "Nauka", Moscow p 173
19. Bigaliev AB, Turebaev MN, Elemesova MS, Bigalieva RK (1977) In: Genetic consequences of environmental pollution. "Mysl", Moscow, p 74
20. Dubinina LG, Bigaliev AB (1978) Test system for detection of mutagenic activity of environmental pollution in human leucocytes, Moscow

Bacterial Mutagenicity Testing
of Polycyclic Aromatic Hydrocarbons

K. Norpoth, G. Djelani, and V. Gieselmann[1]

Widespread literature data (1) as well as specially devised investigations (2) underline the variability of mutagenic effects
seen with polycyclic aromatic hydrocarbons in the *Salmonella*/
oxygenase test. Surprising interlaboratory differences in test
results (1) may be due to a particular influence of some of the
at least 14 major variables of the procedure, recently summarized
by Ashby and Styles (3), on the in vitro activation of PAH compounds. Among the important factors, the balance between activating and detoxifying enzymes present in the S-9 preparation
requires special attention. Evidence has been presented that
only one of the numerous pathways described for benzo(a)pyrene,
B(a)P, leads to most mutagenic and carcinogenic dihydrodiol-
epoxides (4-11) and that their production requires the cooper-
ative activities of monoxygenases and epoxide hydratase (Fig. 1),
the latter enzyme being intensely studied (12-24). In this context it may be pointed out that the initial step of the mentioned activation pathway depends on various forms of oxygenases
which show different catalytic activities and prefer different
positions of the molecule for O_2-dependent transformation (25-
28). Thus not only the activity of the involved epoxide hydrase
but also the activities and relative distributions of at least
13 or more monoxygenases determine mainly the extent of the
carcinogenic action of PAH compounds toward tissues from animals
of different species, age, sex, and nutritional state and explain the striking effects of so-called inducers (2,16,29).

Concerning the *Salmonella*/oxygenase test procedure it may be
helpful to distinguish between these aspects of metabolic activation and factors of the test protocol which can interfere
with in vitro activation of mutagens and mutagenic action. To
investigate influences on the in vitro activation of benzo(a)-
pyrene other than the balanced activities of activating and
detoxifying enzymes, we worked only with liver S-9 preparations
(of Aroclor-1254-treated male mice), which showed in the range
of benzo(a)pyrene levels 0.1-2.0 µg/plate little or no effect
of epoxide hydrase inhibitors, such as cyclohexene oxide and
trichloropropene oxide.[2]

---

[1]Institut für Staublungenforschung und Arbeitsmedizin der Universität Münster,
D-4400 Münster/FRG

[2]Methods of Ames et al. (Ames BN, McCann J, Yamasaki E (1975). Methods for
detecting carcinogens and mutagens with the *Salmonella*/mammalian microsome
mutagenicity test. Mutat Res 31:347-364) with modifications as described in
the text

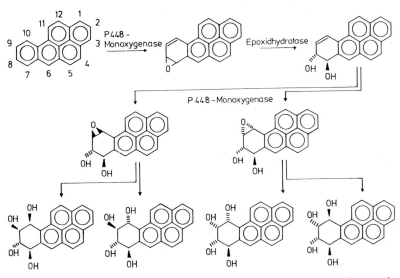

Fig. 1. Formation and degradation of the ultimate carcinogenic B(a)P metabolite (+)-B(a)P-7,8-diolepoxide (*middle row, right*) and (-)-B(a)P-7,8-diolepoxide (*middle row, left*)

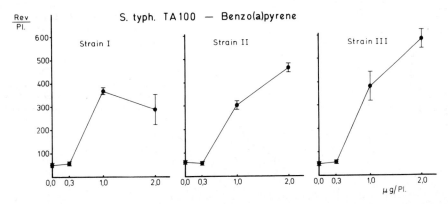

Fig. 2. Mean revertant numbers found in five-plate experiments with B(a)P using liver S-9 preparations of three mouse strains (obtained after Aroclor pretreatment) for Ames test experiments. Tester strain, *S. typhimurium* TA 100; *strain I*, male white NMRI mice; *strain II*, male B6C3F1 mice; *strain III*, male C57 black mice

Figure 2 shows dose-response functions found with *Salmonella typhimurium* TA 100 as the tester strain and S-9 preparations of three different mouse strains. The S-9 fraction of B6C3F$_1$ mice (III) (protein content: 0.9 mg/plate in each experiment) caused markedly higher revertant numbers at the level of 2.0 µg B(a)P/plate than S-9 fractions of C57 black mice (II) and white NMRI mice (I). At levels of 0.3 and 1.0 µg/plate, however, no clear differences were observed.

We tested with these three strains influences of the solvent used, the O_2 pressure, and the composition of the culture medium. In accordance with findings of Wolff (30), we observed less inhibitory solvent effects with methanol and acetone than with DMSO. An example is given in Fig. 3, which demonstrates different B(a)P dose-response functions observed with *S. typhimurium* TA 98 under the influence of B(a)P in presence of liver S-9 from NMRI mice. Anaerobic incubation as well as that under increased O_2 pressure led to a marked decrease of B(a)P-induced back mutations. As shown by Fig. 3, replacement of the air in an incubation chamber by Carbogen, a mixture of O_2 and CO_2 (85:15 v/v), lowered the revertant numbers significantly.

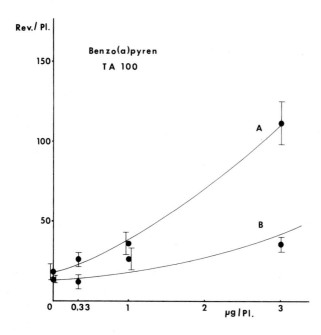

Fig. 3. Mean revertant frequencies found with *S. typhimurium* TA 100 under the influence of B(a)P using the Ames test procedure. Five plates were incubated for each experiment either (A) in normal atmosphere or (B) in an atmosphere of O_2 and CO_2 (85:15 v/v). Liver S-9 preparation of Aroclor-treated male NMRI mice were used for metabolic activation

No improvement could be achieved by changing the O_2 pressure during the incubation time. Therefore, optimal atmospheric test conditions remain unknown, but there were some clear influences of the chosen culture medium. The use of minimal Davis agar instead of agar containing the Vogel-Bonner medium components led to lower revertant number induction not only by B(a)P but also by aflatoxin B_1 and other mutagens. The most suitable agar was the Difco-Bacto-agar. The Difco purified agar showed clear superiority in comparison experiments with purified agars of Oxoid and Merck AG (Fig. 4). When these highly purified agars were employed, dose-response functions were lowered or abolished. We assume from the results that components of the Difco-Bacto-agar are perhaps important cofactors of enzymatic B(a)P activation.

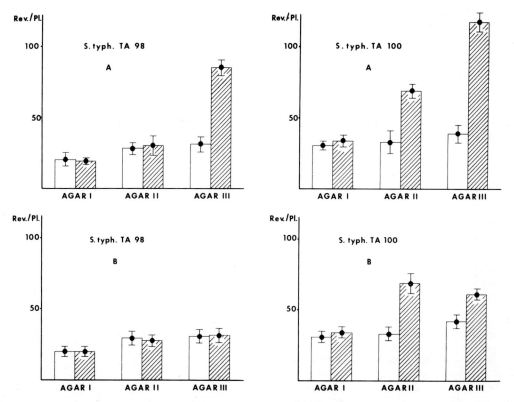

Fig. 4. Mean revertant frequencies found in Ames test experiments with *S. typhimurium* TA 98 and TA 100 as tester strains and 1 µg B(a)P/plate as mutagen. Three plates were incubated in each experiment containing Agar I (Agar Agar "hochrein für die Mikrobiologie" from Merck AG, D-6100 Darmstadt, FRG), Agar II (Difco purified agar), and Agar III (Difco-Bacto-agar), respectively. The amounts of S-9 mix used were $A = 0.05$ ml and $B = 0.1$ ml (mouse liver S-9 mix from male NMRI mice obtained after Aroclor pretreatment)

The experience gained from testing B(a)P was then applied to other PAH compounds. The well-known carcinogens benzo(b)fluor - anthene and benzo(j)fluoranthene (31) as well as benzo(k)- fluoranthene —which is classified as a noncarcinogenic compound (31) —gave positive results with marked dose-response relation- ships (Fig. 5). Single plate experiments with these compounds showed that dose-effect functions can be achieved with limited plate numbers (Fig. 6).

Several groups have investigated filter extracts from urban air samples in order to elucidate whether the mutagenic activity found in the *Salmonella*/oxygenase test reflects carcinogenic activity of the supposed or analyzed PAH contents. Investigations of our group carried out with D. Hoffmann showed clear dose-de- pendent mutagenicity of filter extracts following the passage of about 350 m^3 of air of an industrial urban area. The air com- ponents were collected during a 12-h period each. Filter ex- tracts obtained by Soxhlet extraction with diethyl ether were

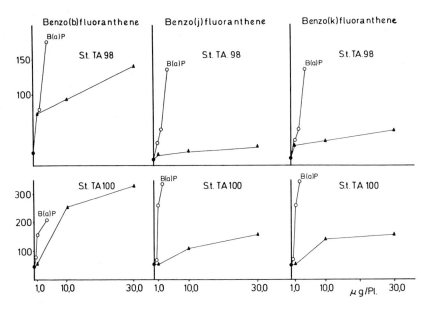

Fig. 5. Mean revertant frequencies found in Ames test experiments with three fluoranthenes using *S. typhimurium* TA 98 and TA 100 tester strains. B(a)P was used as reference mutagen. Five plates were used in each experiment. Metabolic activation: see Fig. 3

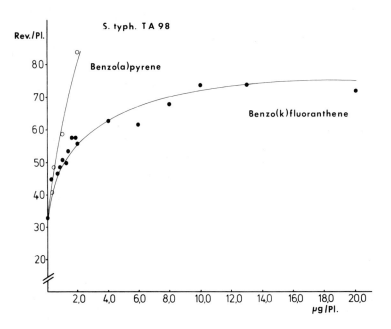

Fig. 6. Revertant frequencies found with *S. typhimurium* TA 98 on single plates containing different amounts of benzo(k)fluoranthene. Activating system: see Fig. 3

then fractionated by procedures to be published in the IARC manual of methods for PAH analyses and kindly communicated to us by G. Grimmer. Thus we could show high mutagenic activity in the acetone water phase which contains the polar components. About half of this activity was caused by directly acting mutagens. No evidence was found for the presence of mutagenic aliphatic or olefinic hydrocarbons since all the activity of the respective cyclohexane phase passed to the nitromethane phase. After Sephadex fractionation of this phase using propanol as solvent, it could be demonstrated that nearly the whole activity of the nitromethane phase was due to 3-6 ring polycyclic hydrocarbons. In agreement with Pitts et al. (32), Tokiwa et al. (33), Talcott and Wei (34), and Dehnen et al. (35), we conclude from these results that mutagenic activities in real urban air as measured by the *Salmonella/* oxygenase test are not only related to the PAH content but also to other air components. These are in part water soluble polar compounds and show reasonable activity even in the absence of metabolic activation. It may be emphasized that no correlation was found between mutagenic activities and the B(a)P contents of the filter extracts, which amounted to values between 2.7 and 27.1 µg/1000 m^3 of air. I wouldn't like to go into a more detailed discussion of the findings mentioned because it seems to me premature to decide whether the new approach of the *Salmonella/*oxygenase test to the problem of carcinogenic compounds in urban air will lead to a total revision of the established view that polycyclic hydrocarbons play a unique role in this context.

Hitherto, 61 homocyclic PAH have been investigated by means of the *Salmonella/* oxygenase test, as reported in the literature (see 1) and here. Of these compounds, 41 are described as carcinogens in animal experiments and 14 have been reported to show no carcinogenic activity. Of the first group, three compounds, and of the second, five gave inverse results in the *Salmonella/*oxygenase test. That means that the number of so-called "false negatives" — whatever it means — is fairly low: about 7%. On the other hand, the number of so-called "false positives" is high: more than 1/3 of the investigated noncarcinogens. It seems therefore that homocyclic aromatic hydrocarbons show more often positive results in the *Salmonella/*oxygenase test than in animal experiments. A preliminary survey of the results obtained with heterocyclic hydrocarbons and other classes of chemicals suggest that this observation reflects a general feature of in vitro mutagenicity test systems for detecting carcinogens.

References

1. Djelani G (1979) Beziehungen zwischen cancerogener and mutagener Wirkung polycyclischer aromatischer Kohlenwasserstoffe im Lichte neuerer Literaturmitteilungen. Inaugural Dissertation, Universität Münster
2. Ashby J, Styles JA (1978) Does carcinogenic potency correlate with mutagenic potency in the Ames assay? Nature 271:452-455
3. Ashby J, Styles JA (1978) Factors influencing mutagenic potency in vitro. Nature 274:20-22

4. Kapitulnik J, Wislocki PG, Levin W, Yagi H, Jerina DM, Conney AH (1978) Tumorigenicity studies with diol-epoxides of benzo(a)pyrene which indicate that (+)-trans-7β, 8α-dihydroxy-9α, 10α-epoxy-7,8,9,10-tetrahydrobenzo(a)pyrene is an ultimate carcinogen in newborn mice. Cancer Res 38:354-358

5. King HWS, Osborne MR, Beland FA, Harvey RG, Brookes P (1976) (+)-7, 8β-Dihydroxy-9β, 10β-epoxy-7,8,9,10-tetrahydrobenzo(a)pyrene is an intermediate in the metabolism and binding to DNA of benzo(a)pyrene. Proc Natl Acad Sci USA 73:2679-2681

6. Koreeda M, Moore PD, Yagi H, Yeh HJC, Jerina DM (1976) Alkylation of polyguanylic acid at the 2-amino group and phosphate by the potent mutagen (+)7, 8β-dihydroxy-9β, 10β-epoxy-7,8,9,10-tetrahydrobenzo(a)pyrene. J Am Chem Soc 98:6720-6722

7. Nakanishi K, Kasal H, Cho H, Harvey RG, Jeffery AM, Jenette KW, Weinstein IB (1977) Absolute configuration of a ribonucleic acid adduct formed in vivo by metabolism of benzo(a)pyrene. J Am Chem Soc 99:258-260

8. Sims P, Grover PL, Swaisland AJ, Pal K, Hewer A (1974) Metabolic activation of benzo(a)pyrene proceeds by a diol-epoxide. Nature 252:326-328

9. Weinstein IB, Jeffery AM, Jenette KW, Blobstein RH, Harvey RG, Harris C, Autrup H, Kasi H, Nakanishi H (1976) Benzo(a)pyrene diol-epoxide as intermediates in nucleic acid binding in vitro and in vivo. Science 193:592-595

10. Wislocki PG, Wood AW, Chang RL, Levin W, Yagi H, Hernandez O, Jerina DM, Conney AH (1976) High mutagenicity and toxicity of a diol epoxide derived from benzo(a)pyrene. Biochem Biophys Res Commun 68:1006-1012

11. Yang SK, Roller PP, Gelboin HV (1978) Benzo(a)pyrene metabolism: mechanism in the formation of epoxides, phenols, dihydrodiol, and the 7,8-diol-9,10-epoxides. In: Jones PW, Freudenthal RI (eds) Carcinogenesis, Vol 3. Polynuclear aromatic hydrocarbons. Raven Press, New York, pp 285-301

12. Bentley P, Oesch F, Glatt HR (1977) Dual role of epoxide hydratase in both activation and inactivation of benzo(a)pyrene. Arch Toxicol (Berl) 39:65-75

13. Oesch F (1974) Purification and specificity of a human microsomal epoxide hydratase. Biochem J 139:77-88

14. Oesch F, Thoenen H, Fahrländer H, Suda K (1974) Epoxide hydratase in human liver biopsy specimens: assay and properties. Biochem Pharmacol 74:1307-1317

15. Oesch F, Glatt HR (1976) Prevention of benzo(a)pyrene-induced mutagenicity by homogeneous epoxide hydratase. Int J Cancer 18:448-452

16. Oesch F, Glatt HR (1976) Evaluation of the importance of enzymes involved in the control of mutagenic metabolites. IARC Sci Publ 12:255-274

17. Oesch F, Glatt HR, Schmassmann H (1977) The apparent ubiquity of epoxide hydrase in rat organs. Biochem Pharmacol 26:603-607

18. Oesch F, Raphael D, Schwind H, Glatt HR (1977) Species differences in activating and inactivating enzymes related to the control of mutagenic metabolites. Arch Toxicol (Berl) 39:79-108

19. Oesch F, Schaßmann H, Bentley P (1978) Specifity of human, rat and mouse skin epoxide hydratase towards K-region epoxides of polycyclic hydrocarbons. Biochem Pharmacol 27:17-20

20. Thakker DR, Yagi H, Lu AYH, Levin W, Conney AH, Jerina DM (1976) Metabolism of benzo(a)pyrene: conversion of (+)-trans-7,8-dihydroxy-7,8-dihydrobenzo(a)pyrene to high mutagenic 7,8-diol-9,10-epoxides. Proc Natl Acad Sci USA 73:3381-3385

21. Thakker DR, Yagi H, Akagi H, Koreeda M, Lu AYH, Levin W, Wood AW, Conney AH, Jerina DM (1977) Metabolism of benzo(a)pyrene. VI. Stereoselective metabolism of benzo(a)pyrene and benzo(a)pyrene 7,8-dihydrodiol to diol epoxides. Chem Biol Interact 16:281-300
22. Lu AYH, Jerina DM, Levin W (1977) Liver microsomal epoxide hydrase. J Biol Chem 252:3715-3723
23. Wood AW, Wislocki PG, Chang RL, Levin W, Lu AYH, Hernandez O, Jerina DM, Conney AH (1976) Mutagenicity and cytotoxicity of benzo(a)pyrene benzo-ring epoxides. Cancer Res 36:3358-3366
24. Wood AW, Levin W, Lu AYH, Conney AH, Yagi H, Hernandez O, Jerina DM (1976) Use of highly purified hepatic microsomal monooxygenase system and epoxide hydrase to metabolically activate and deactivate benzo(a)-pyrene and benzo(a)pyrene derivates. In: Serres FJ de, Fouts JR, Bend JR, Philpot RM (eds) In vitro metabolic activation in mutagenesis testing. Elsevier/North-Holland, Biochemical Press, Amsterdam
25. Huang MT, West SB, Lu AH (1976) Separation, purification, and properties of multiple forms of cytochrome P450 from liver microsomes of pheno-barbital treated mice. J Biol Chem 251:4659-4665
26. Ullrich V, Kremers P (1977) Multiple forms of cytochrome P-450 in micro-somal monooxygenase system. Arch Toxicol (Berl) 39:41-50
27. Welton AF, O'Neal FO, Chaney LC, Aust SD (1975) Multiplicity of cyto-chrome P-450 hemoproteins in rat liver microsomes-preparation and specificity of an antibody to hemoprotein induced by phenobarbital. J Biol Chem 250:5631-5639
28. Warner M, LaMarca MV, Neims AH (1978) Chromatographic and electrophoretic heterogeneity of the cytochromes P-450 solubilized from untreated rat liver. Drug Metab Dispos 6:353-362
29. Nebert DW, Felton JS (1976) Importance of genetic factors influencing the metabolism of foreign compounds. Environmental and genetic factors affecting laboratory animals. Fed Proc 35:1133-1141
30. Wolff T (1977) In vitro inhibition of monooxygenase dependent reactions by organic solvents. Industrial and environmental xenobiotics. Proceedings of an International Conference, Prague, Czechoslovakia, 13-15 September 1977. Excerpta Medica, Amsterdam Oxford, pp 196-199
31. Committee on Biological Effects of Atmospheric Pollutants. Division of Medical Sciences, National Research Council (1972) Particulate poly-cyclic organic matter. National Academy of Sciences, Washington DC,. pp 1-361
32. Pitts JN, Grosjean D, Mischke T, Simmon VF, Poole D (1977) Mutagenic activity of airborne particulate organic pollutants. Toxicol Lett 1:65-70
33. Tokiwa K, Morita K, Takeyoshi H, Takahashi K, Ohnishi Y (1977) Detection of mutagenic activity in particulate air pollutants. Mutat Res 48:237-248
34. Talcott R, Wei E (1977) Brief Communication: airborne mutagens bio-assayed in Salmonella typhimurium. J Natl Cancer Inst 58:449-451
35. Dehnen W, Pitz N, Tomingas R (1977) The mutagenicity of airborne par-ticulate pollutants. Cancer Lett 4:5-12

Studies on Combination Effects
of Chemical Carcinogens in Short-Term Tests

B. L. Pool[1]

Man is exposed to not only one chemical in his environment, but to a great number and variety of different compounds simultaneously. Consequently many malignant tumors of man have been attributed to additive effects of various carcinogenic factors from the environment. Animal experiments which have been performed in our laboratories show that in some cases very low doses of carcinogens given either simultaneously or consecutively have additive effects in the production of tumors (1-5) (Table 1). After giving carcinogens of different chemical structure and same organotropy a synergistic effect is present. The mechanisms of action causing these effects are not known. Short-term tests for mutagenicity are now being used more and more for prediction of effects of chemicals and for the elucidation of their mechanism of action. I will therefore present a few examples of

Table 1. Combination experiments for syncarcinogenesis with different carcinogens in rats or mice, modified after Schmähl (5)

Combination	Organotropy		Syncarcinogenesis
	Same	Different	
DENA			
DAB	+		+
NO-morpholine			
DMNA			
DENA	+		+
DAB			
DENA			
DAST		+	Ø
Urethane			
DMBA		+	Ø

---

[1] Institut für Toxikologie und Chemotherapie, Deutsches Krebsforschungszentrum, Im Neuenheimer Feld 280, D-6900 Heidelberg/FRG

how combination effects have been studied in some short-term
assays by various authors and what is postulated as reaction
mechanisms.

The combination of chemicals may result both in enhancement and
inhibition of effects expected for the individual compounds
when they are tested alone. These effects may be due to following interaction mechanisms: direct chemical interaction; interaction with enzymes; interaction with repair systems; interaction with DNA; interaction with other cell components. In Tables
2 and 3, examples are presented of how inhibiting or enhancing
effects were measured by combining two chemicals in mutagenicity
assays.

For most of the combination effects in short-term tests shown,
no data is known for their effects in long-term carcinogenicity,
experiments. That is why we tried to look for combination effects of compound pairs which have already been investigated
in vivo for elucidation of synergistic effects. Our main aim
was to investigate whether synergistic effects known in vivo are
measurable at all using an in vitro bacterial test system and
to experimentally confirm the awaited methodologic limitations.
These preliminary investigations are the first step in an attempt
to find a relevant and rapid way to study combination effects of
chemical carcinogens as a pretest to long-term in vivo investigations. In order to investigate these aspects we chose the
following experimental procedures.

Methods

Five pairs of compounds were tested for mutagenicity using the
"Ames" assay. Each compound was given in five concentrations,
either along or in combination, whereby one concentration of
one compound was combined with all five of the second partner,
thus resulting in a total of 36 different combination possibilities. The assay was essentially performed according to
the method described by Ames et al. (6) using *Salmonella typhimurium* TA 100 as indicator organism; livers from Aroclor-pretreated Sprague-Dawley rats were used as metabolizing system.
Combinations were tested with and without preincubation (30°C,
25 min). Each experiment was repeated at least twice. In the
following figures of the Results section not all combination
possibilities were plotted. Shown is the concentration response
curve of *one* compound in comparison with its concentration
response curve after addition of one or more concentrations of
the other compound and vice versa. The curves cross the median
values of his$^+$ revertants scored from four plates of each concentration. Also shown are the respective ranges to indicate
possible differences. This form of presentation was chosen
because a statistical evaluation did not seem to be possible, due
to variability and other biological limitations: "Statistical
evaluation as to whether or not the joint action of two mutagens
shows a synergistic (more than additive) effect does not seem
to be worthwhile as long as no evidence for a model of the nor-

Table 2. Inhibiting effects of two chemicals in short-term tests

Compounds		Test organism	Detection by genetic marker	References
A	B			
Dimethylnitrosamine	NO-sarcosine	*S. typhimurium*	Reversion His⁻ → His⁺	Couch and Friedman (10)
Norharman	Benzo(a)pyrene	*S. typhimurium*	Reversion His⁻ → His⁺	Nagao et al. (9)
Norharman	Benzo(a)pyrene	*S. typhimurium*	Reversion His⁻ → His⁺	Levitt et al. (11)
L-Ascorbate	N-Methyl-N-nitro-N-Nitrosoguanidine Dimethylnitrosamine	*S. typhimurium*	Reversion His⁻ → His⁺	Guttenplan (12)
Sodium-flouride	Trenimone	*Phryne cincta*	Dominant lethals	Israelewski and Obe (13)
Dimethylnitrosamine	Reducing agents (sodium ascorbate)	Human fibroblasts	DNA-repair synthesis	Lo and Stich (14)
Diethylnitrosamine	Disulfiram	Rat liver	Strand breaks	Hadjiolov et al. (15)

Table 3. Enhancing effects of two chemicals in short-term tests

Compounds A	B	Test organism	Detection by genetic marker	References
Norharman + harman	Benzo(a)pyrene	*S. typhimurium* high amounts of S-9	Reversion His$^-$ → His$^+$	Nagao et al. (8, 9)
12-O-Tetradecanoyl-phorbol-13-acetate	*N*-Methyl-*N*-nitro-*N*-nitrosoguanidine	*S. typhimurium*	Reversion His$^-$ → His$^+$	Soper and Evans (16)
Benzo(a)pyrene	Methylmethan-sulfonate	Syrian hamster cells	Transformation	Di Paolo and Casto (17)
Chlorpromazine Perphenazine	β-Lactamantibiotics Nalidixic acids	*E. coli* Pseudonomas aeruginosa	Growth inhibition	Yamabe (18)
8-Methoxypsoralen	UV-Light	Lymphocytes	Sister-chromatid exchanges	Wolf-Schreiner et al. (19) Mourelatos et al. (20)

mal (non-synergistic: additive) joint action of two mutagens appears in the results.

The occurring toxic effects together with the different patterns of response in the different experiments requires further investigation of the experimental problems with the Ames test before a solid statistical evaluation can be carried out. This also holds for experiments with only one agent." (Quotation: Dr. J. Wahrendorf).

Results

DENA-DAB

DENA and DAB (Fig. 1) have the same organotropy and mainly induce tumors of the liver. They were shown to have additive effects when applied simultaneously. These effects are such that synergism was observed even at low doses which do not yield tumors when given alone; also noticeable was the shorter period of induction (1).

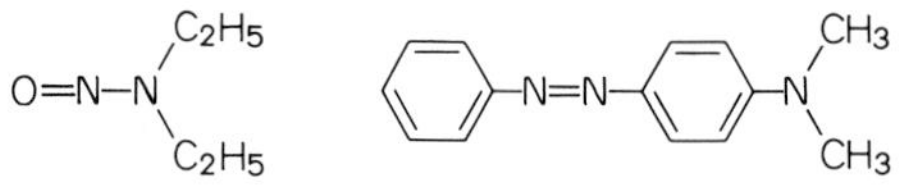

Fig. 1

Figure 2 shows the results obtained in the mutagenicity assay. DENA was dissolved in water, DAB in DMSO. Preincubation was carried out. The graph shows as an example the effect of 25 µg DAB on the mutagenicity of DENA; decrease is present. The effect of DENA is also leveled by addition of 10 or 50 µg of DAB (not shown).

Vice versa, a slight enhancement of DAB mutagenicity is caused by DENA addition — however, this may be not regarded as synergism since the total effect is less than that expected for DENA alone. In other words, DAB decreases the mutagenicity of DENA. This effect is not due to the solvent of DAB, since DMSO was added in the same amount when testing DENA alone.

DENA-BP

BP intratracheally and DENA (Fig. 3) systemically induced squamous cell carcinomas of the tracheobronchial tract in a combination experiment performed by Montesano et al. (7).

Figure 4 shows the results obtained for the combinations of DENA with BP. Plotted again are the mean number of revertants per four plates. DENA was dissolved in water, BP in DMSO. Preincubation was carried out. Both compounds were mutagenic to *S. typhimurium* TA 100 in a dose-response effect. Decrease in number

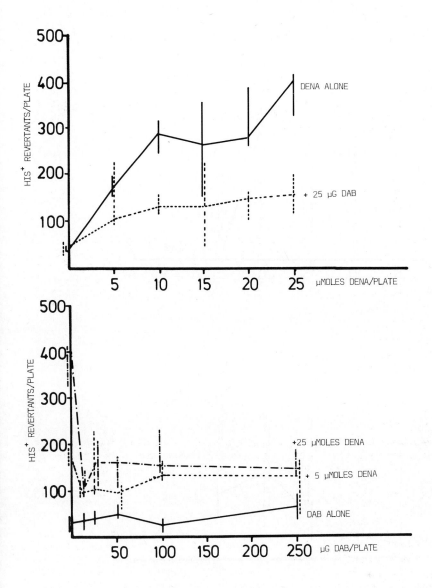

Fig. 2. Combination effects of *DENA* and *DAB* in the *Salmonella*/Ames assay, using strain TA 100, including a preincubation. Shown are the dose response curves through the median value of his[+] revertants scored for four plates and the respective ranges

DENA   BP   Fig. 3

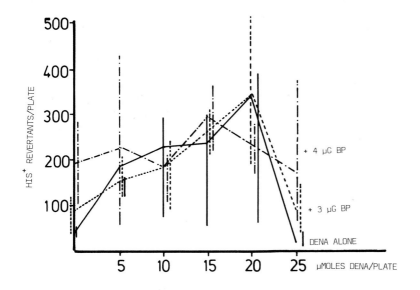

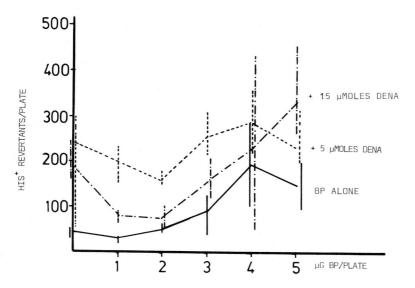

Fig. 4. Combination effects of *DENA* and *BP* in the *Salmonella*/Ames assay, using strain TA 100, including a preincubation. Also see legend of Fig. 2

of revertants is due to toxicity. The first half of the figure shows, as an example, that addition of 3 or 4 µg BP to various concentrations of DENA does not affect the dose-response curve obtained when testing DENA alone. No additive effects are therefore present. Vice versa, when plotting the response of BP and comparing the resulting curve with those including additions of 5 or 15 µmoles DENA, a difference is noticeable. This difference, however, is less than additive, since nonoverlapping

ranges in the separate curves never exceed the values obtained
for DENA alone (*o* value, at the ordinate).

DENA-DAST

DAST (Fig. 5) mainly induces cancer of the auditory canal of
the rat and therefore exerts different organotropic effects
than DENA. No synergism could be detected after giving both
compounds either simultaneously or consecutively to one and the
same animal (3).

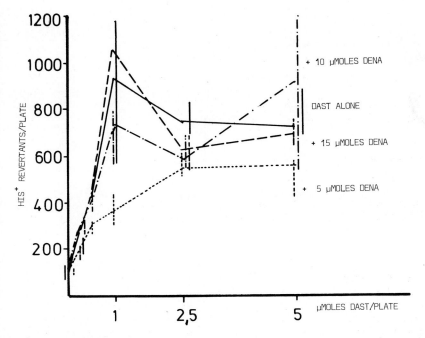

Figure 6 shows results obtained with the combination of DENA
and DAST in the Ames assay. Again solvents were H_2O and DMSO,
respectively. No preincubation was carried out. The addition
of 5, 10, or 15 μmol DENA did not affect the mutagenicity of
DAST, as in almost all cases an overlapping of the ranges is
present. Similarly when carrying out the experiment *with* preincubation (necessary to show mutagenic activity of DENA) no combination effects were visible (results not shown).

Fig. 6. Effect of various *DENA* additions on the mutagenicity of *DAST* in the
Salmonella/Ames assay, using strain TA 100. Also see legend of Fig. 2

Urethane-DMBA

Urethane (Fig. 7) is a systemic carcinogen, which induces cancer
in liver and lung. Dimethylbenzanthracene (Fig. 7) induces
cancer at the site of administration (skin). After simultaneous
application of both compounds to mice, no synergistic effects
were detectable (2). No distinct mutagenicity could be observed
for urethane in TA 100 using Aroclor-induced liver and preincubation. This was to be expected because it is known for its
negative effects in the Ames assay. DMBA, however, was shown to
be the positive previously and only responded here weakly.

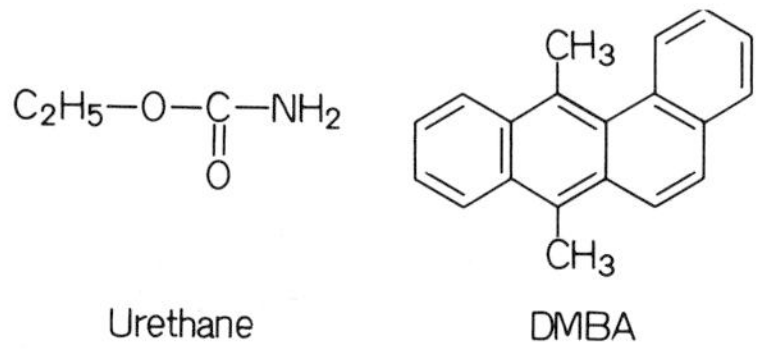

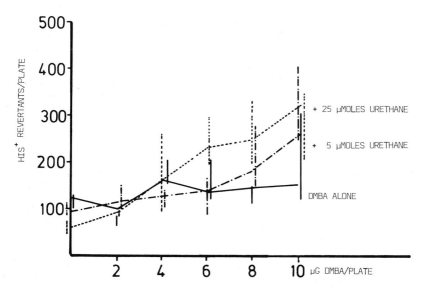

Fig. 7

Figure 8 shows the effect of varying amounts of urethane on the
mutagenicity of DMBA. An enhancement is, however, not present,
therefore no synergistic effect of the two compounds may be
assumed. Also additions of 10 and 15 μmol urethane showed no
effect (results not shown).

Fig. 8. Mutagenicity of *DMBA* alone and in presence of *urethane* in the *Salmonella*/Ames assay, using strain TA 100, including preincubation. Also see
legend of Fig. 2

BP + NO-Morpholine

We also looked for additive effects of these two compounds (Fig. 9) —not knowing their in vivo dispositions when given in combination — since both may be dissolved in DMSO, both need no preincubation and both are distinctly mutagenic to TA 100. Additive effects were therefore expected.

BP   NO-Morpholine   Fig. 9

Figure 10 shows the results obtained for the combination of the two compounds without preincubation. A clear-cut dose-response curve shows the effect of benzo(a)pyrene alone. Additions of a low amounts of nitrosomorpholine (1 µmol) have no effect. The curve is flatter when adding a higher amount of NO-morpholine (10 µmol). This shows enhancement and inhibition also depend on concentration. This is especially evident in the curve for 50 µmol NO-morpholine addition. An enhancement is present for 1 µg BP. Toxicity leads a decrease of response for higher concentrations of BP. The same is true when plotting the data the other way around. Addition of 2 µg and 5 µg BP enhances mutagenicity of NO-morpholine; addition of BP at higher concentrations again results in a nonincreasing response curve.

Discussion

Conclusions which may be drawn from these results are the following. For the two pairs of compounds which showed combination effects in long-term carcinogenicity experiments (DENA-DAB; DENA-BP) no effects were present in the mutation assay. Conversely, both pairs of compounds (DENA-DAST; DMBA-urethane) with no combination effects in carcinogenesis assays also showed no combination effects in the mutation assay.

These negative results do not necessarily support the assumption that no additive effects in the combination of the compounds are actually present. The negative results are probably due to methodologic difficulties: solvent; incubation conditions; dose range; bacterial strain, S-9 concentration. DENA, for example, needs preincubation at room temperature and water as solvent. If this preincubation is omitted, or if different solvents are present, the results obtained with DENA are much lower or even negative. Vice versa, BP or DAB must be dissolved in an organic solvent and respond better without preincubation. Therefore, no optimal conditions may be simulated for both compounds when they are tested together with DENA.

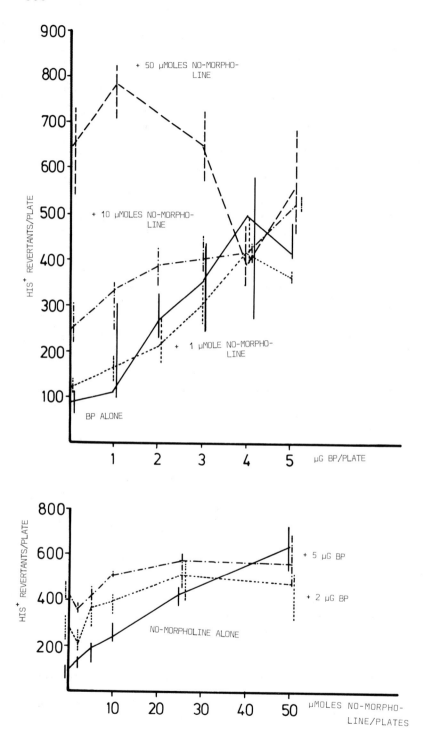

Fig. 10. Combination effects of *BP* and *NO-morpholine* in the *Salmonella*/Ames assay, using strain TA 100. Also see legend of Fig. 2

Also of importance are choice of dose, bacteria, and S-9 concentrations. Additive effects may be observed at lower doses and not at combination of higher ones because of the toxic or inhibiting effect of the compounds on bacteria or S-9 enzymes as was shown for BP and NO-morpholine. Also, in order to even attempt testing combination effects, it is crucial that the chosen indicator organisms are reverted by *both* test compounds, unless compound interaction and influence on enzymes are to be studied. This would explain why urethane, which is not mutagenic to *S. typhimurium* TA 100 had no effect on the mutagenicity of DMBA. However, it also indicates in this system that urethane or its metabolites do not affect the enzymes which activate DMBA. Also crucial is the concentration of S-9, since it is of great importance even when testing one compound alone. Nagao et al. (8,9), for example, demonstrated that harman or norharman can enhance or inhibit the mutagenicity of BP, depending on the amount of S-9 present.

These factors may explain why clear additive effects could only be observed for BP + NO-morpholine in this study. This was the only pair of test compounds which needed nearly the same conditions to exert their mutagenic activity when tested alone. However, even though further additive or even synergistic (more than additive) effects could not be measured, other interactions were seen. This was shown for the example of decreased DENA mutagenesis through DAB. These effects may be due to toxicity or inhibition mechanisms. We are carrying out further experiments for the elucidation of these aspects in order to find out why, for example, inhibition of mutagenesis in vitro may cause enhancement of carcinogenicity in vivo.

We are also presently attempting to investigate combination effects of compounds in the intrasanguine host-mediated assay using *S.typhimurium*, in order to learn more about the mechanisms involved. The *S. typhimurium* indicator organisms promise to be sufficiently sensitive to detect a wider range of known carcinogens/mutagens. The isolation of his[+] revertants from chosen target organs following an analogous application of the carcinogens as in the long-term in vivo experiments are expected to correlate well with tumor occurrence. Many methodological problems we coped with under in vitro conditions will hopefully not be present in this method.

Abbreviations: BP, benzo(a)pyrene; DAB, 4-dimethylaminoazobenzene; DAST, 4-dimethylaminostilbene; DENA, *N*-diethylnitrosamine; DMBA, 9,10-dimethyl-1, 2-benzanthracene; DMSO, dimethyl sulfoxide; NO-morpholine, *N*-nitrosomorpholine

Acknowledgments. I am gratefully indebted to Dr. J. Wahrendorf for advisory help in the statistical evluation of the results. I also thank Ms. S. Serafin and Ms. R. Zimmermann very much for their skilled technical assistance. We thank the Umweltbundesamt for finding this project.

382

References

1. Schmähl D, Thomas C, König K (1963) Experimentelle Untersuchungen zur Syncarcinogenese. 1. Mitteilung: Versuche zur Krebserzeugung an Ratten bei gleichzeitiger Applikation von Diäthylnitrosamin und 4-Dimethylamino-azobenzol. Z Krebsforsch 65:342-350
2. Schmähl D, Thomas C, Brune H (1964) Experimentelle Untersuchungen zur Syncarcinogenese. 2. Mitteilung: Versuche zur Krebserzeugung bei Mäusen bei gleichzeitiger Applikation von Urethan und 9,10-Dimethyl-1,2-benz-anthrazen. Z Krebsforsch 66:297-302
3. Schmähl D, Thomas C (1965) Experimentelle Untersuchungen zur Syncar-cinogenese. 4. Mitteilung: Versuche zur Krebserzeugung an Ratten bei gleichzeitiger oraler Gabe von Diäthylnitrosamin und 4-Dimethylamino-stilben. Z Krebsforsch 67:135-140
4. Schmähl D (1970) Experimentelle Untersuchungen zur Syncarcinogenese. 6. Mitteilung: Addition minimaler Dosen von vier verschiedenen hepato-tropen Carcinogenen bei der Leberkrebserzeugung bei Ratten. Z Krebsforsch 74:457-466
5. Schmähl D (1976) Combination effects in chemical carcinogenesis (experimental results). Oncology 33:73-76
6. Ames BN, McCann J, Yamasaki E (1975) Methods for detecting carcinogens and mutagens with the Salmonella/mammalian-microsome mutagenicity test. Mutat Res 31:347-364
7. Montesano R, Saffioti U, Ferrero A, Kaufman DG (1974) Synergistic effects of benzo(a)pyrene and diethylnitrosamine on respiratory carcinogenesis in hamsters. J Natl Cancer Inst 53:1395-1397
8. Nagao M, Yahagi T, Kawachi T, Sugimura T, Kosuge T, Tsuji K, Wakabayashi K, Mizusaki S (1977) 26. Comutagenic action of norharman and harman. Proceedings of the Japan Academy 53:107-110
9. Nagao M, Yahagi T, Sugimura T (1978) Differences in effects of norharman with various classes of chemical mutagens and amounts of S-9. Biochem Biophys Res Commun 2:373-378
10. Couch DB, Friedman A (1976) Suppression of dimethylnitrosamine muta-genicity by nitroso-sarcosine and other nitrosamines. Mutat Res 38:89-96
11. Levitt RC, Legraverend C, Nebert DW, Pelkonen O (1977) Effects of harman and norharman on the mutagenicity and bindining to DNA of benzo(a)pyrene metabolites in vitro and on aryl hydrocarbon hydroxylase induction in cell culture. Biochem Biophys Res Commun 4:1167-1175
12. Guttenplan JB (1977) Inhibition by L-ascorbate of bacterial mutagenesis induced by two N-nitroso compounds. Nature 268:368-370
13. Israelewski N, Obe G (1977) Suppressive activity by fluoride on the in-duction of dominant lethals with trenimon in spermatozoa of Phryne cincta (Nematocera, diptera). Mutat Res 44:287-290
14. Lo LW, Stich HF (1978) The use of short-term tests to measure the pre-ventive action of reducing agents on formation and activation of car-cinogenic nitroso compounds. Mutat Res 57:57-67
15. Hadjiolov D, Frank N, Schmähl D (1977) Inhibition of diethylnitrosamine-induced strand breaks in liver DNA by disulfiram. Z Krebsforsch 90:107-109
16. Soper CJ, Evans FJ (1977) Investigations into the mode of action of the carcinogen 12-O-tetradecanoyl-phorbol-13-acetate using auxotropic bac-teria. Cancer Res 37:2487-2491
17. DiPaolo JA, Casto BC (1978) In vitro transformation of mammalian cells. In: Slaga TJ, Sivak A, Poutwell R (eds) Sequential treatment with diverse agents. Carcinogenesis, Vol 2. Mechanisms of tumor promotion and car-cinogenesis. Raven Press, New York

18. Yamabe S (1978) Synergistic effects of chlorpromazine and perphenazine on several chemotherapeutic agents. I. General profile of the effects measured by the filter paper strip-agar diffusion method with Escherichia coli and Pseudonomas aeruginosa. Chemotherapy 24:81-86
19. Wolff-Schreiner EC, Carter DM, Schwarzacher HG, Wolff K (1977) Sister chromatid exchanges in photochemotherapy. J Invest Dermatol 69:387-391
20. Mourelatos D, Faed MJW, Gould PW, Johnson BE, Frain-Bell W (1977) Sister chromatid exchanges in lymphocytes of psoriatics after treatment with 8-methoxypsoralen. Br J Dermatol 97:649-654

Mutagenic Activity of Airborne Particulate Pollutants

W. Dehnen[1]

Introduction

Epidemiologic studies suggest that the incidence of lung cancer
might be related to the different levels of air pollution detected in urban and rural areas (1). The assumed causative relationship between pollutants and cancer is based on the fact that
carcinogenic agents are present in air pollutants. Moreover,
airborne particles are composed of a large number of inorganic
and organic substances, which to the greater part have not been
identified, and their possible carciogenic potential is unknown.
These data, however, are needed to provide a basis for epidemiologic analyses of the role of carcinogenic agents in the
causation of cancer.

The bacterial short-term screening test for mutagenicity, introduced by Ames et al. (2), has been used to predict the carcinogenicity of single substances with a reliability of about
90%. Recently this assay has been applied to the complex mixture
of substances present in extracts of particulate airborne pollutants (4-22). It has been suggested that this screening test,
capable of detecting mutagenic agents, would obviate the need
for numerous total analyses of the components present in such
extracts and could be used to identify the substances among the
many others that are carcinogenic (4).

It is the purpose of my short review to discuss the potentialities and limitations of applying the Ames test to extracts from
airborne particulate pollutants.

Factors Affecting the Composition of the Extract

At first I wish to mention some factors affecting the composition
of the extracts. Collecting particles on filters may result in
loss of material due to evaporation (21). The pattern and concentration of the substances retained on the filter depend somewhat on the particle size (18). Chemical reactions between compounds present in the particles and gases may produce artifacts
(14). Finally, the solvent used for extraction may affect the
composition of the extract (17,20). Therefore, the biologic
activity detected in the extract does not necessarily reflect
the activity originally present in the air. The pattern of substances, their concentration, and their chemical properties may
be altered by the collection and extraction. Different samples

---

[1]Medizinisches Institut für Lufthygiene, Gurlittstr. 53, D-4000 Düsseldorf/FRG

should be compared only if the conditions of sampling and extracting are the same.

Conditions of the Assay

The mutagenicity assay has been usually performed according to Ames et al (2) without modifications (7). The aliquots of the extracts have been added in ethanol or dimethylsulfoxide. The mutagenicity has been examined using the *Salmonella typhimurium* strains TA 1537, TA 1538, TA 98, and TA 100. No response was detected when strains TA 1535 and TA 1536 were used (7,17,20). Strains TA 98 and TA 1538 exhibited superior sensitivity to mutagens present in the extracts from airborne particles (4,7, 20) (Fig. 1), combustion emissions (10), and automobile exhaust (22).

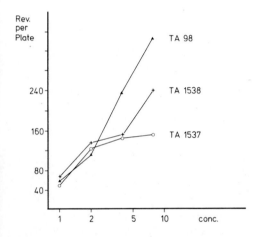

Fig. 1. Mutagenicity of an extract assayed in three *S. typhimurium* strains

Influence of Extract Amount

Another subject of interest is the amount of the extract. In order to obtain dose-response relations, different amounts of the extract have to be added to the test system. A characteristic feature of the extract has to be selected as basis for plotting dose-response curves (Table 1). Most frequently the weight of the residue of the extract or the volume of air from which the extract has been derived is chosen. Two further possibilities are the weight of the particles from which the extract has been derived or a particular compound believed to be representative for a group of important substances, e.g., benzo(a)pyrene, B(a)P, which is related to the other polycyclic aromatic hydrocarbons (PAH), originating from incomplete combustion.

Doses ranging from 50 to 1000 µg of extract residue have been added (Table 2). These doses are equivalent to the weight of airborne particles, from which the extract has been derived,

Table 1. Characteristics of the extracts suited as basis for comparing different samples

1. Weight of the residue of the extract.
2. Volume of air, from which the extract is derived.
3. Weight of particles, from which the extract is derived.
4. Weight of particular compounds believed to be representative for a group of important substances, e.g., BaP.

Table 2. Dosage of the extract

Basis for calculation	Range (per plate)	Reference
Weight of residue of the extract	50 - 1000 µg	Talcott and Wei (17) Tokiwa et al. (20) Dehnen et al. (7)
Equivalent particle weight	100 - 6000 µg	Tokiwa et al. (20) Flessel (8) Commoner et al. (4) Daisay et al. (6)
Equivalent volume of air	1 - 14 m^3	Tokiwa et al. (20) Dehnen et al. (7)

ranging from 100 to 6000 µg. The equivalent volume of air varies from 1 to 14 m^3. The doses of extract added to a single plate thus correspond to a volume of air inhaled during periods lasting from a few hours to 1 day.

Detection of Directly Acting Mutagens

Two classes of agents may be distinguished in the extracts of airborne particulate matter, those mutagenic in the absence of activating enzymes and those requiring metabolic activation by microsomal enzymes. Both kinds of mutagens have been detected in samples derived from airborne particles (4,7), automobile exhaust (22), and combustion emissions (10). It has been reported that the directly acting mutagens can be partly extracted into polar solvents (4). This portion of the mutagens seems to be related to seasonal and meteorologic factors. The origin and chemical nature of the inherently mutagenic agents is not known. They are closely related to levels of lead and other automobile emissions in the air (8) (Table 3). This finding suggests that automobile emissions might be one of the primary sources of this kind of mutagen (14,22). This view is supported by results obtained with automobile exhaust samples (22), which are to a high degree mutagenic in the absence of activating enzymes. It is suggested that nitro-substituted PAH compounds or other nitro compounds might be the active molecules (14,22).

The mutagenicity caused by inherently mutagenic agents can be determined quantitatively, provided no substances interfering with the bacterial growth or the mechanisms leading to mutations in bacteria are present.

Table 3. Correlations between mutagenicity and pollutants

Pollutant	TA 98	TA 100	Reference
Total particulate matter	0.93[a]	0.88[a]	Flessel (8)
Lead	0.85[a] 0.89[b]	0.93[a]	Flessel (8) Wang et al. (22)
Sulfate	0.75[a]	0.81[a]	Flessel (8)
Nitrate	0.83[a]	0.66[a]	Flessel (8)
BaP	0.535[b]		Teranishi et al. (18)

[a] Spearman's rank correlation coefficient
[b] Correlation coefficient r

Detection of Mutagens Requiring Metabolic Activation

The mutagenic activity detectable in the absence of activating enzymes changes if S-9 is included in the assay. The response may increase or decrease, depending on the sample tested. The mutagenicity of automobile exhaust (22) and combustion emissions (10) decreases in the presence of S-9, whereas the mutagenicity of airborne particles usually increases (7,20). The mutagenic activity observed, provided S-9 is included in the assay, is caused in part by inherently mutagenic agents and in part by mutagens requiring metabolic activation (Fig. 2). The relative proportions of these two types of mutagens cannot be determined quantitatively, because an unknown fraction of the mutagens is inactivated or activated by the enzymes present in S-9. Some of the mutagens may be inactivated by binding to components of S-9. Moreover, the enzymes responsible for the activation of mutagenic agents to ultimate mutagens may be inhibited competitively or irreversibly by some of the components present in the extract. Finally, the mutagenicity may be influenced by compounds capable of interfering with the mechanisms leading to mutations in the bacteria. Therefore, quantitative data on mutagenic agents requiring metabolic activation cannot be derived from the Ames assay (see also 4).

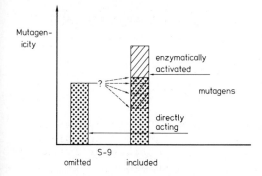

Fig. 2. Relations between directly acting mutagens and enzymatically activated mutagens in an extract containing both kinds of mutagens

Dose-Response Relations

The presence in the extract of substances toxic to bacteria, and of compounds interfering with the activation and inactivation of mutagens, results in varying shapes of dose-response curves (4). The slopes of the curves may decline after an initial rise, or may change continuously. Nevertheless linear or identically shaped dose-response relations are a basic requirement to compare different samples with respect to their mutagenic potential. Comparable quantitative data may be derived from nonlinear dose-response relations according to the method proposed by Commoner et al. (4). The lowest concentration is determined at which twice as many revertants per plate, corrected for a blank, arise as in control samples. The number of revertants detected at this concentration is used as the basis for comparing different samples.

Data on the mutagenicity of extracts of airborne particulate pollutants derived from several publications are shown in Table 4. The results, obtained by several groups, are in good agreement, indicating a similar composition of the extract from different countries. The differences between industrial and rural areas of the mutagenicity calculated per µg residue or m^3 air volume ar obvious. The mutagenicity calculated per nanogram BaP is higher in rural areas than in industrial ones, indicating that mutagenicity in this area is not related to incomplete combustion processes. This result is in good agreement with the finding that the BaP concentration in the air is not correlated or is only weakly correlated with mutagenicity (18).

Table 4. Mutagenic activity in airborne particulate matter

Revertants/µg extract residue	Revertants/m^3	Revertants/ng	Reference
3			Talcott and Wei (17)
0.3 - 2.6 (Industrial)	22 - 445		Tokiwa et al. (20)
0.04 - 1.9 (Rural)	7 - 77		Tokiwa et al. (20)
0.1 - 0.8	1 - 5		Flessel (8)
0.35			Teranishi et al. (19)
0.3 - 0.6 (R) (I)	5 - 16 (R) (I)	6.3 - 17 (I) (R)	Dehnen et al. (7)

The assay was performed with strain TA 98; I, industrial; R = rural.

Summarizing, it can be concluded from this part of the review that:

1. Mutagenicity caused by directly acting mutagens and mutagens requiring metabolic activations can be detected in extracts of airborne particulate pollutants.

2. The proportion of the mutagens requiring metabolic activation
   cannot be determined quantitatively.
3. Dose-response relations for the mutagenic activity in the absence and presence of activating enzymes can be established.

Tracing Mutagenic Agents in Fractions of Extracts

The second part of this review is concerned with the use of the
Ames test for tracing mutagenic agents in subfractions of extracts. Several procedures for fractionating the extracts have
been followed (4,7,19). Applying the fractionation procedure
of Wynder and Hoffmann (23), Teranishi et al. (19) found that
some 15% of the mutagenic activity would be attributed to the
fraction containing the PAH. Almost the same mutagenic activity
was detected in the fractions containing acidic and oxygenated
compounds.

In our own experiments we fractionated the extracts according
to the procedure of Tomingas (7) (Fig. 3). The samples are extracted with methanol. After adding 10% of water, a liquid-
liquid partition is performed between the methanol phase and
cyclohexane. The methanol fraction (MET) contains unknown polar
substances. The cyclohexane fraction is separated by column
chromatography on alumina into the fractions eluted with cyclohexane (CYC) containing the PAH and the fraction eluted with
isopropanol (PRO) containing heterocyclic compounds. The volume
of all fractions is adjusted to the volume of the original
extract.

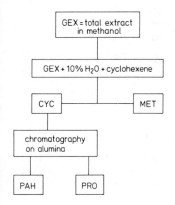

Fig. 3. Fractionating scheme for extracts

Dose-response relations obtained with GEX and its fractions are
shown in Fig. 4. The highest activity is exhibited by the total
extract GEX; the fractions CYC, MET, PRO, and PAH are less active in this order. Extracts and the related fractions derived
from particles collected in an industrial, a residental, and
a rural area were assayed for mutagenicity. The results are
shown in Table 5. The conclusions that may be drawn from the
data are:

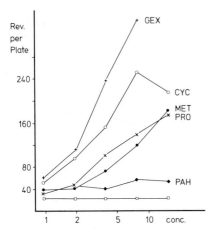

Fig. 4. Dose-response relations obtained with an total extract (GEX) and its fractions. The strain TA 1538 was used. Concentration *1* on the *abscissa* refers to a volume of 14 m^3 air, from which the extract is derived

Table 5. Mutagenicity of the total extract and its fractions in the absence and presence of the indicated additions

	Without addition			+ S-9			+ S-9 + NADPH		
	I	U	R	I	U	R	I	U	R
GEX	89	112	76	58	96	51	205	124	60
MET	55	26	42	71	52	35	63	40	14
CYC	42	24	25	37	21	14	115	59	20
PAH	17	5	3	8	5	0	27	14	0
PRO	21	15	13	17	20	0	100	10	10

Tester strain is TA 98. The number of revertants are corrected for a blank. The amount of extract added corresponds to a volume of 14 m^3 air. I, industrial; U, urban; R, rural.

1. The mutagenic activity present in the total extract GEX without addition of enzymes is reduced if S-9 without NADPH is included but increases after adding the complete activating system. Similar changes in mutagenicity are observed in the fractions CYC, PAH, and PRO, whereas the activity present in the fraction MET is diminished, provided S-9 and NADPH are included, compared with the activity present if S-9 without NADPH is added.
2. The largest increase of mutagenicity dependent on activating enzymes is detected in extracts and fractions originating from the industrial area.
3. The relative mutagenicity present in the PAH-containing fraction shares some 10%-15% of the mutagenicity present in the total extract GEX. PRO is three times as active as PAH. These results indicate that a large number of mutagenic agents dependent on activation by S-9 and NADPH are present particularly in the industrial area. Another part of the mutagenicity present particularly in the fraction MET is inactivated or

activated to varying degrees by S-9 and the complete activating
system. Mutagenic agents requiring metabolic activation are detected in the fractions PAH and PRO.

The Relation of Mutagenicity to Carcinogenicity

Finally, the relation of the mutagenicity to carcinogenicity
detectable in extracts of airborne particles and fractions
will be discussed.

From a theoretic viewpoint, it can be assumed that mutagens
detected by the Ames test are carcinogens with the reliability
of some 90% established for this assay (12). The correlation,
however, between the mutagenic and carcinogenic potencies of
these agents is yet to be investigated. For single substances,
a correlation between carcinogenicity and mutagenicity has been
established in some cases but not in others (3).

Two environmental samples have been tested with respect to the
mutagenic and carcinogenic activity. The first is automobile
exhaust. It has been demonstrated that directly acting mutagens
are present in automobile exhaust and the addition of the complete activating system causes a small increase or a decrease
in the mutagenicity, depending on the machine used as the source
of the exhaust (22). It cannot be concluded that the entire
mutagenicity is caused by directly acting mutagens, because the
proportions of the two classes of mutagens in the presence of
S-9 cannot be determined quantitatively, but it may be assumed
that the greater fraction of the agents is inherently mutagenic
(22). The carcinogenicity of automobile exhaust and its fractions, though derived from other sources than in the mutagenicity
experiments, have been tested after subcutaneous and percutan-
eous application. The fractionation procedure was performed by
the method of Grimmer (9) and the results of the tests are shown
in Figs. 5 and 6 (9,15). The carcinogenicity is detected exclusively in the PAH-containing fractions. As PAH require activating enzymes for their mutagenic action, they are probably
responsible for only the minor part of the mutagenicity detected
in automobile exhaust.

The second kind of samples tested for mutagenicity and carcinogenicity were the extracts of airborne particulate pollutants
and their fractions. In this case the tests were performed on
samples of the same origin. The fractionating procedure and the
results of testing for mutagenicity have been already shown
(Figs. 3 and 4; Table 5). Some 10%-15% of the mutagenicity could
be attributed to the fraction containing PAH.

The carcinogenicity has been determined after subcutaneous application in mice by the method of Pott (16). The results are
shown in Fig. 7. The total extract was more active than the corresponding fraction PAH, except in the rural area. More than
half of the carcinogenic activity was detected in the fraction
PAH. In contrast with the mutagenicity assay, the fraction PAH
shared some 10%-15% of the mutagenicity present in the total extract. The fraction PRO induced 3-4 times as many revertants in

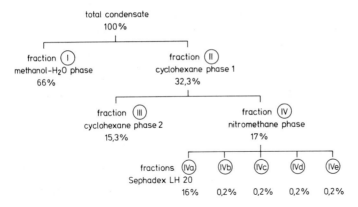

Fig. 5. Fractionating scheme for automobile-exhaust condensate according to Grimmer (9)

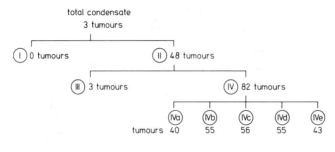

combination of fractions I, III, IVa–IVe : 5 tumours
" " " IVa–IVe : 94 tumours
benzo[a]pyrene : 51 tumours
tricaprylin control : 0 tumours

Fig. 6. Number of tumor-bearing mice after subcutaneous application of automobile-exhaust condensate and its fractions according to Pott (15)

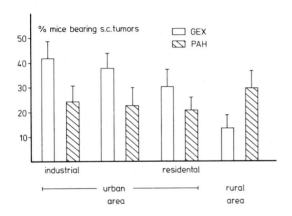

Fig. 7. Carcinogenicity in mice after subcutaneous application of the extracts and the PAH-containing fraction derived from particles collected in industrial, residental, and rural localities (16)

the mutagenicity assay, whereas the carcinogenicity of this fraction was lower than that of the PAH fraction (by F. Pott 1978, personal communication). In the rural area the carcinogenicity of the fraction PAH exceeded that of the total extract, indicating that some constituents of the extract interfere with the process of carcinogenicity in this model. No mutagenicity could be detected in the PAH fraction at concentrations where the total extract is clearly mutagenic.

Conclusions

It can be concluded that the mutagenic potency detected by the Ames test in extracts is not proportionally related to the carcinogenic potency. Two of the facts mentioned above may serve as an explanation:

1. A definite number of revertants can be induced by a different pattern of agents, which are more or less mutagenic or carcinogenic.
2. The large number of compounds present in the extracts influences the activation and inactivation of mutagens in the *Salmonella*/microsome assay, but probably cause more complex reactions in animals under in vivo conditions.

Therefore, it appears that assaying the mutagenicity in unfractionated extracts is not suited to provide a basis for epidemiologic analyses of cancer incidence. On the other hand, the extract can be separated into fractions containing particular classes of compounds such as PAH, thereby reducing the number of agents that may interfere with the mechanisms of mutagenicity and carcinogenicity. Determining the relation of mutagenicity to carcinogenicity should enable one to find those fractions which may serve as indicators for carcinogenicity.

References

1. Stocks P (1960) On the relation between atmosphere pollution in urban and rural localities and mortality from cancer. Br J Cancer 14:397-418
2. Ames BN, McCann J, Yamasaki E (1975) Methods for detecting carcinogens and mutagens with the Salmonella/mammalian-microsome mutagenicity test. Mutat Res 31:347-364
3. Bartsch H (1978) Carcinogenic activity and biological effects in short term tests: quantitative aspects. Staub-Reinhaltung Luft 38:240-243
4. Commoner B, Madyastha P, Bronsdon A, Vithayathil AJ (1978) Environmental mutagens in urban air particulates. J Toxicol Environ Health 4:59-77
5. Chrisp CE, Fisher GE, Lammert JE (1978) Mutagenicity of filtrates from respirable fly ash. Science 199:73-75
6. Daisey JM, Hawryluk I, Kneip TJ, Mukai FH (1978) Mutagenic activity in organic fractions of airborne particulate matter. Conference on Carbonaceous Particles in the Atmosphere, Berkeley, March 20-22
7. Dehnen W, Pitz N, Tomingas R (1977) The mutagenicity of airborne particulate pollutants. Cancer Lett 4:5-12
8. Flessel C (1977) Mutagenic activity of particulate matter in California hi-vol samplers. Third Interagency Symposium on Air Monitoring. Berkeley, May 18-19

9. Grimmer G (1977) Analysis of automobile exhaust condensates. In: Mohr U, Schmähl D, Tomatis L (eds) Air pollution and man. Int Agency for Res on Cancer Lyon, pp 29-40, IARC Scientific Publications No 16

10. Löfroth G (to be published) Mutagenicity assay of combustion emissions. Chemosphere 7:791-798

11. Maxild J, Andersen M, Kiel P (1978) Mutagenicity of fume particles from metal arc welding on stainless steel in the Salmonella/microsmes test. Mutat Res 56:235-243

12. McCann J, Chol E, Yamasaki E, Ames B (1975) Detection of carcinogens as mutagens in the Salmonella/microsome test: assay of 300 chemicals. Proc Natl Acad Sci USA 72:5135-5139

13. Pitts JN, Karel A, Grosjean D, Mischke TM, Simmon VF, Pool D (1977) Mutagenic activity of airborne particulate organic pollutants. Toxicol Lett 1:65-70

14. Pitts JN, Vauwenbergh KA van, Grosjean D, Schmid JP, Fitz D (1978) Chemical and biological aspects of organic particulates in real and simulated atmospheres. Conf on Carbonaceous Particles in the Atmosphere. Berkely, March 20-22

15. Pott F, Tomingas R, Misfeld J (1977) Tumors in mice after subcutaneous injection of automobile exhaust condensates. In: Mohr U, Schmähl D, Tomatis L (eds) Air pollution and cancer in man. Int Agency for Res on Cancer, Lyon, pp 79-88, IARC scientific Publications No 16

16. Pott F, Tomingas R, Brockhaus A, Huth (1980) Studies on the tumourigenicity of extracts and their fractions. Zbl BAKT I Abt ORIG B170:17-34

17. Talcott R, Wei E (1977) Airborne mutagens bioassayed in Salmonella typhimurium. J Natl Cancer Inst 58:449-411

18. Teranishi K, Hamada K, Takeda N, Watanabe H (1977) Mutagenicity of the tar in air pollutants. Proc 4th Int Clean Air Congr Tokyo, May 1977. The Japanese Union of Air Pollution Prevention Association, Tokyo, p 33-36

19. Teranishi K, Hamada K, Watanabke H (1978) Mutagenicity in Salmonella typhimurium mutants of the benzene-soluble organic matter derived from air-borne particulate matter and its five fractions. Mutat Res 56:273-280

20. Tokiwa H, Morita K, Takeyoshi H, Takahashi K, Ohnishi Y (1977) Detection of mutagenic activity in particulate air pollutants. Mutat Res 48:237-248

21. Tomingas R, Voltmer G (1978) Abscheidung von Benzo(a)pyren aus der Atmosphäre auf Glasfaserfiltern. Staub-Reinhaltung Luft 38:216-218

22. Wang YY, Rappaport SM, Sawyer RF, Talcott RE, Wei ET (1978) Direct-acting mutagens in automobile exhaust. Cancer Lett 5:39-47

23. Wynder EL, Hoffmann D (1965) Some laboratory and epidemiological aspects of air pollution carcinogenesis. J Air Poll Contr Ass 15:155-165

Carcinogen Control in the Urine of Dogs

D. Gericke[1], H. Grötsch[1], R. Harzmann[2], and K. H. Bichler[2]

The short-term system for mutagenicity testing developed by Ames
et al. (1,2) uses mutants of *Salmonella typhimurium*. Table 1 shows
the 'Ames' mutants normally used in our laboratory. The *Salmonella/*
microsome assay has been adapted to investigate the mutagenicity
of urine from rats fed 2-acetylaminofluorene (2-AAF) (3,4). A
similar test method has also been described by Marquardt and
Siebert (5) and Siebert (6), using *Saccharomyces cerevisiae*. They
tested the urine of patients given cyclosphamide for mutagenic
metabolites.

Table 1. Ames test I. Genotype of the TA strains used for mutagen
testing[a]

Histidine mutation			Additional mutations		
his G 46	his C 3076	his D 3052	LPS	Repair	R factor
TA 1535	TA 1537	TA 1538	rfa	$\Delta uvrB$	–
TA 100		TA 98	rfa	$\Delta uvrB$	+R

[a] All strains were originally derived from *S. typhimurium* LT 2.
The deletion (Δ), though *uvrB* also includes the nitrate reductase (chl) and biotin (bio) genes

Müller et al. recently reported the identification of two urine
metabolites of vinyl chloride by chemical, not by microbiologic,
methods (7). In attempts to induce urinary bladder carcinomas
in dogs (8), the question arose of how to monitor the excretion
of carcinogens in the urine after subcutaneous (SC) administration. The assays reported there have been developed by us
for this purpose.

Methods

Sixteen femals beagles (breeding colony Hoechst AG, Frankfurt/M.,
Prof. Strasser) received bladder stones by transurethral instal-
lation of fluid Paladur or Technovit 4071 (n = 8 each) (Fa.
Kulzer, Bad Homburg v.d.H.). The material polymerized in the
bladder for 90 and 150 s, respectively (8). Three groups (n = 4

[1] Hoechst AG, D-6230 Frankfurt/Main-80/FRG

[2] Department of Urology, University of Tübingen, D-7400 Tübingen/FRG

each) of dogs were treated twice a week with 2-formylamine-4-
(5-nitro-2-furyl)thiazol (FANFT, 25 mg/kg body weight), with
2-aminodiphenyl (2-ADP, 30 mg/kg body weight), or with a combination of these two compounds (FANFT, 20 mg/kg + 2-ADP,
20 mg/kg + 2-ADP, 20 mg/kg). Four beagles had bladder stones
alone. Every month the dogs were kept in metabolic cages for
24 h to examine the urine.

As mentioned above, the mutagenicity test (1) was used with the
following tester strains: TA 98, TA 100, TA 1535, and TA 1537,
without and with enzymatic activation (S-9 mix). The details
of the methodology are shown in the Figs. 1 and 2. The urine,
collected for 24 h and stored at 4°C, was filtered (Seitz-EK
filter, Seitz AG, Bad Kreuznach). There was no further preparation of the urine before adding it to the upper layer of
the microbiologic test system.

BASISAGAR	TOPAGAR	TESTCOMPOUND	TESTERSTRAIN	S9 - MIX
VOGEL-BONNER- Minimaleagar + 2% Glucose	0.6% agar + 0.5% NaCl + 10% ↳0.5mM L-Histidine ↳0.5mM Biotine	0.1ml (2.5mg-500µg 100µg-20µg-4µg) Diluent: H_2O - DMSO-Ethanol	Brothculture 16h 37°C 0.1 ml	0.5ml S9-Mix contains pro ml: Liverhomogenate - fraction S9 0.04-0.1ml $MgCl_2$ 8µmol KCl 33µmol Glucose - 6 - phosphate 5µmol NADP 4µmol Na_2HPO_4 100µmol

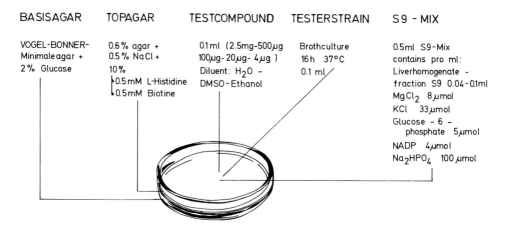

Fig. 1. Ames test II

CULTIVATION   48 h 37°C

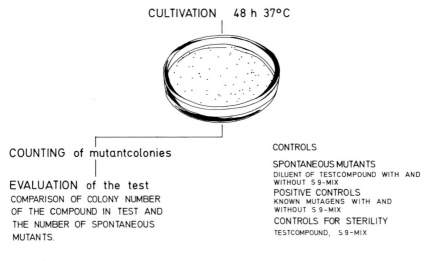

COUNTING of mutantcolonies

EVALUATION of the test
COMPARISON OF COLONY NUMBER
OF THE COMPOUND IN TEST AND
THE NUMBER OF SPONTANEOUS
MUTANTS.

CONTROLS

SPONTANEOUS MUTANTS
DILUENT OF TESTCOMPOUND WITH AND
WITHOUT S9-MIX
POSITIVE CONTROLS
KNOWN MUTAGENS WITH AND
WITHOUT S9-MIX
CONTROLS FOR STERILITY
TESTCOMPOUND, S9-MIX

Fig. 2. Ames test III

Results

Figure 3 shows the results with the four *S. typhimurium* strains
used for the testing of urine from treated dogs. In group 4
(artificial bladder stones + FANFT + 2-ADP), there are ca. 500
mutants/plate with TA 100 without enzymatic activation. The
three other strains did not react at all, neither without nor
with S-9 mix activation. The same results could be achieved with
urine of the dogs in group 3 (artificial bladder stones + FANFT),
as shown in Fig. 4. It seems reasonable that the dogs with
FANFT treatment demonstrate positive results only. However, the
concentration of FANFT in urine is so high that it has to be
diluted. In Fig. 5 the effect of FANFT is shown. It is toxic in
urine diluted 1:2, and the mutagenicity rises with higher dilutions. A 1:10 dilution of urine is the most active; at higher
dilutions the number of mutants decreases again. It was interesting to observe the duration of FANFT excretion in urine after a
single SC injection. The same number of mutants was seen for
each of 4 days after administration and this then dropped to
zero in 72 h. The urine of nontreated controls or of the dogs
with artificial stones only was negative. However, it was very
surprising that the 2-ADP-treated animals did not demonstrate a
positive result since McCann et al. had described this substance
as a weak mutagen (2). We were unable to demonstrate this.
During the course of our studies Donahue et al. (9) published
a reason for the variable 2-ADP response seen with 2-ADP. This
is due to a small percentage of contamination with 4-ADP.
Therefore we were not surprised at all when we had found a
second batch of 2-ADP as mutagenic shown in Fig. 6. Again the
urine concentration 1:2 is toxic for the tester strain TA 98,
but a dilution of 1:10 is positive. The strain TA 100 reacts in
a similar manner.

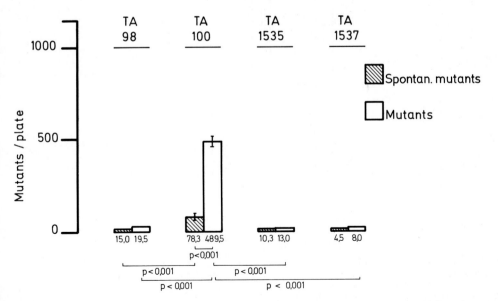

Fig. 3. Ames test (urine) with different tester strains of *S. typhimurium*:
induction of carcinomas in the urinary bladder in dogs ($n = 22$), group 4

398

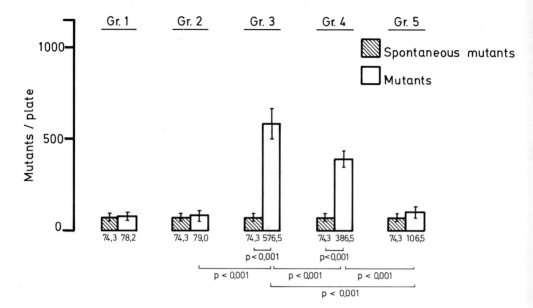

Fig. 4. Ames test (urine), tester strain TA 100: induction of carcinomas
in the urinary bladder in dogs (n = 22)

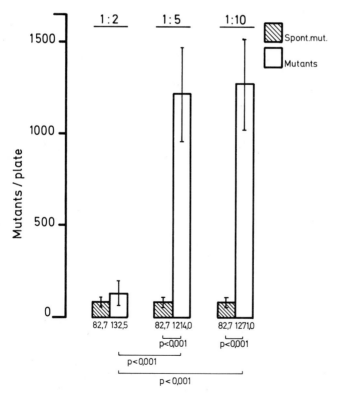

Fig. 5. Ames test (urine) with different urine dilutions: Induction of
carcinomas in the urinary bladder in dogs (n = 22), group 3

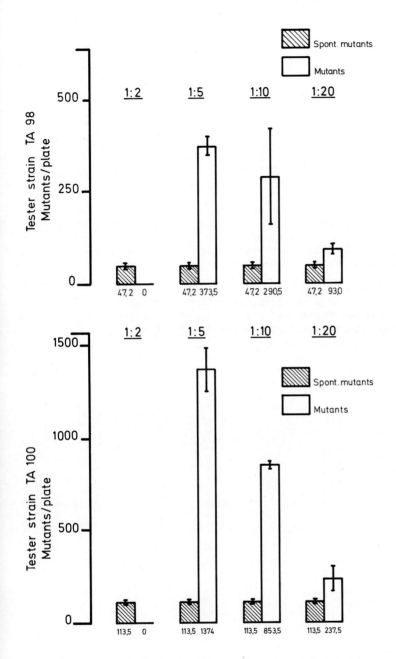

Fig. 6. Ames test (urine) with different urine dilutions: induction of carcinomas in the urinary bladder in dogs ($n = 22$); 2-aminobiphenyl, second batch

Investigations of human beings in different stages of bladder carcinoma are in progress to compare the development of this malignancy with the appearance of mutagens in the urine of the patients.

References

1. Ames BN, Lee FD, Durston EW (1973) Proc Natl Acad Sci USA 70:782, 2281
2. McCann J et al. (1976) Proc Natl Acad Sci USA 72:5153 (1975); McCann J, Ames BN (1976) Proc Natl Acad Sci USA 73:950
3. Durston EW, Ames BN (1974) Proc Natl Acad Sci USA 71:737; McCann J, Ames BN (1975) Ann NY Acad Sci 269:21
4. Commoner B, Vithaysthil AJ, Henry JJ (1974) Detection of metabolic carcinogen intermediates in urine of carcinogen-fed rats by means of bacterial mutagenesis. Nature 249:850
5. Marquardt HH, Siebert D (1971) Ein neuer host mediated assay (Urinversuch) zum Nachweis mutagener Stoffe mit Saccharomyces cerevisiae. Naturwissenschaften 58:568
6. Siebert D (1973) A new method for testing genetically active metabolites. Urinary assay with cyclophosphamide (Endoxan, Cytoxan) and saccharomyces cerevisiae. Mutat Res 17:307-314
7. Müller G, Norpoth K, Eckard R (1976) Identification of two urine metabolites of Vinyl Chloride by GC-MS-investigations. Int Arch Occup Environ Health 38:69
8. Harzmann R (1978) Habilitationsschrift, Universität Tübingen
9. Donahue EV, McCann J, Ames BN (1978) Detection of mutagenic impurities in carcinogens and non-carcinogens by high-pressure liquid chromatography and the Salmonella/microsome test. Cancer Res 38:431-436

Subject Index

Lymphocyte Hybridomas

Second Workshop on "Functional Properties of Tumors of T and B Lymphocytes"
Sponsored by the National Institute (NIH) April 3–5, 1978 Bethesda, Maryland, USA
Editors: F. Melchers, M. Potter, N. Warner

Reprint. 1979. 85 figures, 86 tables. XXI, 246 pages
ISBN 3-540-09670-1
(Originally published as **Current Topics in Microbiology and Immunology, Vol. 81**)

Plasma cell-plasmacytoma hybrids are a unique source of homogeneous antibodies with extraordinary specificity. Since the original discovery by Köhler and Milstein, many laboratories have become actively engaged in making lymphocyte hybrids of normal and malignant cells, mainly to produce homogeneous antibodies specific for a wide variety of interesting antigens. In addition, these hybrids have become useful as models for studying T-cell functions and lymphocyte growth regulation and differentiation, as a means for studying the location of genes expressed in lymphocytes, immunoglobulins, and for study of the biochemical basis of neoplastic change.

The second workshop on "Functional Properties of Tumors T and B Lymphocytes" was held in April 1978 at the National Institutes of Health, Bethesda, Maryland, USA, bringing together the world's leading experts in this field. This book publishes the proceedings of that workshop and represents an impressive summary of the scientific progress and the technical know-how of many laboratories working on lymphocyte fusions, a technique which is currently gaining wide interest in immunology, molecular and cellular biology, biochemistry and medical research.

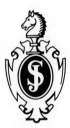

Springer-Verlag
Berlin
Heidelberg
New York

Recent Results in Cancer Research/

Fortschritte der Krebsforschung/

Progrès dans les recherches sur le cancer

Editor in Chief:
P. Rentchnick

Co-editor: H. J. Senn

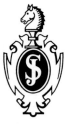

Springer-Verlag
Berlin
Heidelberg
New York